ISCHAEMIC HEART DISEASE

BOERHAAVE SERIES
FOR POSTGRADUATE
MEDICAL EDUCATION

PROCEEDINGS OF THE BOERHAAVE COURSES
ORGANIZED BY
THE FACULTY OF MEDICINE, UNIVERSITY OF LEIDEN
THE NETHERLANDS

ISCHAEMIC HEART DISEASE

EDITED BY

J. H. DE HAAS, M.D., H.C. HEMKER, M.D., AND
H. A. SNELLEN, M.D.

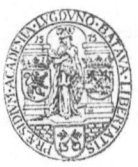

LEIDEN UNIVERSITY PRESS

1970

SOLE DISTRIBUTOR FOR JAPAN
NANKODO COMPANY LIMITED/TOKYO

SOLE DISTRIBUTOR FOR THE UNITED STATES OF AMERICA AND CANADA
THE WILLIAMS AND WILKINS COMPANY / BALTIMORE

Library of Congress Card Number 70-125958
ISBN-13:978-94-010-3349-7   e-ISBN-13:978-94-010-3347-3
DOI: 10.1007/978-94-010-3347-3

Jacket design: E. Wijnans GVN

© 1970 Leiden University Press, Leiden, The Netherlands
Softcover reprint of the hardcover 1st edition 1970

PREFACE

The Boerhaave Courses in Cardiology have been held once or twice a year since 1955. For the greater part they were meant for specialists in Cardiology, Pediatrics, and Internal Medicine, who wished to hear about recent advances in Cardiology and in its anatomical and physical basis.

For some time the courses reflected mostly the work in Leiden, especially on congenital heart disease, but soon the highly valuable cooperation of other centres was obtained on subjects in which they had more experience.

In later years speakers from abroad were also invited and they contributed greatly to the wider scope of the courses. It was thus possible to organize detailed discussions on special subjects by panels of experts for an audience of interested clinical specialists. General reviews were also given for widely varying groups including general practioners and health officers. The special courses were usually given in English and were international in character, while the general courses were given in Dutch.

This book reports on a course that united both trends. It was held entirely in English mainly because it was combined with a meeting organized by the Dutch Heart Association and because of the support given by the Secretary of Health who opened this meeting personally and by the European branch of the World Health Organization which was represented by Dr. Pisa.

The choice of the subject of Coronary Heart Disease was in keeping with this setting because it represents a subject with considerable general interest and because it concerns almost all doctors. However, it requires specialized information from experts on an international level.

It is certainly not the first time, nor will it be the last, that this subject will be treated in a review, but it was felt that a report should be published in order to make this review accessible to a larger medical audience both in Holland and elsewhere.

J. H. DE HAAS, H. C. HEMKER, H. A. SNELLEN

CONTENTS

CHAPTER III

DIAGNOSTIC METHODS IN ISCHAEMIC HEART DISEASE

LIST OF ACTIVE PARTICIPANTS

F. H. Bonjer, Netherlands Institute for Preventive Medicine, Leiden, Netherlands

C. J. F. Böttcher, Gaubius Institute, State University, Leiden, Netherlands

A. V. G. Bruschke, Department of Cardiology, St. Antonius Hospital, Utrecht, Netherlands

Ch. Dubost, Department of Cardiac Surgery, Broussais Hospital, Paris, France

J. E. French †, Sir William Dunn School of Pathology, University of Oxford, U.K.

M. H. Frick, Cardiovascular Laboratory, University Central Hospital, Helsinki, Finland

J. J. Groen, Department of Methodology of Psychobiological Research, University Hospital, Leiden, Netherlands

J. H. de Haas, Netherlands Heart Foundation, The Hague; University of Leiden, Netherlands

H. K. Hellerstein, Department of Medicine, Case Western Reserve University, Cleveland, Ohio, U.S.A.

H. C. Hemker, Laboratory of Cardiovascular Biochemistry, University Hospital, Leiden, Netherlands

R. E. B. Hudson, Department of Pathology, National Heart Hospital, London, U.K.

P. G. Hugenholtz, Department of Cardiology, Dijkzigt Hospital, Rotterdam, Netherlands

J. V. Joossens, Department of Cardiology, St. Raphaël University Clinics, Louvain, Belgium

W. B. Kannel, Department of Health, Education and Welfare, Public Health 'Service, Framingham, Mass. U.S.A.

M. J. Karvonen, Institute of Occupational Health, Helsinki, Finland

P. Lichtlen, Medical Clinic, Kantonspital, Zürich, Switzerland

E. A. Loeliger, Department of Research in Haemostasis and Thrombosis, University Hospital, Leiden, Netherlands

E. F. Lüscher, Theodor Kocher Institute, University of Bern, Switzerland

S. L. Morrison, Department of Social Medicine, Usher Institute, Edinburgh, U.K.

C. L. C. van Nieuwenhuizen, Department of Cardiology, St. Antonius Hospital, Utrecht, Netherlands

M. F. Oliver, Department of Cardiology, The Royal Infirmary, Edinburgh, U.K.

S. Paulin, Department of Radiology, University of Göteborg, Sweden.

Z. Pisa, World Health Organization, Regional Office for Europe, Copenhagen, Denmark

J. Pool, Department of Cardiology, University Hospital, Leiden, Netherlands

J. P. Roos, Department of Cardiology, University Hospital, Leiden, Netherlands

G. Rose, London School of Hygiene and Tropical Medicine, London, U.K.

W. Schweizer, Department of Cardiology, University Clinic, Bügerspital, Basle, Switzerland

A. Senning, Department of Cardiac Surgery, University Clinic, Kantonspital, Zürich, Switzerland

W. van der Sluys, Department of Cardiology, University Hospital, Leiden, Netherlands

H. A. Snellen, Department of Cardiology, University Hospital, Leiden, Netherlands

J. Stamler, Chicago Health Research Foundation, Chicago, Ill., U.S.A.

E. Varnauskas, Department of Cardiology, Medical Department I, Sahlgrenska Sjukhuset, University of Göteborg, Sweden

A. J. Vergroesen, Unilever Research Laboratory, Vlaardingen, Netherlands

H. W. H. Weeda, Department of Cardiology, University Hospital, Leiden, Netherlands

L. Werkö, Department of Cardiology, Medical Department I, Sahlgrenska Sjukhuset, University of Göteborg, Sweden

S. A. G. J. Witteveen, Department of Cardiology, University Hospital, Leiden, Netherlands

CHAPTER I

ASPECTS OF PATHOGENESIS

PATHOLOGY OF ISCHAEMIC HEART DISEASE

R. E. B. HUDSON

Ischaemic heart disease may occur whenever the blood supply to the heart is deficient in *quality* (as in severe anaemia or in ordinary transposition of the great vessels) or in *quantity* (as in coronary artery obstruction, aortic valve disease, or severe hypotension).

In infancy, it may be due to congenital anomalous origin of the left coronary artery from the pulmonary trunk (fig. 1) or to atresia of the left artery beyond its ostium from the aorta. Other causes of coronary artery disease in infancy include arteritis with aneurysm formation and thrombosis (possibly a hypersensitivity reaction), gargoylism, calcification, and non-specific aortitis and arteritis; some of the last-mentioned cases may be due to congenital rubella, in which intimal thickening of systemic and pulmonary arteries has been described. It should also be remembered that in the evolution of the post-natal intima of the arteries, a thick, complex, musculo-elastic layer is formed and this may persist in some infants more than in others, causing stenosis of the lumen; this persistence has been noted among Askenazi Jewish babies (1).

When infancy and childhood are passed, the usual cause of ischaemic heart disease is coronary artery atheroma (atherosclerosis). This is a degenerative disease of the intima of arteries, associated with focal deposition of lipid containing cholesterol; this evokes fibrous thickening of the intima into plaques, which eventually calcify, develop haemorrhages, ulcerate and thrombose. At the same time, the media beneath the lesions becomes thinned and the adventitia develops lymphocytic infiltration, which may be marked. Two typical stenotic arteries are shown in figs. 2 and 3; the former illustrates lipid deposition, fibrosis and haemorrhage of the intima, thinning and destruction of the media, and thrombosis of the lumen; the latter shows an advanced stage of massive intimal fibrosis with reduction of the lumen to two tiny recanalization spaces. It is obvious that coronary vasodilating

3

agents can have no action at the site of such lesions; the undoubted benefits of amyl nitrite, glyceryl trinitrate and other remedies must therefore arise indirectly, probably through a lessening of the work of the heart by generalised vasodilatation of healthy segments of arteries of the body.

In the writer's opinion, atheroma is fundamentally a *congenital* (and possibly inherited) disease of the arterial wall determined *at birth* by the particular way in which the post-natal intimal and medial layers of the wall are evolved from the musculo-elastic and medial complex; this view is complementary to the well-known involution of the pulmonary arteries which occurs in the first few months of life, in conformity with the fall of pressure in the lesser circuit as the lungs expand at birth. It is reasonable to suppose that points of variable structure will evolve at awkward junctions in the systemic arterial tree, namely at branchings and bifurcations (as has been demonstrated in the circle of Willis); these sites are physically 'weaker' in some people than in others and become foci for atheroma. The higher the blood lipids (and the blood pressure), the more will fatty material seep into these sites; this is borne out by the 'galloping' atheroma which occurs in young people, including young women, suffering from type 2 familial hyperlipoproteinaemia, which may cause fatal coronary artery obstruction. Again, when the integrity of the intimal lining is broken, platelet accumulation and thrombosis occur to cover the area, and even block the lumen; this process will be aggravated in states of hypercoagulability.

This view can account for most of the known aetiological facts about atheroma eg. the constant occurrence at certain sites; the presence of lesion in people with *normal* blood lipids and pressure, and their aggravation by hypercholesterolaemia and hypertension; the variations between individuals, races, and the sexes (before the menopause, at any rate), and the tendency to affect families.

Unhappily, it also means that prophylactic 'correction' of blood lipids and blood pressure and the application of long-term anticoagulant therapy of any kind, can offer only partial benefit, merely delaying a process, the course of which is inexorably determined at birth by the inherited soundness or otherwise of the evolving arterial tree.

Other causes of coronary artery obstruction are relatively rare, and include embolism, syphilis, dissecting aneurysm and trauma. *Embolism* in a coronary artery may derive from thrombus or vegetations in the

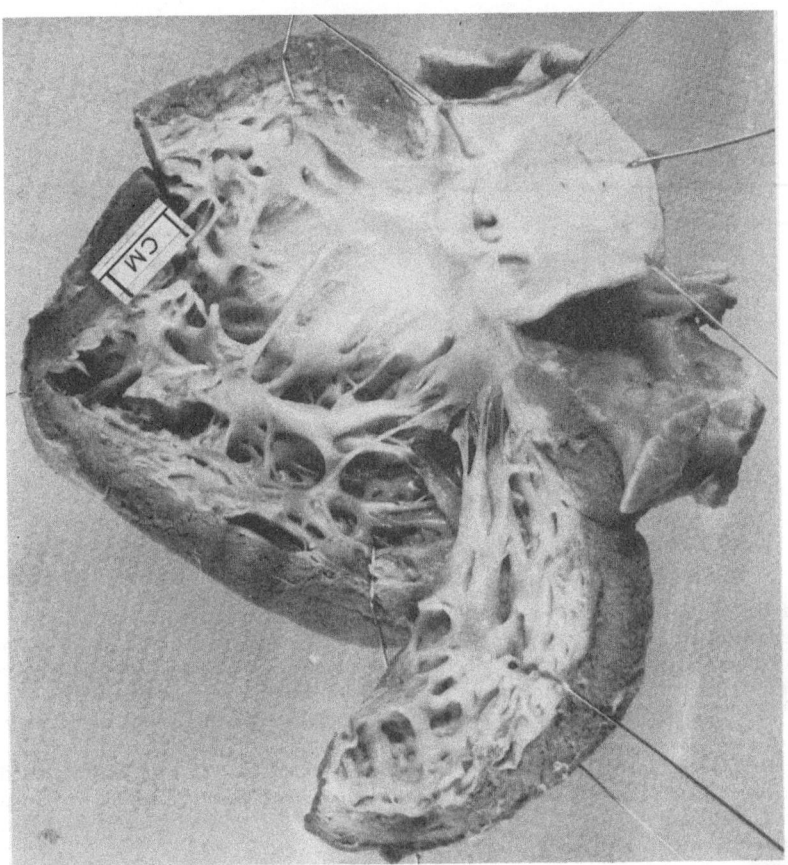

Fig. 1. Endomyocardial fibrosis due to the left coronary artery arising from the pulmonary trunk in a female infant of 6 months.

Acknowledgment: The illustrations are adapted trom the writer's monograph 'Cardiovascular Pathology' by courtesy of Edward Arnold (Publishers) Ltd.

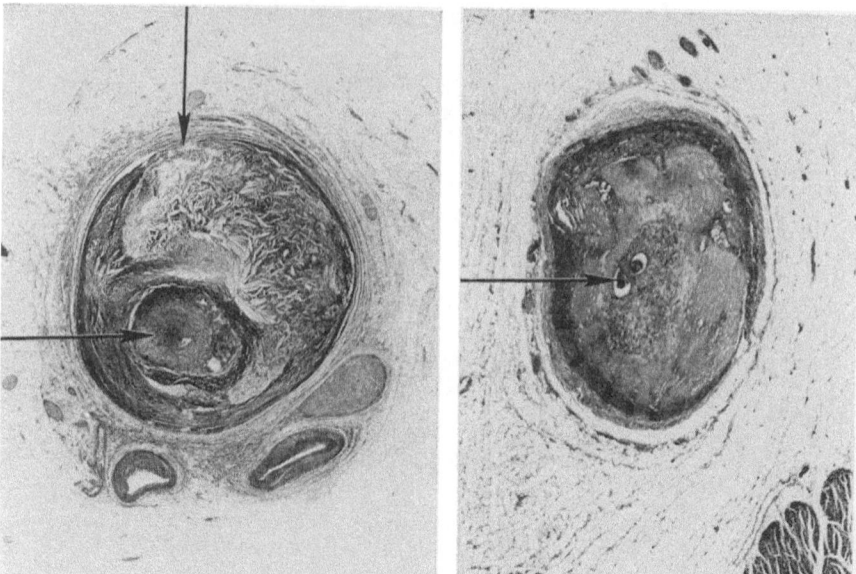

Fig. 2. (left) Thrombus (left arrow) occluding the lumen of the anterior descending branch of the left coronary artery, already stenosed by severe classical atheroma, in the heart of a man of 60 years. The media is greatly thinned, and at the site of the upper arrow, it is actually destroyed. Inside the media, the intima is fibrotic and packed with lipid containing cholesterol esters (which occupied the elliptical clefts). Heamorrhage and some calcification were also present in the intima. (Elastic-van Gieson × 10).

Fig. 3. (right) Right coronary artery in the heart of a woman of 60 years virtually occluded by intimal fibrosis; the lumen is reduced to 2 small recanalization spaces (arrow) in the organising final occluding thrombus. The media (the dark ring) is thinned to a tenuous membrane at bottom right.

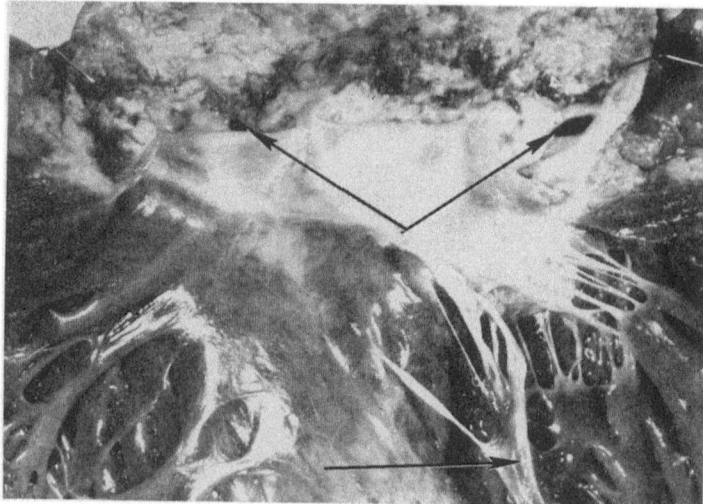

Fig. 4. Coronary ostial stenosis in syphilitic aortitis; the upper arrows indicate the points of black probes inserted into the ostia from the arteries. There is very severe aortic atheroma just above the valve; and there is also necrotic atrophy of a papillary muscle (lower arrow). From a man aged 55 years.

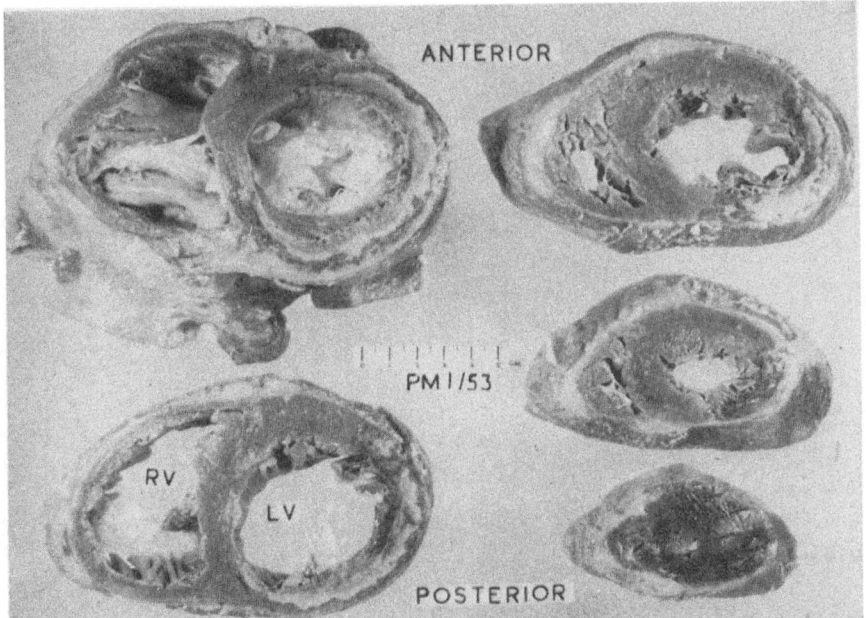

Fig. 5. Acute myocardial infarction, chiefly posterior, about 1 week old, in the heart of a man of 53 years. The infarcted area is creamy coloured, and surrounded by a zone of haemorrhage. The lesion is most extensive in the basal slice (top left).

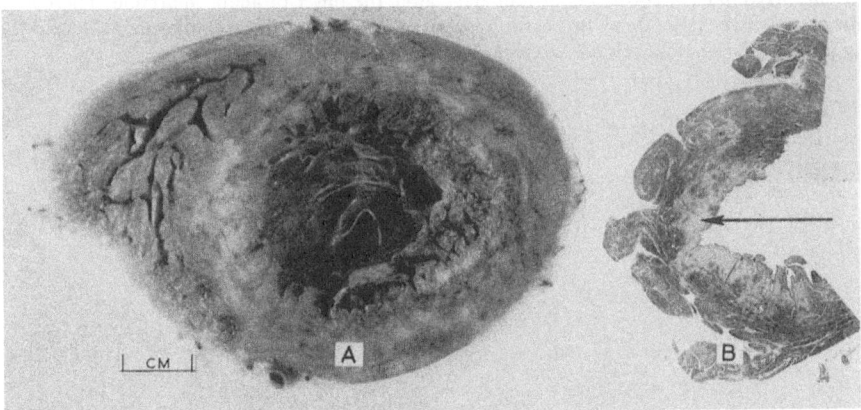

Fig. 6. Subendocardial infarction due to stenosis of the epicardial portions of all three main coronary arteries in the heart of a woman of 69 years.

A. Macroscopic appearance; the lesions are circumferential. The anterior surface is below.

B. Microscopic appearance; the arrow indicates the subendocardial zone of replacement fibrosis in the interventricular septum. (Haematoxylin-eosin × 2).

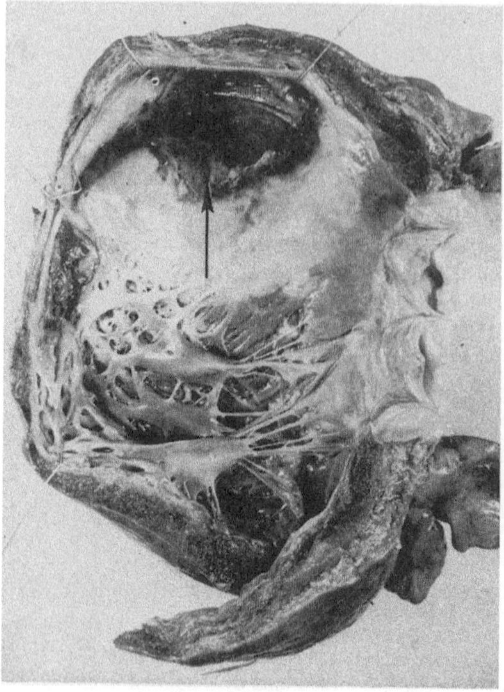

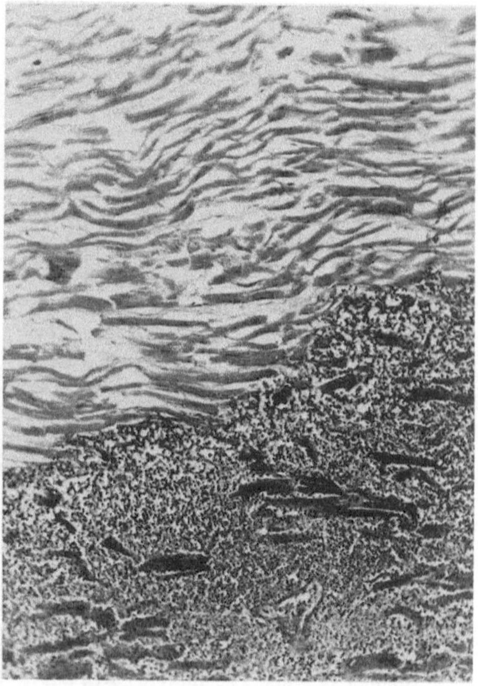

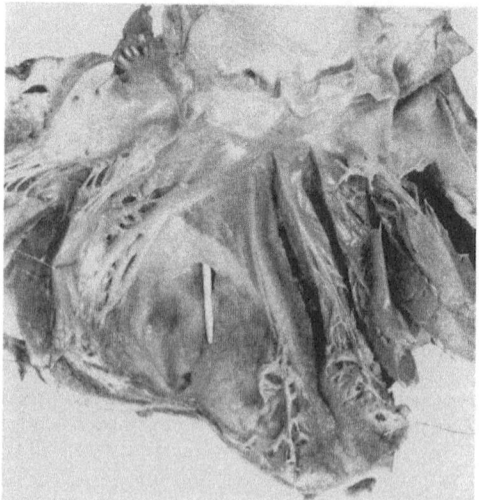

Fig. 7. (left) Anteroseptal infarction – aneurysm lined with friable thrombus (arrow) in the heart of a man of 54 years.

Fig. 8. (richt) Myomalacia cordis about four days after the onset of acute infarction. There is a distinc junctional zone between the dead myocardium above and the massive polymorphonuclear cell exudate engulfing muscle debris below. (Haematoxylin-eosin × 75).

Fig. 9. Healed infarction-perforation of the inter-ventricular septum (white probe), seen from the left ventricle.

left side of the heart, or in the pulmonary veins; the writer has encountered two examples of fatal acute myocardial infarction due to thrombo-embolism from the left atrial appendage in patients with rheumatic mitral valve disease. Occasionally, embolism is due to particles of tissue freed during surgery of the left heart valves; if this is suspected at necropsy, it is a good plan to make a plain radiograph of the heart and to look for calcified particles before cutting open the coronary arteries. Rarely, the embolism is paradoxical, originating in the systemic veins and reaching the left heart via a right-to-left shunt in the heart. It is not always easy to decide whether a thrombotic occlusion in a main coronary artery is embolic or merely complicating a focus of atheroma; in both cases the lesion is commonest in the anterior descending branch of the left artery.

Syphilitic aortitis is unique in causing ostial stenosis (fig. 4); indeed it may be difficult to locate the ostia, and in the example shown, it was necessary to probe the 2 arteries from *outside* the aorta. The arteries distal to their ostia are usually normal so that surgical relief of the obstruction may cure ischaemic symptoms.

Trauma of the coronary arteries can be caused by a blow on the chest but usually, it is due to cannulation during investigatory or surgical bypass procedures. Excessive perfusion pressures may cause coronary artery stenosis manifesting several weeks after operation.

Two main types of lesion may result from coronary artery obstruction. The *first* type is due to sudden occlusion of one main artery of a coronary tree unprepared for such a disaster; this causes regional infarction. In general, anterior descending artery obstruction causes anteroseptal infarction, and circumflex artery obstruction (right or left) causes posterior infarction. An example is shown in fig. 5. Although death may be sudden, the early myocardial lesion may not be visible at necropsy; the dead tissue releases its enzymes into the circulation quite early however, and this may be detected within 3 to 4 hours, if the victim survives, or may be demonstrated in the myocardium at necropsy. Other useful, but non-specific signs of myocardial damage are anisotropism (best seen in the fibres sectioned lengthwise), and fuchsinophilia.

The *second* type of lesion is the result of gradual stenosis of all three main coronary arteries, which allows full development of the arterial tree. This postpones and modifies final disaster, when the ischaemic myocardium cannot withstand the further deprivation caused by another minor stenosis or obstruction. There is a long history of angina pectoris but no discrete infarction; instead, there is widespread necrosis and fibrosis of the subendocardial myocardium (fig. 6); the innermost narrow rim of muscle escapes destruction, being nourished by blood in the chamber.

Cardiac infarction can occur without marked coronary artery obstruction in haemorrhagic shock, especially if their is already some coronary artery or valvar disease.

The chief complications of myocardial infarction are dysrhythmias, pericarditis, thrombo-embolism, aneurysm formation and cardiac rupture (external or internal).

Dysrhythmias are the most deadly of the complications because they are unpredictable and occur most commonly at the start of the attack. It is no exaggeration to say that sudden death in a person who has coronary artery stenosis but no other necropsy abnormality may be attributed to ventricular fibrillation or to cardiac standstill; this is on the evidence from continuous monitoring of patients in 'coronary' intensive care units. Heart block may occur, but in the writer's experience, this is due usually to involvement of the branches, rather than to lesions of the atrioventricular node of the bundle of His; it can however, occur with extensive anteroseptal infarction (when it is serious and persistent) or with posterior infarction (when it is transient).

Pericarditis together with fever, leucocytosis and electrocardiographic changes, form the classical tetrad of acute myocardial infarction. Sometimes the pericarditis becomes chronic as part of Dressler's syndrome of recurrent fever, chest pain, pleuropericarditis and pneumonitis with haemoptysis, and raised erythrocyte sedimentation rate; it is probably an autoimmune reaction to the damaged myoepicardium.

Thromboembolism is a constant menace to life and limb; the thrombus covers the endocardial surface of the damaged myocardium, and in the early stages, it is friable and may embolize anywhere in the systemic arteries e.g. the limbs, brain, kidneys, spleen, gut, or the myocardium itself. Occasionally, the thrombus is massive and virtually fills the left ventricle, seriously hindering proper contraction of the chamber.

Aneurysm formation is not uncommon and is due to bulging of a wall severely damaged throughout its thickness. The lesion is a source of thromboembolism (fig. 7) and may lead to rupture of the chamber or to chronic heart failure if the patient survives long enough. This has encouraged surgeons to amputate or invaginate the aneurysm. Occasionally however, survival is so prolonged that calcification of the lesion occurs. This is therefore, a relatively benign finding; one of Sir John Parkinson's patients had a calcified aneurysm for at least 20 years.

Rupture of the heart is most common in the first week after the heart attack, when the myocardial damage and cell infiltration are at their maximum, justifying the term *myomalacia cordis* (fig. 8). The rupture may be external or internal.

External rupture of the heart is one of the 2 main causes of fatal haemopericardium and tamponade (the other being dissecting aneurysm). The rupture track through the necrotic wall is usually tortuous and the epicardial lesion may be inconspicuous.

Internal ruptures may involve the chordae tendineae or papillary muscles of the mitral valve, causing acute mitral regurgitation and volume overload of the unprepared left atrium, resulting in acute pulmonary oedema, and death in some cases. Alternatively, the rupture may perforate the interventricular septum, leading to acute overload of the right ventricle and congestive heart failure. If the patient survives long enough, however, the scarring around the orifice (fig. 9) may permit successful surgical closure, if considered necessary.

Perhaps I might end in philosophical vein. There seem to be three unattainable essentials in the prophylaxis of ischaemic heart disease. *Firstly*, we must choose our parents carefully, just as a man should if he wants a good head of hair. *Secondly* it is better to be borne a female; one Professor of Medicine, hearing this advice, commented that if he had to choose between having ischaemic heart disease and being a woman, he would, with deepest respects to the ladies, prefer to have ischaemic heart disease. *Thirdly*, we should live as primitively as possible, eschewing tobacco, consuming only Nature's foodstuffs and spending our days in vigorous exercise; this would ensure healthy ventilation and physiological levels of blood lipids and of fibrinolytic mechanisms; stressful situations would be plentiful and accepted without harm quite naturally – unlike our civilization, in which deep emotion often leads to a fatal heart attack if the coronary arteries are stenosed. Indeed, the writer recalls the case of the husband who came rushing to this hospital in a taxi on learning of his wife's death from ruptured heart. On arrival, he too was dead, and so I had husband and wife together and speechless, probably for the first time, in my mortuary.

All that most of us can do is to avoid overweight and over smoking, take plenty of exercise, keep the mind (and the bowels) open and trust in our Maker.

REFERENCE

1. Neufeld, H. Structural changes of coronary arteries in early life. *Communication to the Second Symposium on Current Aspects of Cardiology*, Institute of Cardiology, London, June 16-18.(1969).

ANATOMY OF THROMBUS FORMATION

J. E. FRENCH †

A thrombus resembles a blood clot as formed in vitro in that it consists entirely of blood constituents, but its distinctive anatomy depends on the ordered rather than random arrangement of these constituents and on their relative proportions. In particular, the blood platelets, which tend to be inconspicuous in the clot, make up a major proportion of at least some parts of the thrombus.

These distinctive features can largely be explained in terms of the effect of blood flow on the solidification of the blood. It has sometimes been lost sight of by those who study the coagulation of blood in vitro that the normal state of the blood is one of movement. Blood in repose, to use Welch's phrase, is an unnatural state brought about by removing blood from the body, or by cessation of the heart's action or by local obstruction or impairment of the circulation. It is in relation to this last situation that the distinction between clotting and thrombosis becomes of major importance. Whereas clotting is likely to be a *consequence* of local arrest of flow, thrombosis is often its *cause*.

It has been known for a long time that two interlinked though separable processes are concerned in the solidification of blood: coagulation of plasma and aggregation of formed elements, represented in mammals by the blood platelets (1). Coagulation involves a series of time-consuming reactions and is at a disadvantage in free flowing blood since a local threshold concentration of the coagulation factors cannot be built up if they are continually washed away and diluted in the passing stream. On the other hand the aggregation process is relatively favoured since it occurs rapidly at a site of local stimulation and the platelets taking part in it are continually replenished from the passing stream. It follows that while flow continues platelets will be the dominant element in the mass which forms. As flow is reduced or stopped the contribution of the two processes is reversed; fibrin formation becomes pronounced and platelets, either individually or in small clumps, are

9

merely dispersed randomly in the fibrin net. Thus the typical thrombus is made up of two more or less different parts. The part that forms first in flowing blood contains a high proportion of platelet material usually as a central branching framework, covered over by a layer of condensed fibrin strands and leucocytes. The part that forms secondarily as blood flow is reduced or stopped consists of a looser network of fibrin with red cells, leucocytes and platelets randomly distributed in it; it fills in the spaces between the branches of the platelet framework and sometimes extends far beyond it when occlusion of the lumen has caused stagnation in a column of blood (2).

The general principles involved in the formation of a thrombus apply at all sites in the circulation though the actual proportions of the different components within it depend on the size and configuration of the vessel in which the thrombus is formed and on the local conditions of blood flow. The classical description of the anatomy of a thrombus was based on the appearance of the long occluding thrombi which occur in the veins of the leg with their characteristically sluggish flow. Here it is possible to distinguish a small pale head, made up predominantly of platelet material at the point where the thrombus first began to grow; a neck, which shows pale rib-like markings where the branching arms of the platelet framework reach the surface; and a red tail often of considerable length which forms later as a stagnant column of blood, distal to the point of occlusion, undergoes coagulation (3). It is unlikely, however, that a single histological section can be taken through the head and neck to show an axial view of the platelet framework in such diagrammatic form. More commonly it will show the framework cut transversely or obliquely so that it appears as islands or strands of granular platelet material, often with leucocytes packed around them, and with fibrin and red blood corpuscles filling the intervening spaces.

In arteries, where if thrombi are to form they must do so in the presence of more vigorous flow, there is relatively more platelet material and relatively less fibrin coagulum. These thrombi tend to be short and condensed, with alternating laminae of pale and dark red material but without an obvious distinction between head and tail. Mural thrombi, in which blood continues to flow past the free border, will also be expected to consist largely of platelet material and indeed in some early forms of mural thrombi, platelets may be the only blood constituent that can be identified.

Although the anatomy of a thrombus can be described in terms of the events which take place during its development, it is doubtful if this information could all have been deduced from the examination of natural thrombi in man. The thrombi which are seen at post mortem, or even the fresher specimens obtained from surgical material, may have been present *in situ* for days or weeks before they are examined histologically and may have undergone degenerative changes which obscure many of their early features. Much of the detailed information has therefore been obtained from observations on thrombosis in injured vessels in experimental animals where events can be observed directly in living preparations, or in which the thrombus can be fixed at chosen intervals for histological examination. The classical experiments of this type were carried out by Bizzozero, Eberth and Schimmelbusch, and Welch at the end of the last century and established many of the points on which modern knowledge of thrombus structure is based. This early work has been reviewed elsewhere (4), and will not be described in detail. More recently much of this work has been confirmed by the use of improved techniques for viewing living preparations and by electron microscopy, and it is now possible to depict the events much more clearly than previously and so to provide a more firm structural basis on which to build the explanation of the formation of thrombi in physiological and biochemical terms.

THE INITIAL STAGES
Platelet adhesion

The first change that can be observed in the development of an experimental thrombus is that platelets begin to accumulate in the lumen of the vessel at the injured site (5). These platelets are at first loosely arranged, have retained their normal discoid shape and appear to touch one another only at a few points. Some may be in contact with the endothelium lining the vessel, but there is no convincing evidence that they will adhere tenaciously unless the endothelium has been completely destroyed or has developed microscopic defects as a result of the injury (6). Thus in experimental arterial thrombi it is usual to find that the endothelium is missing completely from the sites where the thrombus is attached (fig. 1). In veins, platelet accumulation can be induced by much milder forms of injury, but even in such cases it is usual to find a loss of endothelial continuity in the region where the platelets are attached to the wall (7).

It seems probable that the adhesion of platelets is stimulated by contact with the sub-endothelial connective tissue which is exposed to the blood when the endothelium is lost. It is known that platelets will adhere readily to collagen fibres in vitro, and to extravascular collagen fibres during the formation of a haemostatic plug, and it is probable that exposed collagen on the inner surface of the vessel wall would have a similar effect. It is difficult, however, to be certain from transverse sections that collagen is always present at the sites where platelets adhere and the properties of elastic tissue and intimal ground substance would merit further investigation in this regard. In man, the contact of the blood with components of the diseased intima which occurs when the surface of an atherosclerotic plaque is ulcerated or broken appears to be an important factor leading to thrombosis (8).

In arteries, thrombosis may develop no further than the stage of platelet adhesion if the flow remains rapid and linear. It is this fact that allows the operation of thrombo-endarterectomy or the insertion of an arterial graft of foreign material to be carried out in man. Although these procedures involve the destruction of the inner part of the wall of an artery or leave an area denuded of endothelium, they are not usually followed by significant thrombosis provided that a rapid blood flow is restored. This point is illustrated by experiments in rabbits in which a region in the abdominal aorta is denuded of endothelium by passing a roughened probe into the lumen (9). When flow is restored little more than single platelets or small platelet clumps adhere and appear scattered over the bare area (fig. 2). Under these circumstances the adherent platelets can be viewed en face by scanning electron microscopy as well as in section by transmission electron microscopy since they are not obscured by an overlying mass of thrombus material. It can then be seen that the adherent platelets have undergone morphological changes which include swelling and formation of pseudopodial projections, but it is still not clear whether they are clinging specifically to the network of fibres or more generally to the inner surface of the internal elastic lamina (10).

Platelet aggregation

When flow is conducive to the further growth of the thrombus, more platelets adhere to those already attached to the wall and, apparently, a chain reaction is set in motion which builds up a predominantly platelet mass. It used to be thought from observations with the light

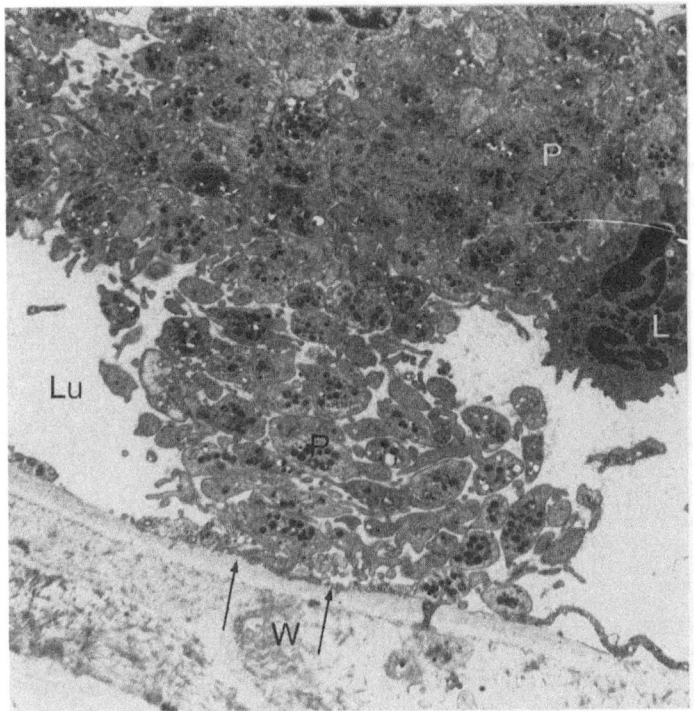

Fig. 1. A mass of platelets (P) in the lumen (LU) of an injured artery in the rabbit cerebral cortex is adherent to the wall (W) at a site where the endothelium has been destroyed (arrows). A single leucocyte (L) is seen at the edge of the mass. Electron micrograph. × 6000.

Acknowledgement. Figs. 1, 2 and 4 are taken from unpublished experiments carried out jointly with A. J. Honour and B. L. Sheppard.

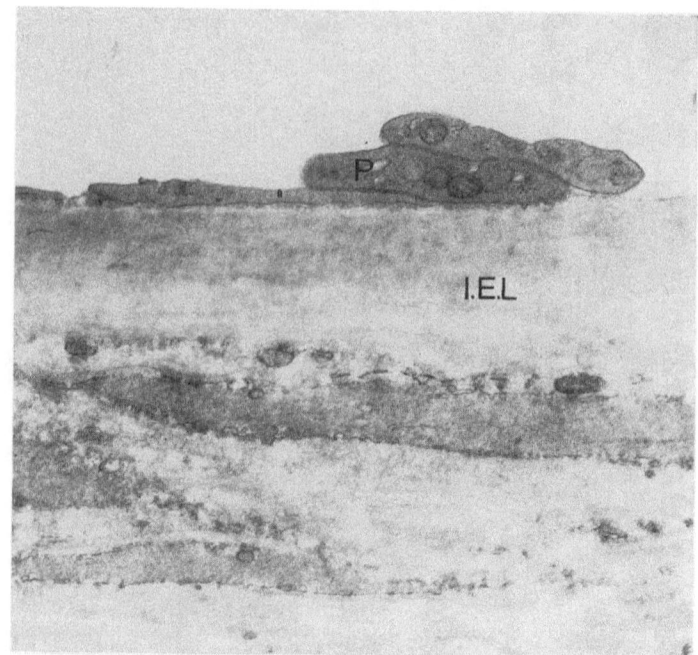

Fig. 2. A group of platelets (P) is adherent to the inner surface of the internal elastic lamina (I.E.L.) in the aorta of a rabbit at a site where the endothelium has been destroyed. Electron microgaph. × 30,000.

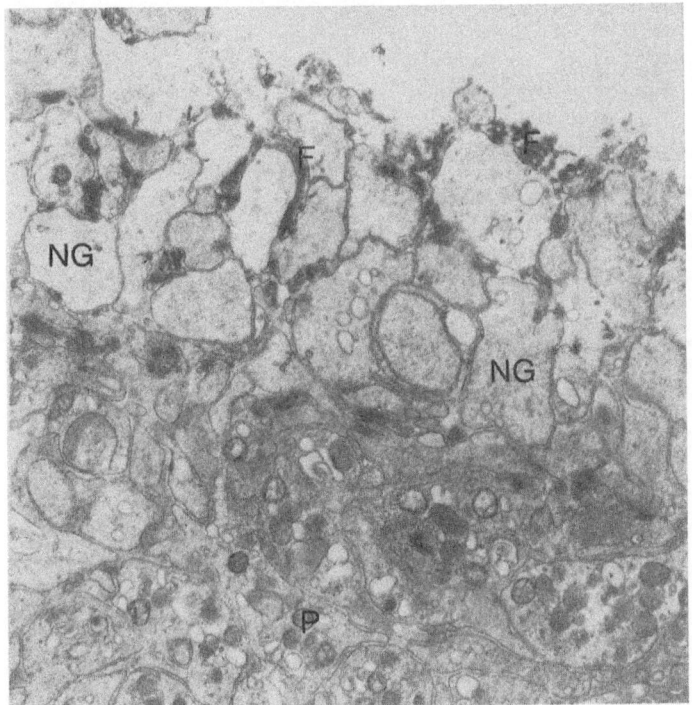

Fig. 3. The periphery of a platelet aggregate (P) in an 'artificial thrombus' shows the presence of fibrin (F) as fine strands around the edges of non-granular bodies (NG). Electron micrograph. × 18,000.

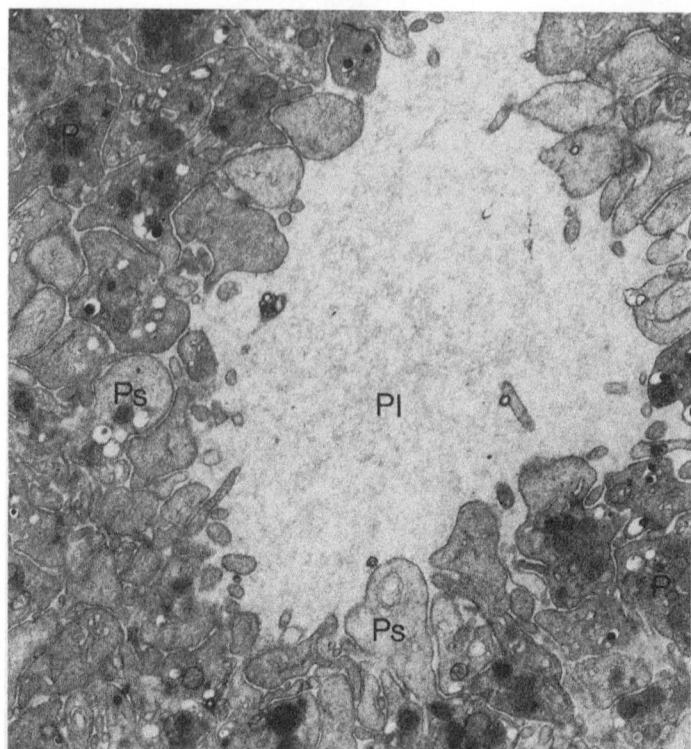

Fig. 4. Part of a platelet mass (P) in a small thrombus in an injured cerebral artery in a rabbit. The platelets at the edges of a space containing plasma (PL) are swollen and have formed outward projections or pseudopodia (PS). Electron micrograph. × 18,000.

microscope that the platelets fused together at this stage, but by electron microscopy it can be seen that this is not so. Although the platelets become very tightly packed together, their boundary membranes are intact and show a fairly regular spacing of about 200 A° from those of adjacent platelets. This gives to the platelet mass a very characteristic mosaic pattern as seen in transverse section (7). Within the limitations of such a compact structure, the platelets appear swollen and some have formed outward projections of their hyaloplasm. With standard methods of electron microscopy, no material has been clearly identified in this narrow gap between the platelet membranes and, as with the gap of similar dimensions which can be seen between the plasma membranes of other types of cell in contact, its nature is not fully understood. Recent evidence indicates that platelets have a surface coating of material rich in carbohydrate which can only be shown up by special staining methods. It is therefore probable that the gap is more apparent than real and is in fact occupied by this outer coating of the plasma membranes (10).

Usually no fibrin can be detected in the growing thrombus at this stage and without this added support it is inherently unstable. Small or larger fragments may be detached from it and be swept away by the blood-stream and sometimes this platelet embolism followed by regrowth of the aggregate is repeated over quite prolonged periods. A natural counterpart in man of this phenomenon observed in experimental animals is the formation of platelet emboli from mural thrombi in the carotid arteries and their subsequent lodgement in vessels of the retina or brain (11).

The growing platelet mass will eventually form the framework of the fully developed thrombus, but its size and configuration will depend on a number of local factors. While rapid flow will tend to wash it away, slowing of flow or whirling or eddying currents in the stream will make more platelets accessible to it. This is not the place to discuss the chemical mediators of platelet aggregation but it can be pointed out that if such factors were released from the damaged vessel wall at the site of injury their local concentration could also affect the extent and rate of growth of the platelet mass which was formed. It has been shown, for example, that when adenosine diphosphate is applied to the surface of moderately injured arteries in the cerebral cortex of the rabbit the size of the platelet aggregates in the lumen is much greater than would otherwise be formed (12).

Stabilization of platelet thrombi

Under conditions where the platelet mass can grow to sufficient size to impede blood flow without being dislodged it undergoes a series of changes beginning at its edges which serve to increase its stability. The peripheral platelets lose their granules and undergo marked swelling so that the platelet aggregates come to be surrounded by a fringe of relatively translucent non-granular bodies. Concurrently fibrin makes its first appearance as a network of fine strands around the non-granular bodies at the periphery; this network extends inwards a short distance from the edge but it does not at this stage penetrate the central parts of the mass (fig. 3). These changes can be attributed to the action of thrombin which is probably first formed in pockets of plasma within the interstices of the platelet mass (fig. 4). It is at this stage too that leucocytes, which had not taken part in the earlier development, begin to adhere around the edges of the platelet mass, apparently attaching specifically to the non-granular bodies rather than to intact platelets.

As the flow is further reduced fibrin formation extends into the plasma spaces between the branches of the platelet framework and may spread further into the stagnating column of blood distal to the obstruction of the lumen. It has been pointed out that this wider extension of the clotting process may occur before the circulation has been brought entirely to a halt. Thus the coagulation part of a thrombus may show, in contrast to a clot formed *in vitro*, an arrangement of fibrin in coarse bands or membranes. This streamline pattern of the fibrin suggests that it may begin to form along the contact surfaces of laminae of flow in the sluggish stream (13).

The later stages

Many of the natural thrombi observed at post mortem do not show the platelet material so clearly as in the fresh experimental thrombi and they may contain a much greater relative proportion of fibrin and of leucocytes. These differences were used at one time as a reason to question whether natural and experimental thrombi could be formed in the same way. Since, however, it is by no means certain that the thrombi observed at post mortem are newly formed it is important in making such comparisons to look at the experimental thrombi also at later intervals. Welch (14) carried out such observations and effectively countered the arguments of his critics, but it is of interest to consider this problem again with the aid of the electron microscope.

It has been shown that with time the platelet aggregates become less densely packed and show a varying degree of degeneration of internal structure. With the separation of the platelets or platelet remnants there is a gradual extension of fibrin into the spaces between them and, eventually, permeation of the whole mass (15). This fibrin is probably derived from the plasma which infiltrates the platelet mass as it shrinks or breaks up, but since the platelets themselves are known to contain fibrinogen, some may be derived from this source. This change accounts for the apparent transformation of platelets to fibrin which may be observed by the light microscope (13). It is not entirely clear how long platelets can persist as identifiable structures. The point is difficult to answer since the growth of a thrombus can be episodic with accumulation of fresh platelets on the surface of an older deposit. Thus the age of a particular platelet observed in the thrombus at the time of sampling does not necessarily correspond to the age of the thrombus as a whole.

In addition to the leucocytes which are incorporated in the thrombus as it grows, others invade it later from the surrounding blood and vessel wall. Granulocytes rapidly show degenerative changes and by release of their lytic enzymes aid in the gradual digestion of the mass. Macrophages, derived from blood monocytes, which are incorporated or migrate into the thrombus, are active in the removal of cell debris. Several reports have indicated that macrophages are capable of ingesting platelets (16) and, since these have a high lipid content, it is probable that this is one of the ways in which the foam celles may be formed in ageing thrombi (17).

The final stage in the natural history of a thrombus is organisation, with penetration of its substance by mesenchymal cells and growth of endothelium over its free surfaces. Many of the mesenchymal cells have the morphological features of vascular smooth muscle but since these cells have apparently the ability to synthesise collagen and elastic tissue the mass is gradually transformed into musculo-elastic tissue, with an end result that is hard to distinguish from other types of thickening in the wall. The organisation of an occluding thrombus may lead to the permanent obliteration of the segment in which it was formed or, if recanalised, to a thickened segment with a drastically reduced lumen. The growth of endothelium over the free surface of a mural thrombus results in effect in the incorporation of the thrombus

into the intima and the formation of a raised plaque that may repro-
duce in arteries many of the features of the atherosclerotic lesion (18).
This process provides the basis for the so-called encrustation theory of
atherosclerosis.

REFERENCES

1. Silberberg, M. *Physiol. Rev.* 18, 197 (1938).
2. French, J. E. & R. G. Macfarlane. in *General Pathology*, edit. Lord Florey. 4th Edit., Chap. 9. Lloyd-Luke, London. – in press.
3. Hadfield, G. *Ann. Roy. Coll. Surg. Engl.* 6, 219 (1950).
4. Poole, J. C. F. & J. E. French, *J. Atheroscler. Res.* 1, 251 (1961).
5. Poole, J. C. F., J. E. French, & W. J. Cliff. *J. clin. Path.* 16, 523 (1963).
6. French, J. E. *Internat. Rev. exper.* Path. 5, 253 (1966).
7. French, J. E., R. G. Macfarlane & A. G. Sanders *Brit. J. exp. Path.* 45, 467 (1964).
8. Friedman, M. & G. J. van den Bovenkamp. *Amer. J. Path.* 48, 19 (1966).
9. Poole, J. C. F., A. G. Sanders, & H. W. Florey. *J. Path. Bact.* 75, 133 (1958).
10. French, J. E. *Proc. Conference on Thrombosis*, Washington 1967 – in press. (1969).
11. Gunning, A. J., G. W. Pickering, A. H. T. Robb-Smith & R. W. Ross-Russell. *Quart. J. Med.* 33, 155 (1964).
12. Honour, A. J. & J. R. A. Mitchell. *Brit. J. exp. Path.* 45, 75 (1964).
13. Jørgensen, L. *Acta path. microbiol. scand.* 62, 189 (1964).
14. Welch, W. H. Reprinted in William Henry Welch Papers and Addresses, Baltimore: Johns Hopkins Press .1, 47 (1887).
15. Jørgensen, L., H. C. Rowsell, T. Hovig, & J. F. Mustard. *Amer. J. Path.* 51, 681 (1967).
16. Poole J. C. F. *Quart. J. exp. Physiol.* 51, 54 (1966).
17. Hand, R. A. & A. B. Chandler. *Amer. J. Path.* 40, 469 (1962).
18. Woolf, N., J. W. P. Bradley, T. Crawford & K. C. Carstairs. *Brit. J. exp. Path.* 49, 257 (1968).

BIOCHEMISTRY OF PLATELETS AND
THROMBUS FORMATION

E. F. LÜSCHER

Platelets are formed by fragmentation of the cytoplasm of the mega-karyocyte; they contain no nucleus and not long ago were thought to be rather primitive structures. In fact they are highly differentiated and specialized cellular elements. This is indicated by their intricate subcellular structure (for a review see 1): in addition to the usual equipment which includes lysosomes (2, 3), mitochondria, vacuoles, a complex microcanalicular system with indications of structures resembling a Golgi-apparatus (4, 5, 6, 7), more specialized elements are also found. These include storage organelles for biologically active amines (8, 9) and, most likely, adenine nucleotides, as well as a marginal bundle of microtubules running along the cytoplasmic membrane in the equatorial plane of the disc-shaped, circulating platelet (10, 11, 12, 13, 14, 15, 16).

Platelets play an important role under physiological as well as under pathological conditions: they adhere and aggregate at the site of a vascular injury, thus forming a hemostatic plus essential in the physiologic arrest of hemorrhage. Under pathological conditions, basically the same process is responsible for the formation of platelet aggregates which may lead to vascular occlusion and thrombus formation. As exemplified by the increased vascular fragility in thrombocytopenia, platelets also bear a hitherto poorly understood relationship to the vascular wall. They act as storage organs for several biologically active amines which may be released under certain conditions and finally they form an integral part of the intrinsic pathway of thrombin formation. As will be discussed later, all these different aspects of platelet function are intimately linked by a rather uniform reactivity of the platelets to a variety of external stimuli.

PLATELET 'METAMORPHOSIS'

Platelets circulate as inert disks with a life span of about 7-11 days (cf. 17). They show glycolytic as well as respiratory activity and are comparatively rich in adenosine-triphosphate (ATP). In order to play their role in hemostasis or in thrombus formation they have to undergo a series of profound alterations involving their morphology and biochemical properties and which furthermore are characterized by the formation of tight and irreversible aggregates, by release reactions whereby certain substances are liberated from the platelets in a rather specific way, and by the appearance of material with procoagulant activity which usually is present in a masked form. These alterations are accompanied by first an activation, and later the decline of metabolic activity. The total of all these changes is observed in the course of the coagulation of platelet-rich plasma; it has been termed the 'viscous metamorphosis' (VM) of the platelets (cf. 18).

Agents capable of inducing VM: The typical alterations observed in platelets in the course of blood coagulation can also be brought about by the addition of the enzyme thrombin to washed platelets in the absence of plasma, provided an adequately buffered solution containing Ca^{2+}-ions is used as the suspension medium (19). Further work has shown that besides thrombin several other enzymes with specificities related to trypsin are equally capable of inducing VM; this is particularly the case for certain snake venom proteases (20. 21). On the other hand, plasmin, the most abundant plasma protease, proves inert. There exists no correlation between fibrin formation and the effect of these enzymes on platelets, making it rather unlikely that fibrinogen is the essential substrate on the platelet surface. Platelets contain other thrombin-labile substrates besides fibrinogen (22, 23), and it remains to be seen whether one of those is involved in the induction of VM.

Another agent which is quite unrelated to proteolytic enzymes and which again in the presence of Ca^{2+}-ions induces platelet changes closely resembling VM is collagen (24, 25, 26, 27, 28, 29). Platelets adhere rapidly to connective tissue or to collagen fibers, and *in situ* to the basement membrane; in the presence of Ca^{2+}-ions this is followed by their mutual aggregation and by a release reaction. This as yet poorly understood reaction is of great importance since by initiating platelet deposition on sites of vascular injury and subsequent events it may trigger thrombus formation.

Immune complexes are also capable of initiating a reaction resembling VM. It is unnecessary that their components cross-react with platelet constituents; the only prerequisite for their activity seems to be their complement – activating capacity (30, 31). On the other hand, the addition of serum complement proves unnecessary for the induction of this reaction. As yet the question remains open whether platelets contain themselves the essential constituents of the complement system or whether they possess membrane receptors of a different character which are capable of reacting with the complement-activating sites of immunoglobulins.

Platelets are known to display phagocytic activity (32, 33). If brought together with gammaglobulin-coated latex particles, a type of reaction resembling VM is again observed. This 'opsonization' of the latex is intimately linked to the aquisition by the gamma globulin of complement-activating properties (34); thus the basic mechanism of this reaction obviously is the same as the one involved in platelet reactivity towards immune complexes.

It is rather remarkable that unrelated materials such as proteases, collagen or immune complexes induce in platelets quite comparable reactions. It seems logical to look for a common denominator, i.e. a factor, or factors, which are put into action in the very first phase of VM and which determine the further course of events. Such a factor has indeed been found in the form of adenosine-5-diphosphate (ADP).

THE ROLE OF ADP IN PLATELET AGGREGATION

Gaarder et al. (35) were the first to identify as ADP a low molecular substance, first isolated from red cells (36) which acted as a powerful aggregating agent for blood platelets. As shown shortly afterwards, ADP is released from blood platelets in the course of VM in sufficient amounts to account for their mutual aggregation (37).

Added to platelets suspended in citrated, but not in EDTA-plasma, minute amounts of ADP will cause aggregation; this effect depends upon the presence of a plasmatic cofactor which was found to be fibrinogen (38, 39, 40). This type of aggregation is reversible; ADP does not enter the cell and is rapidly degraded, whereupon the aggregates fall apart. Such platelets remain morphologically intact. Larger amounts of ADP have a different effect; before the nucleotide disappears by enzymatic cleavage it is capable of initiating far-reaching alterations in the platelets: their storage organelles disappear (41) and adenine nucleotides, including ADP, as well as biologically active amines are released from them (42). This implies that after the addition of threshold concentrations of ADP to platelets this additional, released nucleotide induces the irreversible formation of platelet aggregates (43).

Adrenaline by itself is also capable of causing platelet aggregation; in amounts as small as 10^{-8}M it is furthermore a potentiator of ADP-induced aggregation (44). Serotonin may act in a similar way, except that its effect is time- and concentration dependent (45). Both amines are taken up by platelets and stored in strongly osmiophilic granules; they are released from them in the course of the socalled 'degranulation', which always accompanies VM.

The release reaction therefore is of prime importance for platelet functions; it is an active, energy-dependent and highly specific process (46, 47, 48). Thus it is of interest that the released adenine nucleotides are not derived from a metabolically active pool, but from a special one with a rather slow turnover (49). Degranulation, i.e. the disappearance of typical dense bodies, occurs simultaneously with the release reaction and it therefore seems not unlikely that nucleotides are stored together with biologically active amines in the same storage organelles.

The special role of ADP suggests that most of the observed platelet reactions, in particular VM, including irreversible aggregation, will be observed whenever a suitable agent brings about the release reaction. The ADP thus made available would then be responsible for all subsequent alterations, in particular for irreversible aggregation. Haslam (50) has indeed shown that in the presence of agents capable of rapidly eliminating ADP from the system, platelets will not aggregate even after the addition of thrombin.

Several hypotheses have been proposed in order to explain the dramatic and highly specific effect of ADP on platelets. Most of them start with the assumption that the nucleotide interferes with the activity of a membrane-located ATPase. The characteristics of this enzyme exclude the Na^+/K^+-dependent membrane-ATPase and point to the possibility that the contractile protein of the blood platelets, thrombosthenin, is involved (51, 52, 53).

Thrombosthenin is an actomyosin-like protein; it represents up to 15 percent of the platelets total protein (for a review see 54). It can be dissociated into actin-, and myosin-like moieties (thrombosthenin A and M; cf. 55). The possibility has to be taken into account that thrombostenin A bears a close relationship to the microfilaments which form the structural subunits of the microtubules (5, 56), the latter disappearing at the expense of contractile microfibrils whenever platelets undergo VM. Thrombosthenin M is a weak ATPase; its activity is enhanced by the combination with the actin moiety (57). Inhibition of the myosin ATPase-activity by ADP has been described for muscle myosin (58).

The ADP-inhibition of the thrombosthenin ATPase would lead to structural changes of the platelet membrane, or, according to some authors, to a dissociation of thrombosthenin into its components by accumulation of ATP (51). Aggregation is thought to result either from alterations in charge distribution on the cell surface, or from the formation of new actin-myosin complexes between adjacent platelets. It should be noted that all these theories imply that thrombosthenin in located on the platelet surface; up to now convincing evidence for this assumption is still missing.

On the other hand, there can be little doubt that contractile activity plays a major role in platelet function. Platelet aggregates show spontaneous, active contraction, and this may be a decisive factor in the formation of firm, mechanically resistant platelet thrombi. Most likely, the release reaction is also linked to contractile activity; as stated before it is an energy-dependent process, perhaps involving the active participation of a contractile micro-canalicular system. Not unexpectedly, several of the many substances known to interfere with platelet activity are also capable of interaction with the isolated contractile protein (cf. 59).

PLATELET ACTIVITY AND THROMBUS FORMATION

Any endothelial lesion which leads to the availability of connective tissue, in particular to the denudation of the basement membrane, will result in the deposition of platelets. These adhere at first passively; they will then undergo VM under the influence of collagen. Theoretically the subsequent release reaction should lead to the incorporation of new platelets into this primary mixed aggregate, and these platelets in turn should develop VM, because of a critical ADP-concentration in their environment. Thus, an ever growing aggregate should form. Under experimental conditions this prediction has been verified many times; however, the formed platelet masses remain fragile and as a rule are easily fragmented and carried away by the blood stream in the form of harmless micro-emboli. For the formation of a solid, obstructing thrombus some additional event must obviously enter into play, and there is some evidence that this might be the activation of the blood clotting system. As discussed before, thrombin is a powerful initiator of vm. Any disruption of tissue leads to the appearance of tissue activator, and the vascular wall is particularly rich in tissue thromboplastin. Thus, thrombin will almost invariably be formed by the extrinsic pathway of the blood clotting system at the site of vascular injury. This must be considered an additional factor, besides collagen in the initiation of vm in the first, adhering platelets.

More important, however, is the appearance of platelet procoagulants, in particular of platelet factor 3 in the course of vm. This factor, a phospholipoprotein, is essential for the formation of activator complexes in the intrinsic pathway of thrombin formation. Again, the formed thrombin will cause vm in adhering or already aggregated platelets. It forms an alternative pathway to platelet aggregation in addition to the ADP-mechanism discussed above. It is the thrombin formed by this pathway which finally leads to fibrin formation, i.e. the formation of a red thrombus, which as a rule follows serious impairment of circulation by established platelet masses.

Thrombus formation must be looked-at as a dynamic process: the released ADP which is essential for platelet aggregation, may become degraded before critical concentrations are reached; thrombin is constantly inactivated by antithrombins, and the circulating blood not only dilutes activators of vm and coagulation, but also disrupts formed, unstabilized thrombi by sheer mechanical force. Factors favoring thrombus formation therefore are all the cofactors of platelet aggregation, to mention first adrenalin; the higher incidence of thrombus formation in stress situations may be explained this way. Not less important is the often discussed 'hypercoagulability', i.e. a condition characterized by a higher tendency to thrombin formation, be it because of the presence of activators, or a decrease of inhibitors in circulation. Finally the flow conditions are of marked influence – a stagnant or slowed-down circulation, for reasons given above, facilitating platelet aggregation and fibrin formation.

CONCLUSIONS

The study of the biochemical background of platelet function has already led to interesting results: the transformation of the circulating, inert platelets to aggregated platelet masses is a complex, energy-dependent process, in which the platelet release reaction and ADP in particular play an essential role. This transformation is brought about by thrombin, by collagen, by complement-activating immune complexes, by adrenaline, under certain conditions by serotonin, and most important, by ADP. Many aspects of the reactions involved are as yet poorly understood. Nevertheless, some insight into a most complex multicomponent system has already been gained, and it can be hoped that an even better knowledge of the basic mechanisms will open the way to new approaches to the prevention of thrombus formation.

REFERENCES

1. Schulz H., *Thrombocyten und Thrombose im elektronenoptischen Bild*. Springer, Berlin, Heidelberg, New York. (1968).
2. Marcus A. J., W. Zucker-Franklin, L. B. Safier, H. L. Ullman, Studies on human platelet granules and membranes. *J. clin. Invest.* 45, 14 (1966).
3. Siegel A., E. F. Lüscher, Non-identity of the α-granules of human blood platelets with typical lysosomes. *Nature*, Lond. 215, 745 (1967).
4. Behnke O., Electron microscopic observations on the membrane systems of the rat bloot platelet. *Anat. Record*, 158, 121 (1967).
5. Bettex-Galland M., E. F. Lüscher, E. R. Weibel, Thrombosthenin – Electron microscopical studies on its localization in human blood platelets and some properties of its subunits. *Thrombos. Diathes. haemorrh.* (To be published).
6. White J. G., Effects of ethylenediamine tetracetic acid (EDTA) on platelet structure. *Scand. J. Haemat.* 5, 241 (1968).
7. Zucker-Franklin D., Ultrastructural analysis of transport and storage by a platelet membrane system. Abstr. XII. *Congr. int. Soc. Haemat.* 205 (1968).
8. Davis R. B., J. G. White, Localization of 5-hydroxytryptamine in blood platelets: An autoradiographic and ultrastructural study. *Brit. J. Haemat.* 15, 93 (1968).
9. Prada, da, M., A. Pletscher, J. P. Tranzer, H. Knuchel, Subcellular localization of 5-hydroxytryptamine and histamine in blood platelets. *Nature*, Lond. 216, 1315 (1967).
10. Behnke O., T. Zelander, Substructure in negatively stained microtubules of mammalian blood platelets. *Exper. Cell Research*, 43, 236 (1967).
11. Haydon G. B., A. Taylor, Microtubules in hamster platelets. *J. Cell Biol.* 26, 673 (1965).
12. Sandborn E. B., J. J. Le Buis, P. Bois, Cytoplasmatic microtubules in blood platelets. *Blood* 27, 247 (1966).
13. Silver M. D., J. E. Mc Kinstry, Morphology of microtubules in rabbit platelets. *Z. Zellforsch.*, 81, 12 (1967).
14. Sixma J. J., I. Molenaar, Microtubules and microfibrils in human platelets. *Thrombos. Diathes. haemorrh.* 16, 153 (1966).
15. White J. G., The substructure of human platelet microtubules. *Blood* 32, 638 (1968).
16. Zucker-Franklin D., R. L. Nachman, Microtubules and microfilaments of blood platelets. *J. Cell Biol.* 35, 149 A (1967).
17. Cooney D. P., B. A. Smith, D. E. Fawley, The use of ^{32}diisopropylfluorophosphate (32DFP) as a platelet label: Evidence for reutilization of this isotope in man. *Blood*, 31, 791 (1968).

18. Roskam J., Proposals for certain definitions in haemostasis and thrombosis in 'Diffuse Intravascular Coagulation'. *Thrombos. Diathes. haemorrh.*, suppl. 20, 317 (1966).
19. Lüscher E. F., Viscous metamorphosis of blood platelets and clot retraction. *Vox sang* 1, 133 (1956).
20. Davey M. G., E. F. Lüscher, Actions of thrombin and other coagulant and proteolytic enzymes on blood platelets. *Nature*, Lond. 216, 857 (1967).
21. Davey M. G., E. F. Lüscher, Effects of some coagulant snake venoms upon human platelets. *Proc. 10th Congr. europ. Soc. haemat.* 2, 1118 (1967).
22. Davey M. G., E. F. Lüscher, Platelet proteins. *Biochemistry of blood platelets*, E. Kowalski, S. Niewiarowski, Ed.; page 9, Academic Press, London, NY (1967).
23. Ganguly P., Studies on platelet proteins II. Effect of thrombin. *Blood* 33, 590 (1969).
24. Caen J. P., Y. Legrand, Analyse des fonctions plaquettaires – Adhésion et agrégation des plaquettes du collagène purifié lyophilisé. *Rev. franç. Et. Clin. Biol.* 13, 1028 (1968).
25. Hovig T., L. Jørgensen, M. A. Packham, J. F. Mustard, Platelet adherence to fibrin and collagen. *J. Lab. clin. Med.* 71, 29 (1968).
26. Loder P. B., J. Hirsh, G. C. de Gruchy, The effect of collagen on platelet glycolysis and nucleotide metabolism. *Brit. J. Haemat.* 14, 563 (1968).
27. Lüscher E. F., Les mécanisms de l'activation des plaquettes sanguines. *Path. Biol.* 14, 224 (1966).
28. Puszkin E., Z. Jerushalmy, Effect of connective tissue and collagen on platelet lactate. *Proc. Soc. exper. Biol.* NY 129, 346 (1968).
29. Wilner G. D., H. G. Nossel, E. C. Le Roy, Aggregation of platelets by collagen. *J. clin. Invest.* 47, 2616 (1968).
30. Bettex-Galland M., E. F. Lüscher, Untersuchungen über die Auslösung der viskösen Metamorphose der menschlichen Blutplättchen durch Immunkomplexe. *Path. Microbiol.* 27, 533 (1964).
31. Mueller-Eckhardt Ch., E. F. Lüscher, Immune reactions of human blood platelets. I. A comparative study on the effects of heterologous antiplatelet antiserum, of antigen-antibody complexes, of aggregated gamma-globulin, and of thrombin on platelets. *Thrombos. Diathes. haemorrh.* 20, 152 (1968).
32. Glynn M. F., H. Z. Movat, E. A. Murphy, J. F. Mustard, Platelet phagocytosis. *Blood* 25, 603 (1965).
33. Glynn M. F., R. Herren, J. F. Mustard, Adherence of latex particles to platelets. *Nature*, Lond. 212, 79 (1966).
34. Mueller-Eckhardt Ch., E. F. Lüscher, Immune reactions of human blood platelets. II. The effect of latex particles coated with gamma globulin in relation to complement activitation. *Thrombos. Diathes. haemorrh.* 20, 168 (1968).
35. Gaarder A., J. Jonsen, S. Laland, A. Hellem, P. A. Owren, Adenosine diphosphate in red cells as a factor in the adhesiveness of human blood platelets. *Nature*, Lond. 192, 531 (1961).
36. Hellem A. J., The adhesiveness of human blood platelets in vitro. *Norwegian Monographs on Med. Science* (1960).
37. Käser-Glanzmann R., E. F. Lüscher, The mechanism of platelet aggregation in relation to hemostasis. *Thrombos. Diathes. haemorrh.* 7, 480 (1962).
38. Cross M. J., Effect of fibrinogen on the aggregation of platelets by adenosine diphosphate. *Thrombos. Diathes. haemorrh.* 12, 524 (1964).
39. Deykin D., G. R. Pritzker, E. M. Scolnick, Plasma cofactors in adenosine diphosphate – induced aggregation of human platelets. *Nature*, Lond. 208, 296 (1965).
40. McLean. J. R., R. E. Maxwell, W. Hertler: Fibrinogen and adenosine diphosphate-induced aggregation of platelets. *Nature*, Lond. 202, 605 (1964).
41. Sixma J. J., J. J. Geuze, Degranulation of human platelets during ADP-induced aggregation. *Vox sang.* 10, 309 (1968).

42. Zucker M. B., J. Peterson, Serotonin, platelet factor 3 activity, and platelet aggregating agent released by adenosine diphosphate. *Blood* 30, 556 (1967).
43. Macmillan D. C., Secondary clumping effect in human citrated platelet-rich plasma produced by ADP and adrenaline. *Nature*, Lond. 211, 140 (1966).
44. Thomas D. P., Effect of cathecholamines on platelet aggregation caused by thrombin. *Nature*, Lond. 215, 298 (1967).
45. Baumgartner H. R., G. V. R. Born, Effects of 5-hydroxytryptamine on platelet aggregation. *Nature*, Lond. 218, 137 (1968).
46. Davey M. G., E. F. Lüscher, Platelet release reactions. *Biochim. Biophys. Acta* 165, 490 (1968).
47. Holmsen H., H. J. Day, Thrombin-induced platelet release reaction and platelet lysosomes. *Nature*, Lond. 219, 760 (1968).
48. Mürer E., A. J. Hellem, M. C. Rozenberg, Energy metabolism and platelet function. *Scand. J. clin. Lab. Invest.* 19, 280 (1967).
49. Holmsen H., Adenine nucleotide pools in platelets. *Abstr. XII Congr. int. Soc. Haemat.*, 202 (1968).
50. Haslam R. J., Role of adenosine diphosphate in the aggregation of human blood platelets by thrombin and by fatty acids. *Nature*, Lond. 202, 765 (1964).
51. Booyse F. M., M. E. Rafelson, jr., Hypothesis: Studies on human platelets. III: A contractile protein model for platelet aggregation. *Blood*, 33, 100 (1969).
52. Salzman E. W., D. A. Chambers., L. L. Neri, Possible mechanism of aggregation of blood platelets by adenosine diphosphate. *Nature*, Lond. 210, 167 (1966).
53. White J. G., The muscular system of platelets. *Blood* 30, 539 (1967).
54. Bettex-Galland M., E. F. Lüscher, Thrombosthenin, the contractile protein from blood platelets, and its relation to other contractile proteins. *Advanc. Protein Chem.* 20, 1 (1965).
55. Bettex-Galland M., E. F. Lüscher, H. Portzehl, Dissociation of thrombosthenin into two components comparable with actin and myosin. *Nature*, Lond. 193, 777 (1962).
56. Zucker-Franklin D., Microfibrils of blood platelets: Their relationship to microtubules and the contractile protein. *J. Clin. Invest.* 48, 165 (1969).
57. Bettex-Galland M., H. Portzehl, E. F. Lüscher, Dissoziation des Thrombosthenins in seine zwei Komponenten. Untersuchung ihrer Adenosintriphosphatase-Aktivität. *Helv. Chim. Acta* 46, 1595 (1963).
58. Kiely B., A. Martonosi, The binding of ADP to myosin. *Biochim. Biophys. Acta* 172, 158 (1969).
59. Lüscher E. F., Report of the Subcommittee on Current Concepts of Hemostasis. Platelets, their role in hemostasis and thrombosis. *Thrombos. Diathes. haemorrh*, suppl. (1969).

BIOCHEMICAL CHANGES IN THE MYOCARDIUM DURING THE REPARATIVE PROCESSES FOLLOWING CORONARY ARTERY OCCLUSION

W. BRAASCH, S. GUDBJARNASON, R. J. BING

The mechanism of tissue repair in infarcted heart muscle consists of two parallel phases, the catabolic phase of degradation of dead and severely damaged heart muscle cells and the anabolic phase of fibroblastic proliferation and synthesis of scar tissue replacing the necrotic muscle.

After an acute coronary occlusion there is a rapid response of the infarcted tissue to the injury. The reparative processes, as manifested by incorporation of glycine-2-C^{14} into cellular subfractions from normal and infarcted heart muscle, are associated with an early increase in nucleolar ribosomal RNA-and protein synthesis. These synthetic processes require oxygen and substrates, that cannot be readily transported into the ischaemic area. The primary question concerning tissue repair therefore is that of energy production, since the energy for synthetic reparative processes must be made available in the infarcted and hypoxic muscle.

The purpose of our studies was to examine alterations in the metabolism of infarcted cardiac muscle, particularly with respect to pathways of energy production and the mechanism of fatty degeneration or accumulation of lipids in the ischaemic tissue.

The metabolic changes of the non infarcted left ventricle were also of interest because a rapid loss of contractility and even passive bulging of the ischaemic area results in an increased workload for this portion of the heart, which again can lead to a compensatory hypertrophy.

Methods

Myocardial infarctions were produced in dogs by ligating branches of the descendens and circumflex left coronary arteries. (fig. 1).

Between 48 hours and 6-9 months after occlusion the thoracic wall and pericardium were reopened and biopsy samples taken from the periphery and the center of the infarct and from the non-infarcted part of the left ventricle, immediately frozen in precooled freon® and trans-

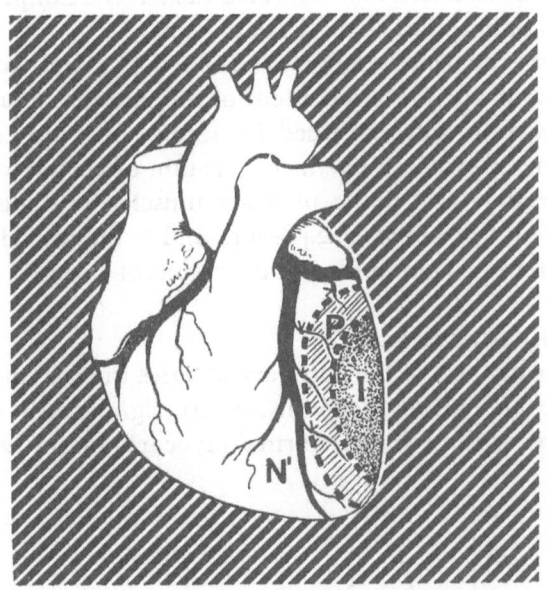

Fig. 1. Scheme of experimental procedure. Production of infarct by ligating branches of the left descendens and circumflex coronary artery. Muscle samples were taken from the center (I) and the periphery (P) of the infarcted part and from the non-infarcted part (N') of the left ventricle.

ferred to liquid nitrogen. The tissue samples were pulverized and homogenized and the content of ATP, creatine phosphate and lactate determined enzymatically.

After removing the hearts about 1 g of muscle was taken from the corresponding areas and deep-frozen. Enzyme activities from the glycolytic and the oxidative pathway and from the hexose-monophosphate shunt were then determined the next day. The following enzymes from the glycolitic pathway and the oxidative metabolism were used: phosphofructokinase, fructose-1,6-diphosphate aldolase, glyceraldehyde-phosphate dehydrogenase, α-glycerophosphate dehydrogenase, lactate dehydrogenase, malate dehydrogenase, NAD and NADP specific isocitrate dehydrogenase and glutamate oxaloacetate transaminase.

The hexose-monophosphate shunt was represented by glucose-6-phosphate dehydrogenase and 6-phosphogluconate dehydrogenase. The creatine phosphokinase was also determined.

Lipid synthesis was studied by incorporation of acetate-C^{14} into the lipids of infarcted and non-infarcted tissue. The samples were taken 2 hours after i.v. injection of 30 µC/kg of acetate.

The substrate concentrations were related to g wet weight, the enzyme activities to the protein content of the samples, determined with the biuret reaction and expressed in µmole substrate converted per minute per mg of protein. The incorporation of acetate was expressed in µmole acetate-1-C^{14} per g of heart muscle. The mean values of the different groups between 24 hours and 6 months after coronary artery ligation were compared with the results of a control group.

RESULTS AND DISCUSSION

24 hours after ligation of the coronary arteries the enzyme activities of the oxidative and glycolytic pathway are significantly lower in the ischaemic myocardium than in normal myocardium (fig. 2).

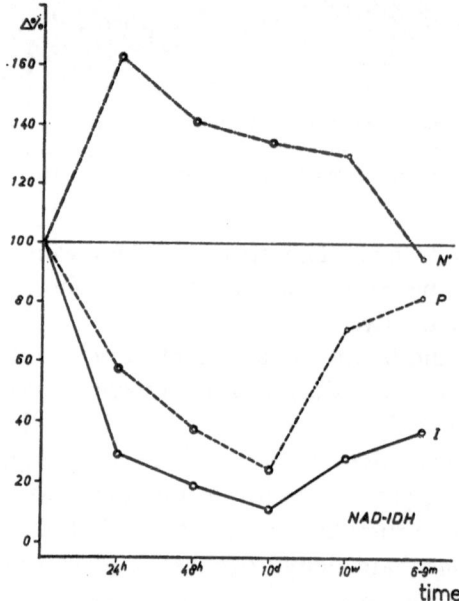

Fig. 2. Changes, as percent of normal, of the NAD-dependant isocitric dehydrogenase in the center (I) and periphery (P) of the infarct and in non-infarcted left ventricle (N') between 24 hours and 6-9 months following coronary artery ligation.

The lowest values are reached after 10 days in the center of the infarct with 11-15% for the oxidative and 5-30% for the glycolytic pathway and 21% for the creatine phosphokinase compared with the mean values of the control group. This decline is followed by a gradual increase, so that normal levels are reached after 6 months in the periphery of the infarct. In the center, however, the enzyme activities remain significantly reduced.

In the non-infarcted part of the left ventricle we observe an increase of glycolytic and oxidative enzyme activities, which also return to normal after 6 months.

Fig. 2 demonstrates as example the percent changes of the NAD-specific isocitric dehydrogenase, a mitochondrial enzyme from the oxidative pathway.

The changes in the concentration of ATP, creatine phosphate and lactate in the center and the periphery of the infarct and in the non-infarcted part of the left ventricle 2 and 10 days and 6-9 months after onset of ischaemia are illustrated in fig. 3.

The mean content of creatine phosphate is reduced from 8,5 to 1,5

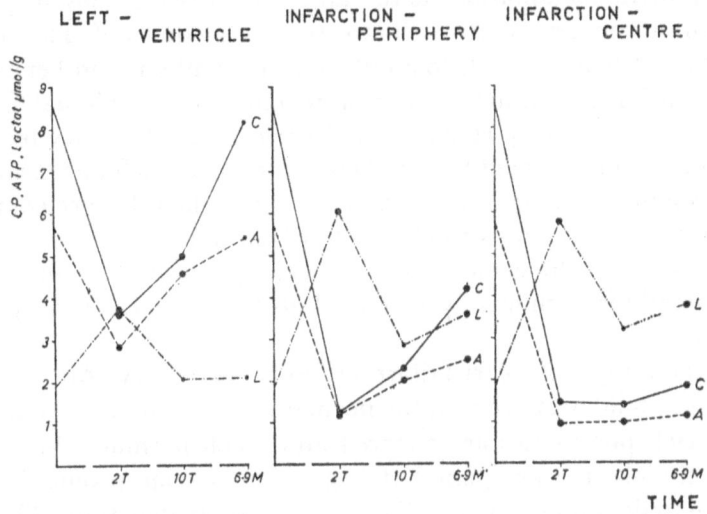

Fig. 3. Mean values of creatine-phosphate (c), adenosinetriphosphate (A) and lactate (L) in μmol/g in the center and periphery of the infarction and in the non-infarcted left ventricle, two (2 D) (n = 5) and ten days (10 D) (n = 6) and 6-9 months (6-9 M) (n = 9) following onset of ischaemia. Big dots indicate significant differences (P < 0,05) with respect to a normal control group (n = 14).

and that of ATP from 5,7 to 0,9 μmol/g in the center of the infarct 48 hours after coronary artery occlusion (fig. 3). There is no change at the 10th day and only a slight increase 6 months later.

In the periphery of the infarct the energy rich phosphates are also significantly reduced at the end of the second day. They, however, show a marked increase at the 10th day and reach about 50% of the control values at the end of the 6-month period.

The mean lactate level has increased 3-fold after 48 hours and is still significantly higher after 6-9 months in the center as well as in the periphery of the infarct.

But also in the *non-infarcted* part of the left ventricle we see the creatine phosphate and ATP content significantly reduced 48 hours after coronary artery ligation. The concentration of lactate is significantly higher than in the controls. The energy rich phosphates markedly increase again until the 10th day and reach the control levels after 6-9 months. The lactate concentration is normal again at the end of the 10th day.

The decrease of ATP and creatine phosphate in the non-infarcted left ventricle is explained by a functional overloading as a result of a loss of contractility of the infarcted area. Despite activation of the oxidative and glycolytic metabolism the resynthesis of creatine phosphate is not sufficient to compensate for the increased energy demand. The creatine phosphate deficiency leads to a reduced ATP synthesis and hence to an 'energy deficiency failure' according to Fleckenstein. Similar findings have been reported by Hochrein and coworkers, when they increased the work-load of isolated hearts. According to Gerlach and Thorn the heart muscle shows signs of congestive failure when the ATP content of the myocardium is reduced below 50% of normal.

The mean enddiastolic left ventricular pressure of our animals consequently is significantly increased 48 hours after coronary artery ligation.

But these signs of heart failure are only temporary. After 10 days the enddiastolic pressure is in the normal range again and the levels of energy rich phosphates are restored and reach normal values at the end of the observation period (fig. 3). The enzyme profile does not show an activation of myocardial metabolism at that time. The non-infarcted left ventricle seems to have compensated for the loss of contractility of the ischaemic myocardium.

In contrast to the diminished activity of glycolytic and mitochondrial enzymes there is a significant rise in the activity of the hexose-monophosphate shunt enzymes (fig. 4). The changes in activity of the glucose-6-phosphate dehydrogenase are most pronounced in the center of the infarct, where the activity has increased 30-fold at the end of the 10th day. In the periphery of the infarct the activity has increased 20-fold and in the non-infarcted left ventricle it is still 250% higher than that of the control group. The activities of the glucose-6-phosphate dehydrogenase then decline again and approach normal levels 10 weeks after infarction, 6-9 months after coronary artery occlusion, however, the activity of the glucose-6-phosphate dehydrogenase is still significantly higher in the scar tissue of the healed infarct than in the normal cardiac muscle (fig. 4).

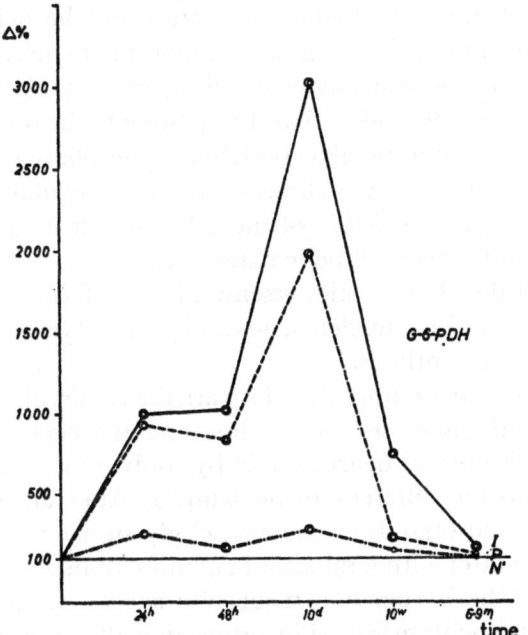

Fig. 4. Percent changes of the hexose-monophosphate-shunt enzyme glucose-6-phosphate-dehydrogenase in the non-infarcted left ventricle (N') and the periphery (P) and center (I) of the infarct between 24 hours and 6-9 months following coronary artery ligation. 100% = mean value of the control groups.

The enhanced formation of $C^{14} O_2$ from glucose-1-C^{14} in infarcted tissue, also reflects an increased activity of the hexose-monophosphate shunt. Our assay system did not contain exogenous NAD or NADP. The increase in C 1/C 6 ratio from 3,5 in normal heart muscle homogenate to 9,8 in homogenate from infarcted tissue is of significance because those tissue samples are obtained from the left ventricle of the same hearts and so reflect alterations due to coronary occlusion.

The activation of the hexose-monophosphate shunt seems to be ATP dependant with an increase in activity at lower ATP levels, since the $C^{14} O_2$ production of glucose-1-C^{14} is reduced, when ATP is added to the homogenate of the infarcted tissue with no change in the normal heart muscle sample.

A relative increase in activity of glyceraldehyde-phosphate dehydrogenase in infarcted tissue indicates that anaerobic phosphorylation of ADP to ATP can continue at a relatively high level in the ischaemic area, if the substrate glyceraldehyde-phosphate can be provided. A continuing supply of glyceraldehyde-phosphate could be delivered by the shunt since the activity of the glucose-6-phosphate dehydrogenase and also of the 6-phosphogluconate dehydrogenase continues to increase for at least 10 days after infarction. In addition to the role of the hexose-monophosphate shunt in glyceraldehyde phosphate-production and potential ATP-formation the shunt enters as a regulative device into the overall energy production of the cell through its numerous interconnections with other metabolic pathways.

The role of the shunt is also essential for the formation of ribose-5-phosphate required for nucleic acid- and protein synthesis and also for NADPH dependent synthesis.

In line with these findings therefore are the results about the changes of protein synthesis in the border-line and the center of the infarct compared with normal heart muscle by studying the incorporation of glycin-C^{14} into the different tissue samples. After an initial decrease to 70% of normal there is an increase of glycin incorporation into the center of the infarct with a maximum of more than 200% at the end of the 4th day. The border-line tissue also shows an early increase in protein synthesis with maximal incorporation 48 hours after infarction. These changes are paralleled by an increase in RNA- and DNA concentration.

Studies about the incorporation of glycin-C^{14} into the subcellular fractions showed an early renewal of cell material in the infarcted area. Incorporation into nuclear ribosomal fraction increased first, followed by mitochondria and microsomes. The incorporation into contractile proteins however remained subnormal.

The decrease in oxidative metabolism of infarcted and non-infarcted muscle is accompanied by a significant increase in lipid synthesis in the energy deficient muscle (fig. 5). Two days after infarction the incorporation of acetate $1\text{-}C^{14}$ into lipids is greatest in the periphery of the infarct, but at the 10th day the increase in lipid synthesis in the center of the infarct exceeds that of the periphery.

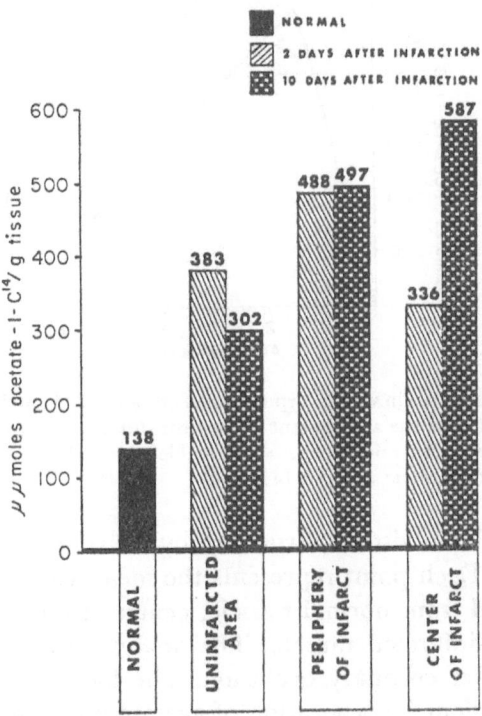

Fig. 5. Incorporation of acetate-1-c^{14} into lipids of infarcted and uninfarcted heart muscle two days (n = 4) and ten days (n = 6) after coronary artery occlusion compared to normal (n = 10).

The increased lipid synthesis is also associated with an alteration in the fractional distribution of acetate into the various lipids. In infarcted tissue the relative incorporation of labeled acetate into the triglycerid fraction is significantly increased, whereas the relative incorporation into phospholipids is markedly diminished. In order to relate the rate of lipid synthesis to energy metabolism the incorporation of acetate into myocardial lipids was studied in vitro as a function of the ATP-concentration. Our experiments indicate that myocardial lipid synthesis is strongly dependent upon cellular ATP content with maximal incorporation at the relatively low ATP level of one μmol/g of tissue. The incorporation diminishes with increasing ATP-concentration reaching the lowest rate of synthesis at physiological ATP-concentration of 6-8 μmol.

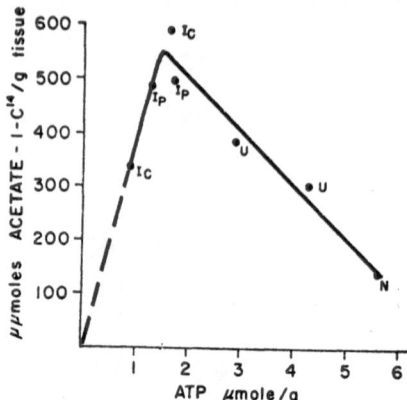

Fig. 6. Relationship between in vivo incorporation of acetate-1-C¹⁴ into lipids of normal and infarcted heart muscle and the ATP content of the tissue (μmol/g). Biopsy samples were obtained two and ten days after infarction. N = normal left ventricle, U = non-infarcted muscle, IP = periphery of infarct, IC = center of infarct.

Fig. 6 confirms the in vitro observations by the results of the analysis of biopsy samples. Each point represents the mean values of 6-10 biopsy samples removed from normal muscle, center of infarct, periphery of infarct and non-infarcted muscle. The analyses were performed two and ten days after coronary occlusion. The figure illustrates an ATP or energy dependent incorporation of acetate into lipids. The acetate incorporation into lipids reaches a maximum in infarcted muscle at an ATP level of 1-2 μmol/g. The incorporation diminishes significantly with increasing ATP content of the tissue and reaches the lowest level in the normal heart muscle not subjected to myocardial infarction (fig. 6).

The increase in fatty acid and lipid formation seems to serve two functions, first to regenerate NADP required for continuous operation of the hexose-monophosphate-shunt and second to remove the products of the glycolytic pathway in the ischaemic tissue.

The activation of the hexose-monophosphate-shunt, only of minor importance under normal conditions in the myocardium, seems to be an adoptive mechanism of the ischaemic tissue as well as of the non-infarcted left ventricle, subjected to an increased workload. It is known from the literature, that this direct oxidative pathway is mainly used when new cell material is needed. In the infarcted myocardium too there are an increased proliferation of cells and a renewal and transformation of necrotic tissue into connective scar tissue.

The activation of the hexose-monophosphate-shunt and the increased protein synthesis in the non-infarcted part of the left ventricle makes possible the compensatory hypertrophy of the infarcted heart.

It was possible to influence these reparative processes in the myocardium following coronary artery occlusion. When the tissue repair was stimulated and the animals treated with anabolic agents such as insulin, growth hormone or dianabol there was a significant increase in protein synthesis of non-infarcted as well as infarcted heart muscle. When this treatment was continued for several weeks the development of left ventricular aneurysms in these animals could be completely prevented.

The role of protein intake in tissue repair and cardiac hypertrophy or adaptation after myocardial infarction was examined by feeding the animals a protein free diet. These animals showed the very low rate of survival of 33% against a survival rate of 70-80% in the group on a regular diet. A significantly impaired tissue repair, as illustrated in the formation of a very thin scar and frequent development of aneurysms was also observed in the animals on a protein deficient diet.

By a stimulation of the reparative processes in the ischaemic myocardium with a quicker and improved scar formation and a better adaptation of the non-infarcted left ventricle to the increased workload we one day hope to be able to decrease the mortality, prevent complications and reduce the time of rehabilitation of our infarct patients.

Literature on request from the author.

Medizinische Universitäts-klinik
6900 Heidelberg 1
Bergheimerstraße 58
W.-Germany

QUANTITATION OF ENZYME RELEASE FROM INFARCTED HEART MUSCLE

S. A. G. J. WITTEVEEN, W. TH. HERMENS, H. C. HEMKER,
L. HOLLAAR

Although the determination of serum enzyme levels in patients with a myocardial infarction has been a more or less standard procedure for many years, it is surprising that these determinations are used mostly to establish a diagnosis. Among the abundant literature (1, 2, 3, 4, 5) on enzyme elevations after myocardial infarction in man there are only a few articles in which the authors try to use a quantitative approach by comparing for example the maximal enzyme elevations with the death rate after infarction (6, 7) or with the electrocardiographic changes (8). As is to be expected some correlation was found.

In animal experiments good correlations were found between the size of the infarction at autopsy and the maximal serum enzyme levels determined after the infarction (9).

One of the main reasons why the quantitative approach has not been used frequently in man is probably because a thorough analysis of enzyme levels is possible only when significantly more data are collected than is done in actual clinical practice. This makes it difficult to find the maximum of the enzyme levels attained in an individual patient as well as to estimate the disappearance rate of the enzyme from the plasma. Also one has to know the distribution volume, i.e. the volume of fluid into which the enzymes are diluted after having leaked out of the necrotic cells. From animal experiments it is known that intravenously injected enzymes are rapidly divided over plasma and extravascular space (10, 11).

Our aim has been to find a method by which the total amount of enzyme freed into the circulation can be estimated and hence the extent of the infarcted area can be assessed. In our experiments we tried first of all to get an accurate picture of the course of the enzyme levels after an infarction. In view of this it was necessary to take bloodsamples every four hours during the first three days, after that time fewer samples were taken for eight to fourteen days.

The plasma-activity of the following enzymes was measured: Glutamic-oxaloacetic transaminase, glutamic pyruvic transaminase, lactate dehydrogenase, alpha-hydroxybutyrate dehydrogenase, phospho-hexose-isomerase, creatine phosphokinase.

In doing this we were able to collect a great number of data for each patient, (fig. 1, 2). With the aid of an IBM 1800 computer these data were analysed for the following parameters: half life time of the enzymes in the plasma release-curve in international units per hour per liter of distribution volume (I.U./h.L.) and cumulation curve of enzyme release in I.U./L. This was done in the following way:

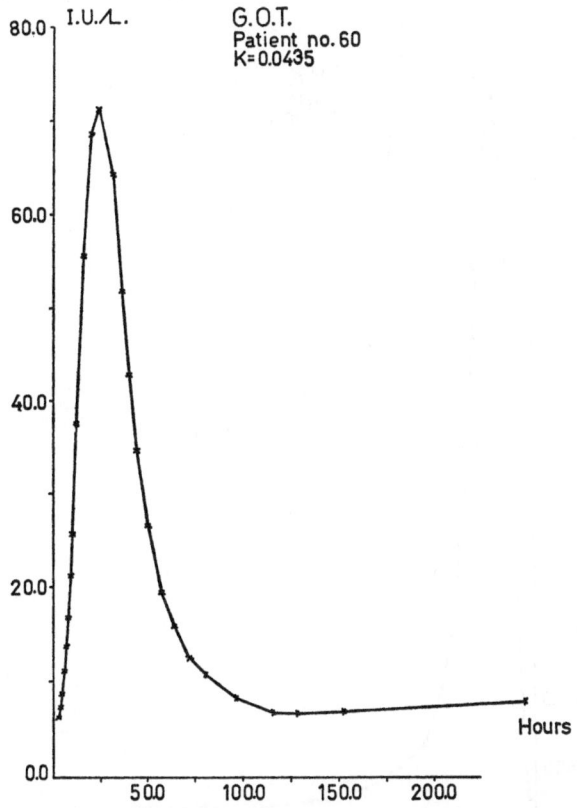

Fig. 1. Plasma-glutamic-oxaloacetic transaminase levels after a myocardial infarction. Plasma-enzyme-activity in I.U./L. time in hours. o hours moment at which infarction occurs. k = rate constant of disappearance of the enzyme from the plasma.

First of all it is assumed that the change in concentration P of the enzyme in the plasma at each instant $\left(\dfrac{dP}{dt}\right)$ is a function of input and output

$$\frac{dP}{dt} = F(t) - k_1 P(t) \tag{1}$$

F(t) is the rate of release of the enzymes from the dead cells into the plasma. It is important to note that no assumption has to be made as to the form of this function. $k_1 P(t)$ is the rate of elimination of the enzymes from the plasma; this elimination in good approximation is a first order process and therefore its velocity is proportional to the

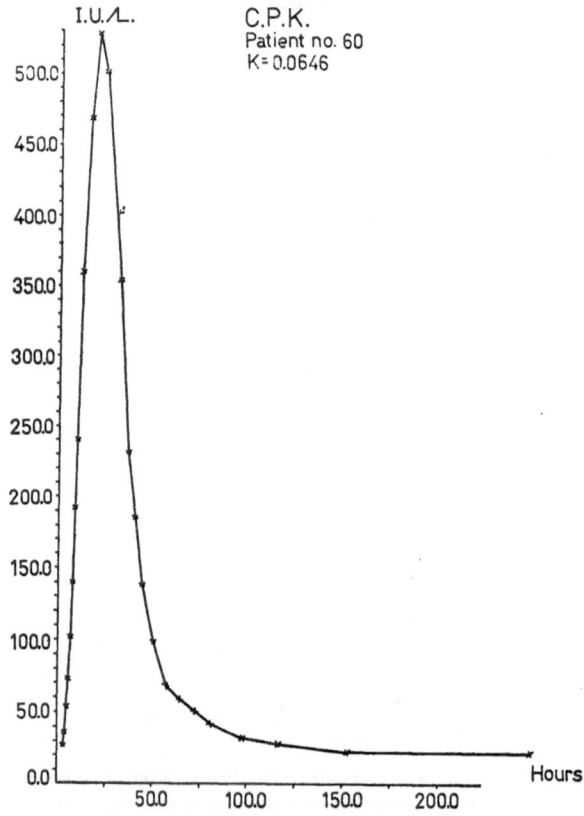

Fig. 2. Plasma-creatine-phosphokinase levels after a myocardial infarction.

amount present at each instant; k_1 is a rate constant and $P(t)$ is the concentration of the enzyme at time t.

Formula (1) is the general formula which applies to the ascending part and the top of the curve (fig. 1, 2) where there is a shed out of enzymes from some source (in this case from the necrotic tissue in the infarcted area) as well as in the downslope. At a certain instant, however, no more leakage takes place, so $F(t) = 0$ and the instantaneous charge in plasma enzyme activity is:

$$\frac{dP}{dt} = -k_1\, P(t) \tag{2}$$

This equation has as its solution

$$P = P_0.\, e^{-k_1 t} \tag{3}$$

The disappearance of the enzymes from the plasma then is described by an exponential decay.

The validity of formula (3) was assessed and the reaction constant k was calculated by using the downslope of the curve that renders plasma enzyme activity as a function of time.

In this traject the semilogarithmic plot proved to be approaching linearity very closely as was shown by a correlation coefficient of 0.990-0.999 in most cases. The slope of the semilogarithmic plot equals $-k_1$; the rate constant.

After having calculated this k_1, it was possible to calculate the rate of release $F(t)$ of enzymes from the infarcted area into the plasma by using formula (1).

In this way a curve could be constructed of the quantity of enzyme released per hour against time. In figs. 3 and 4 this curve (lower curve) is given together with the serum enzyme-concentration curve (upper curve). In the upper curve the plasma-enzyme-activity is plotted, in the lower curve the quantity of enzyme that is discharged into the plasma per hour.

As can be seen, the release of the enzyme (in this case C.P.K.) starts very early: at about 3 hours after the infarction. It increases rapidly to reach its maximum at 10 hours. It declines after that time gradually and after 30 hours no release of C.P.K. takes place any more. For G.O.T. and PHI approximately the same values are found.

The release curves of LDH and in consequence of alpha-HBD, which represents the same enzyme start at about 4 to 5 hours, reach their maximum at about 15 hours and are again at zero level at 40 hours. These values depend somewhat on the size of the infarction. If the patient has high plasma-enzyme levels the top and the end of the release-curve will be a few hours later, indicating that from a large infarcted area it takes more time for the enzymes to diffuse out.

All plasma-enzyme activities are expressed in I.U./liter. Therefore the 'release-curve' is expressed in the same units. It gives the amount of enzyme that is discharged per hour into one liter of plasma or extravascular fluid; as yet we have no determinations of the distribution volume. The total amount of enzyme released into one liter of the distribution volume can be calculated very easily by integrating the release curve.

As the release curve has more or less the same form in different

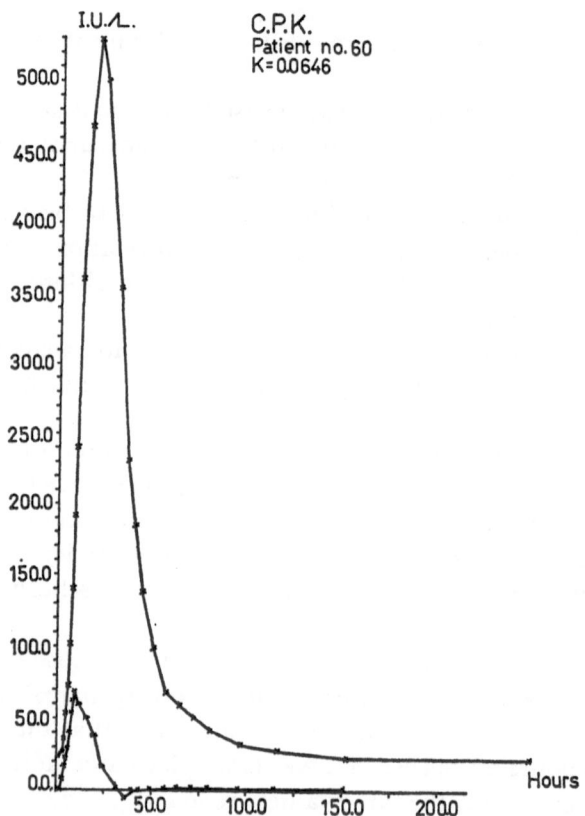

Fig. 3. Glutamic oxaloacetic activity in the plasma (I.U.) after an infarction (upper curve). Release-curve of G.O.T. from the infarcted area into the plasma (same units), (lower curve).

patients for a given enzyme the integration of this curve might be done in practice with much less points on the curve, and therefore with much less plasma samples than was done on our experiments, provided one takes a few bloodsamples on the first day after the infarction and sufficient samples at 24 to 72 hours for calculation of the rate constants of the breakdown of the enzymes in the plasma. As the latter values determined in 10 patients appeared to be rather variable, the latter determinations can never be omitted. The amount of enzyme calculated in the way indicated is the amount per liter of distribution volume. Therefore it does not yet give us a measure for the extent of the infarcted area. To be able to know this we should know the tissue activities of the myocardium and the distribution volumes (i.e. plasma

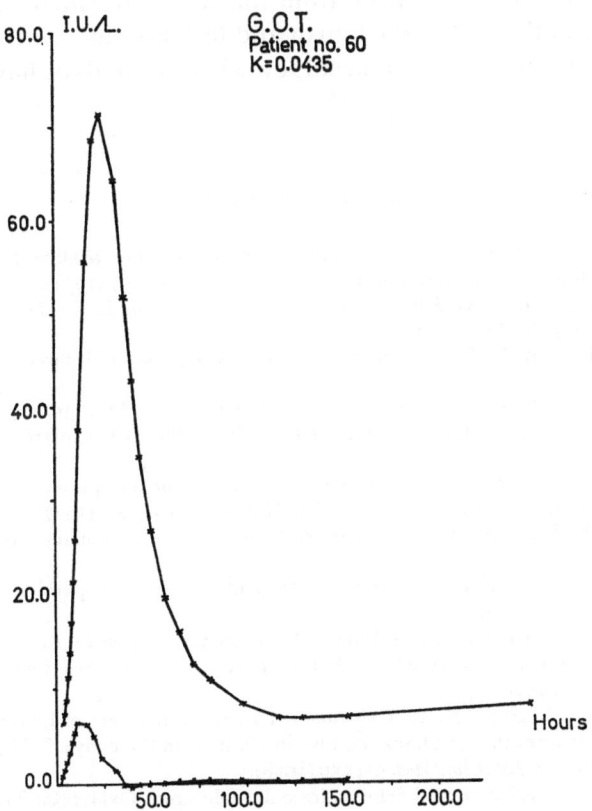

Fig. 4. Plasma levels and release curve of creatine-phosphokinase after a myocardial infarction (upper and lower curve respectively).

+ extravascular space) of the different enzymes after their release. At present studies are under way to assess these parameters.

IN CONCLUSION:

One can get a reasonably exact measure of the size of myocardial infarction in man, when one knows:

a. the plasma-enzyme levels four times daily
b. the half-life time of the different enzymes in the plasma
c. the general features of the release-curve
d. the distribution volume of the enzymes
e. the normal content of the enzymes in the heart.

Only the first of these data has to be assessed in each patient. The second and third can be taken from the data presented and preliminary results indicate that the fourth and fifth are sufficiently invariable to be given with reasonable accuracy when more data have been obtained.

REFERENCES

1. LaDue, J. S., F. Wroblewski, A. Karmen, Serum glutamic oxaloacetic transaminase activity in human acute transmural infarction. *Science* 120, 497 (1954).
2. Agress, C. M., J. H. C. Kim, Evaluation of enzyme tests in the Diagnosis of Heart Disease. *Am. J. Card.* 6, 641 (1960).
3. Batsakis, J. G., R. O. Briere, Enzymatic Profile of Myocardial Infarct. *Am. Heart J.* 72, 274 (1966).
4. Hamolsky, M. W., Enzymes in acute myocardial infarction. *Circ.*: 35, 427 (1967).
5. Coodley, E. L., Evaluation of Enzyme Diagnosis in Myocardial Infarction *Am. J. Med. Sci.* 256, 300 (1968).
6. Kibe, O., N. J. Nilsson,: Observations on the diagnostic and prognostic value of some enzyme tests in myocardial infarction. *Acta Med. Scand.* 182, 597 (1967).
7. Smith, A. F., Diagnostic value of serum-creatine-kinase in a coronary care unit. *Lancet* 2, 178 (1967).
8. Forster, G., Zur Enzymdiagnostik von Herzinfarkt und Myopathien. *Schweiz. Med. Wochenschr.* 97 ,329 (1967).
9. Nydick, I., F. Wroblewski, J. S. LaDue, Evidence for increased serum glutamic-oxalo-acetic transaminase (SGOT)-activity following graded myocardial infarction in dogs. *Circ.*, 12, 161 (1955).
10. Dunn, M., J. Martins, K. R. Reissmann, Disappearance rate of glutamic oxalacetic transaminase from the circulation and its distribution in the body's fluid compartments and secretions. *J. Lab. Clin. Med.* 51, 259 (1958).
11. Massarrat, S., Verhalten und Schwundrate der Glutamat-Oxalacetat-Transaminase in der Blutbahn. *Z. ges. Exp. Med.* 148, 56 (1968).

PANEL DISCUSSION ON ASPECTS OF PATHENOGENESIS

MODERATOR: C. F. J. BÖTTCHER

Böttcher: The members of the panel have agreed that we should concentrate the discussion on the later stages of the sequences of events which start with the earliest signs of arterial disease and proceed to thrombotic complications, impaired circulation, and finally myocardial necrosis. If time permits we shall go back to the earlier events. The first problem for discussion is the pattern of myocardial necrosis as it evolves from the study of plasma enzyme levels.

Hemker: As you have seen from the simulation curves presented by Dr. Witteveen the plasma enzyme levels that evolue after myocardial infarction cannot be completely explained by the assumption that the infarcted area is a bag of enzymes which becomes leaky about eight hours after the vascular occlusion. Our best estimate of the situation at the present time is that the individual cells in the area shed out their contents randomly distributed about a given mean. This would give the upslope of the appearance curve the shape of an integrated Gaussian.

Braasch: The release of enzymes in the necrotic tissue is of course influenced by the remaining blood supply in the infarcted part of the heart. A blood supply is necessary for the transport of the enzymes in the systemic circulation where they can be detected later. To correlate the size of an infarct with the enzyme levels detected in venous blood, is a difficult task because precise information on the blood supply to the infarct is not known.

Witteveen: It is indeed difficult to know if all the enzymes have been released by the infarcted area. You can never be sure that some of the enzymes are not left at the site of the infarction because the vascular supply to the infarcted area is insufficient. On the other hand the enzymes can be transported by diffusion.

Böttcher: I would like to go on to the next topic for discussion. What is the role of thrombosis in impairing the circulation in acute myocardial infarction? I will refer two questions which came from the audience to Dr. Hudson and ask him to first reply briefly to them.

Hudson: The first question is a very important one and one which we cannot answer. It is: could not thrombosis be a complication rather than a cause of acute cardiac infarction? The point is this: do we get a clot in a coronary artery because the heart is infarcted or does the clot cause the cardiac infarction? There is no possible way of answering this question truly but I think that where the artery is occluded, the affected area becomes infarcted. There is enough experimental evidence to support this. So I think that the thrombosis comes before the infarct and not vice versa.

The next question is similar to the previous one. It is: from your experience what is the incidence of coronary thrombosis in patients who die of myocardial infarction? The answer is: as carefully as we look for it. We know only in recent years that there is a difference between a clot, which is what the blood looks like if it clots in a tube, and a thrombus, which is a mass of platelets with or without fibrin. At routine necropsy we shall not find these thrombi in small vessels. The vessel is narrowed down to a small lumen, and we may not find the occluding thrombus itself. Nevertheless, people who have sectioned the heart after death into thin slices 2 or 3 millimeters thick and have examined the slices with great care, have found an occluding thrombus in over 80% of hearts with acute myocardial infarction.

Böttcher: We come now to what may be called the heart of the matter. We agree that thrombi play an important role here, but how does a diseased arterial wall cause thrombosis? This question has five subdivisions. The first one is: what is the relative importance of thrombocytes and coagulation factors? The second question is: is there in this respect a difference between arteries and veins? The third is: how can we imagine the action of oral anticoagulant therapy? The fourth is: is it feasible to develop drugs that directly influence platelets? The last question is: is there a place for fibrinolytic or fibrinogenolytic therapy in prevention?
I would like to ask Dr. Lüscher to make a few comments on the first question.

Lüscher: It should be made clear in the first place that the thrombocytes themselves form part of the clotting system because they contribute an essential phospholipid component called platelet factor 3 to the intrinsic mechanism of prothrombin activation. The extrinsic system which is independent of platelets may be of importance in the initiation of thrombin formation; for its propagation however, the participation of platelets is essential. The formation of a hemostatic plug or of a white thrombus must be explained in terms of an interplay between thrombin formation and other factors involved in platelet aggregation. Hageman factor (factor XII) is remarkable in several respects. In vitro, blood deficient in this factor shows a prolonged clotting time and consequently individuals with this deficiency would be expected to be perfectly safe from incidents of intravascular activation of the clotting system. However, Mr. Hageman, the first person described with this condition, died last year of thrombosis. It therefore appears more appropriate to consider the role of the contact factors as a whole, and perhaps Dr. Hemker would like to make a few comments.

Hemker: It is obvious that the soluble blood clotting factors in plasma are of some importance otherwise we could not imagine that anticoagulant therapy would have any effect. There are still two strange observations. In the first place it has already been mentioned that factor XII, which starts the process of intrinsic coagulation, obviously has not too much of an effect on thrombus formation. On the other hand, Ingram has described several patients with congenital afibrinogenaemia or hypofibrinogenaemia who developped full blown thrombosis. Somehow, the beginning and the end of the pure coagulation process are not of too much importance, but those factors which are affected by vitamin κ deficiency do have some importance. I think that very probably the main connection between plasmatic coagulation and thrombocytes is the generation of thrombin which subsequently affects the thrombocytes. This explains why fibrinogen is not involved. The role of contact activation remains obscure, however.

Böttcher: The next question is whether there is any difference between arteries and veins with regard to the coagulation factors and thrombocytes. I must say that from experiments by members of our own institute in collaboration with Prof. Butterfield's group in London we have the impression that there are certainly differences, particularly as far as platelet behaviour is concerned. I would like to know the opinion of other members of the panel on this point.

Lüscher: Lasch, Roka and coworkers have shown already several years ago that venous blood appears to have a higher content of activated clotting factors than arterial blood and that it looses this increased coagulability on passage through the liver. In more general terms this might mean that a slowed-down circulation must lead to an increasing hypercoagulability and to a more rapid thrombin formation whenever other prerequisites are fulfilled. It is difficult to assess the importance of this possibility for ischaemic heart disease, but it may be essential for the understanding of certain forms of venous thrombosis.

Loeliger: Perhaps I could add a remark from the clinical point of view. Possible differences in venous and arterial blood were mentioned which could contribute to differences in the prevalence of venous and arterial thrombosis. Evidence against such influences may be the fact that intracardiac thrombosis after myocardial infarction is encountered at equal frequency in both the right and left ventricle. Anticoagulants counteract thrombus formation in both ventricles powerfully. This implies that there is no clinically important difference in thrombogenetic and thrombolytic activity of venous blood (right ventricle) and arterial blood (left ventricle and coronary arteries).

Böttcher: We can now proceed to the question: how can we imagine the action of oral anticoagulant therapy?

Lüscher: There can be no doubt that efficient anticoagulation prevents the formation of obstructing thrombi, although it does not necessarily prevent the formation of loose, fragile platelet aggregates. Several workers believe that thrombin formation is not essential in the formation of dense platelet aggregates. According to the scheme shown this morning it is indeed possible to explain platelet aggregation exclusively by the ADP-mechanism in combination with the effect of collagen. On the other hand, experience shows that excessive anticoagulation will finally interfere with normal hemostasis and therefore also with the formation of consolidated platelet masses in general. Thrombin formation therefore appears essential for the formation of a solid, obstructing platelet thrombus under in vivo conditions. It is obvious of course, that depression of clotting activity leads also to impaired fibrin formation.

Böttcher: We will continue on the question of therapy and consider whether it is feasible to develop drugs that directly influence platelet aggregation. About three or four years ago this possibility looked very promising, at least from in vitro experiments. In particular the group of Prof. Born in London was working in that direction. I have the impression that the hope is fading gradually. We might discuss the present day situation, and I call on Dr. Lüscher to discuss this point.

Lüscher: An amazing number of sometimes quite unrelated drugs have been found to affect platelet aggregation. Thus, certain tranquilizers, anti-inflammatory agents and antihistaminics, to mention but a few, will act as inhibitors. In only a few cases ideas as to a possible mode of action have been developed. Thus, adrenalin aggregates platelets, and in such small amounts as may appear in circulation under stress conditions it still is a powerful potentiator of ADP-induced aggregation. It seems plausible that drugs capable of competing for its receptor sites on the cell will inhibit its action on platelets. The prolonged inhibitory effect of therapeutic doses of aspirin most likely is due to the acetylation of essential primary amino groups in platelets. Accordingly salicylates show no comparable activity. Thrombosthenin, the contractile protein of thrombocytes is thought by several authors to be the target of ADP in the induction of aggregation. Although in somewhat higher concentrations, many of the inhibitory drugs are equally capable of interfering with the contraction of isolated thrombostenin. Quite a few among them were also found to damage platelets at concentrations slightly above the one required for optimal inhibition of aggregation; this could mean a rather limited therapeutic range.

Vergroesen: I would like to comment on this subject of drugs influencing platelet aggregation and adhesion by mentioning prostaglandin. Up to now we have not observed any side effects of dosages of prostaglandin E 1, which could completely inhibit platelet aggregation both in vivo and in vitro. These prostaglandins are synthesized in the body from dietary linoleic acid, which is one of the naturally occurring polyunsaturated fatty acids. These fatty acids have a well proven beneficial effect on the inhibition of atherosclerotic disease. We think that probably there is a direct correlation between the beneficial effects of linoleic acid and these prostaglandins via the effect of the latter on the inhibition of platelet aggregation.

Böttcher: I would like to say that, although prostaglandins are extremely interesting compounds, there is still a tremendous amount of research necessary before there will be any certainty that they could exert a role in influencing platelet aggregation or any other thrombotic phenomenon. I agree with Dr. Vergroesen, that there are some vague indications in that direction but I am really convinced that we are in the very early stages of investigation. This is meant as a slight warning to those who might want to start using these compounds tomorrow.

Vergroesen: I do not think that the relation between prostaglandin and thrombocyte aggregation is vague at the moment. I am convinced that it has been well proven. It has also been well proven that the body is capable of synthesizing prostaglandins from essential fatty acids very efficiently.

Böttcher: It is obvious that there is a difference of opinion on this subject among the members of the panel. This would require us to go into too much detail here.

Hudson: I do not quite know what we are trying to do now. We have had some superb papers this morning, telling us that platelets can seal imperfections in vessels, a miraculous process. We are now trying to stop this happening, and I am not quite sure of what we are up to. We do not seem to be advancing at all. All anticoagulation puts the patient on a tight rope as it were. On the one hand the patient may bleed to death from overdosage, and on the other hand, underdosage will be completely useless. In the recent MRC trial, none of the patients was properly anticoagulated. And here we are again trying to stop a natural process by interfering with platelet aggregation, which we know is a protective mechanism. I suspect that if we do find a really efficient drug to do this, the patient will either bleed to death or not have enough to have any effect.

Lüscher: I would not close this part of the discussion on such a pessimistic note. It is of course possible that an effective inhibitor of platelet aggregation might as well interfere with hemostasis. However, the experiments by Born and coworkers with adenosine derivatives have shown that this is not necessarily the case. It is quite possible that further work will lead to the development of substances with satisfactory activities and a useful therapeutic range.

Böttcher: There was another question on therapy. It is: is there a place for fibrinolytic therapy and/or prevention or even fibrinogenolytic therapy and/or prevention?

Hemker: People who cannot synthesize fibrinogen because of an inborn error of metabolism show thrombosis. It is obvious that there is little reason for inducing fibrinogen deficiency, for instance with snake venoms (Arvin) and then hoping that they will not show thrombosis. This is apart from all of the complications which are seen when you infuse snake venom into people.

Lüscher: Degradation of fibrinogen may lead to split products with antithrombin activity which also interfere with platelet aggregation. Nevertheless, the induction of fibrinogenolysis appears indeed as a complicated and inconvenient way to the prevention of thrombosis.

French: Is the platelet fibrinogen still present in these patients who get thrombosis without circulating fibrinogen?

Lüscher: The platelets from patients with congenital afibrinogenaemia don't contain fibrinogen. Since normal platelets suspended in afibrinogenaemic plasma behave abnormally, plasmatic, much more than platelet fibrinogen seems to be of importance for normal platelet function.

Böttcher: The following question is addressed to Dr. French: can diseased platelets cause thrombosis in a normal vessel? In other words, does hypercoagulability exist? This is related to the general problem of wether or not thrombosis in arteries is always caused by arterial disease.

French: I wonder if I might refer briefly to the concept of Virchow's triad in thrombosis, that is: change in the vessel wall, change in the blood flow, and change in the constituents of the blood. These are the predisposing factors. In any situation you have to take all these factors into account though they may operate in many different proportions. In many experimental arterial thrombi, the most striking change is a severe mechanical injury to the vessel wall; in natural arterial disease the severe lesions of atherosclerosis are the most prominent factors. Nevertheless, the other factors can come into play too. With relatively small changes in the wall, one can understand, that if the platelets are increased in number, or are more adhesive, a thrombus is more likely to form or to be more extensive. Hypercoagulability is a difficult state to define in this context since it concerns the actual circulating blood rather than the sample one can observe in a test tube.

Hudson: I agree with Dr. French on this matter. I think that there must always be a lesion although we may not be able to identify it.

Lüscher: Mustard has described the presence in human platelets of peptides with an effect on vascular permeability. This author thinks that this material, originating from platelet aggregates deposited in circulation will induce endothelial damage. Could you believe in such a concept?

Hudson: I cannot believe or disbelieve it; I prefer to wait for further evidence.

Böttcher: We can now take time to discuss the early stages of arterial disease, questions about the causative factors of arterial disease, particularly questions about the primary changes in the vessel wall. One could consider changes in the vessel wall in the beginning which are unrelated to lipids. For instance, a disequilibrium between filtrating plasma protein and the vessel wall mucopolysaccharides and changes in transport phenomena in general.

A second possibility is that of a cellular reaction. Then of course Duguid's theory about microthrombic sedimentation has to be considered. Finally, one could consider as a primary change, disturbances in lipid metabolism. I would like to start this part of the discussion by making a few remarks about the viewpoint of my group. I wish to emphasize that there are differences in this respect between atherosclerosis in humans, and in animals, with lesions similar to atherosclerotic lesions in humans. We believe that in experimental animals the conditions are usually so unphysiologic that the process begins with a simple physico-chemical phenomenon, the adhesion to the arterial wall of lipid loaded phagocytes from the blood stream followed by endothelial growth over the adhered cells. In our opinion the earlier stages of atherosclerosis in experimental animals resemble a much later stage of atherosclerosis in man, where at sites where there has already been damage to the endothelium, adhesion of platelets, formation of microthrombi and adsorption of lipids occurs. This sequence of events has been well described by Hubert. We believe that the earliest changes have nothing or little to do with lipids, but have to do with changes in the subendothelial layer, changes in the network of mucopolysaccharides leading to permeability changes and similar phenomena. I am sure that there are other opinions among the panel members.

Vergroesen: From your own work and publications, there is a much quoted communication that in atherosclerotic lesions there is deposition of cholesterol linoleate suggesting that an increased intake of linoleic acid might be unfavourable. I should like to ask you if you still have this opinion? Secondly I should like to ask you: what do you think of these cholesterolester deposits in the arterial wall? Are they the cause or are they the result of atherosclerotic disease?

Böttcher: I would like to slightly correct the quotation you made. In very early lesions, that is when the so-called streaks and spots are observed, there is first of all an increase of cholesterol oleate. That is the earliest cholesterol ester which starts to accumulate. We find the strong predomenance of cholesterol linoleate in the advanced lesions. We have never stated that, from this, one could immediately draw the conclusion that one should not use linoleate-rich food, because there would be some cause and effect connection between an excessive linoleate intake in the food and the deposition of cholesterol linoleate in the vascular wall. The biochemistry of this situation is more complicated than that. However, one must at least consider it as one of the many possibilities. We must still take into account the fact that we do not know why the blood level of cholesterol in humans is lowered after the ingestion of a linoleate-rich diet. The possibilities are a more rapid excretion, a decreased synthesis, or a deposition of cholesterol somewhere in the body. As far as we can judge from the latest experimental results, particularly those of Prof. Ahrens in New York there is still a great deal of uncertainty about the possible mechanism. As long as this question has not been settled, it is practically impossible to reply to Dr. Vergroesen's remark. I believe that as long as we do not have a definite reply, it means that one should not exaggerate the intake of linoleate-rich food until its fate in the body is known. If I may quote what Prof. Hudson said this morning about what one should or should not do, I am quite convinced that one should avoid foods that are deficient in those lipids. The choice lies midway between these two.

Vergroesen: Referring to the work by Ahrens, I would like to state that he followed the cholesterol shift only for 10 days after a change in the fat composition of the diet. He observed, in fact, a shift into the tissues for the first 10 days. If we assume that this shift will continue throughout the experiment, I wonder where all this cholesterol will be deposited if you treat an animal or human being for years with this unsaturated fatty acid diet. If you accept this shift, as constantly occurring during a period of years, the subject would be one cholesterol crystal: I think that the better explanation of the effects of polyunsaturated fatty acids is an increase in the excretion of cholesterol in the bile, which has been demonstrated to occur in several wellplanned and controled experiments such as these by Dr. Thomassen and coworkers.

Böttcher: Shortly after we found the accumulation of cholesterol linoleate in the arterial wall particularly in the advanced stage of arteriosclerosis Ahrens and coworkers performed post-mortem examinations on subjects who had died after long-term dietary experiments with controlled fat intakes. They found that in the atherosclerotic lesions, not only the cholesterol esters but even the triglycerides and the phospholipids were mainly linoleates. This does not prove anything, but at least it suggests a connection between food intake and what is deposited in the arterial wall. I would also like to comment on the simple calculation of Dr. Vergroesen, that if the deposition in tissues takes place for years, it would mean that at some time the entire body would be one large cholesterol crystal. You must agree that this is a slight oversimplification. There are a few other biochemical phenomena occurring in the body, particularly there is a continuous decomposition of deposited material. Therefore, a simple calculation cannot be made in such cases.

French: I cannot see that we can assign an order of priority to the possible causes of arterial disease. Each one of the processes that have been mentioned by Prof. Böttcher is going on in the arterial wall and they could all be adding up and contributing together to the development of the lesion. I think that this does not in any way detract from the importance of investigating each of these processes, but we might do this more satisfactorily without prejudging the issue of which is the first or the most important. One more small point on the criticism of the relevance of some work in experimental animals, the lesions not being the same as in men. I would agree with Prof. Böttcher's remark with regard to certain features of the lesion in rabbits and in other small laboratory animals, but there is a remarkable similarity between the lesions that are produced in larger animals, particularly in primates and swine, and the lesions in men. Too harsh a criticism of the animal experiments on this ground is not justified.

Böttcher: I quite agree with that remark. In particular, I would like to state that as soon as the lesions become more advanced, even in rabbits or other animals, they resemble the lesions in humans more closely. Still Prof. Constantinides warns that even if the appearance is similar it does not mean that they have been caused by the same agent or initial factor. We must always keep in mind that even in those animals which are phylogenetically close to human beings the chemical composition of the blood, the ratio between different lipoproteins, lipid composition, etc. are so different that one must be very careful in drawing conclusions as to the causative initial factor of these lesions.

CHAPTER II

THE EPIDEMIOLOGICAL APPROACH

ACUTE CORONARY HEART DISEASE IN A COMMUNITY

S. L. MORRISON

Ischaemic Heart Disease can be investigated in populations as well as in individuals. The study of its manifestations in patients presenting themselves to clinicians, or being presented to pathologists, has certain limitations and the application of epidemiological methods is complementary to clinical and pathological studies. Epidemiology is concerned with the distribution and determinants of disease in human populations and one of its essential features is the discovery of *all* the cases in a defined population. Such studies can therefore test hypotheses derived from the clinical study of those patients who happen to be seen in a particular clinic. Ideas generated in the clinic – for example, about the characteristics of patients developing the disease – can be tested by comparing the occurrence of these factors in all patients in a given population with a control group in that population. Much more importantly, epidemiological studies can extend beyond patients to include those with pre-symptomatic disease and can thus enlarge our knowledge about the natural history of a disease and about its precursors.

The most readily available, and in some ways the 'hardest' epidemiological data about IHD are derived from death certificates. Analyses of mortality rates from IHD have certainly been useful; in particular, they have focussed attention on this disease as a major, and increasing, cause of premature death in most western countries. Mortality analyses have also indicated areas for further research by contrasting the experience in different countries, in different areas of the same country, in the two sexes, in different age groups and in different occupations. Analysis of the actual place of death and of its circumstances have highlighted the problem of sudden, unexpected death and have thus shown the urgent need for preventive measures.

A more sophisticated level of epidemiological study concerns morbidity as well as mortality. Some of the most valuable investigations have been long-term studies of carefully defined populations. These prospective, or cohort, studies have measured and recorded many characteristics of all the individuals in a population and have then related the occurrence of IHD to these characteristics. (The well-known Framingham, Tecumseh and London Transport studies are all examples of excellent cohort studies.) From work of this kind, we are now well aware of the importance of raised blood pressure, raised serum cholesterol, smoking habits and physical activity in affecting the risk of subsequent manifestations of IHD. Cohort and other studies have led to the concept of high risk groups and to the possibility of early intervention before a heart attack has occurred. Careful prevalence surveys of various manifestations of IHD are also important in enlarging our understanding of this disease.

One cannot overestimate the importance of these and other kinds of epidemiological studies aimed at increasing knowledge about many aspects of IHD and especially looking towards its prevention. However, hypotheses about preventive measures must be rigorously tested and large scale action is still only a possibility for the future. In the meantime, existing knowledge about the immediate treatment of acute attacks must be applied efficiently to the highest possible proportion of patients suffering a heart attack in a community. If this is to be done, then a detailed picture of the occurrence of acute IHD must be built up in the community. This requires the gathering of detailed information about every patient suffering an acute heart attack and the events surrounding that attack. This kind of study has been described by Morris (1964) as 'completing the clinical picture' by moving outside the hospital or clinic and studying *all* those affected in the population. In the context of IHD it can be described as 'action research' – using epidemiology to provide the basis for action in a given community to see that existing knowledge is properly applied in that community.

In Edinburgh, discussions between clinicians and epidemiologists about ways of measuring the effectiveness of a new Coronary Care Unit exposed our ignorance about the total attack rate of this disease in the City, about the proportions of patients treated at home and in hospital and the outcome of that treatment, and about the timing of events after symptoms began. We began to realise the importance of finding out what was happening in our own community. It was therefore decided that a study should be carried out in which an attempt would be made to record data about every occurrence of acute IHD in the city over a period of one year. The objective was to provide a factual basis for planning, evaluation, and further research.

THE EDINBURGH STUDY

The setting of the study is a city with a total population of approximately 500,000 persons, in a country with a very high death rate from ischaemic heart disease. The medical services are organised in a comprehensive National Health Service; virtually all the inhabitants are registered with general practitioners and, except in emergency, reference of patients to hospital-based consultants is through a general practitioner. There are two major hospitals, both teaching hospitals and both having new Intensive Care Units, and eight other hospitals. Simple routine information is available about every patient discharged from hospital, through the Scottish Hospital In-Patient Enquiry. All death certificates pass through the hands of the City's Medical Officer of Health and all sudden deaths of persons not being attended by a doctor are reported to the Police Surgeon.

The study was based on notification by general practitioners of every patient in whom acute IHD was suspected. To ensure the fullest possible notification, practitioners were encouraged to notify any patient in whom there was any suspicion of an acute attack – we were not worried about false positives but we did want to keep the number of false negatives, or missed cases, to a minimum. Notification was made by telephone to the Study Office at any time of the day or night, calls being recorded by Robophone out of office hours. At the time of notification, the general practitioner completed a short and simple questionnaire, recording the findings of his clinical examination. If the patient was to be admitted to hospital, the GP's responsibility then ended (except for providing follow-up information six months later). The study team obtained further clinical details from the hospital doctor and the case notes, and basic demographic and social data from the patient; information about the times at which events occurred was also recorded. If the patient was being kept at home, a doctor from the team visited the patient, usually within 12 hours, recorded an ECG, withdrew a quantity of blood for enzyme measurement, and obtained the demographic, social and timing information. The general practitioner was informed by telephone of the interpretation of the ECG, and the results of enzyme tests. He was then asked to record further brief clinical details of the patient's progress between the 2nd and 4th days.

General practitioners also notified cases of sudden death in their practices; further notifications came from the Police Surgeon. Unfortunately the medico-legal system in Scotland is such that an autopsy is performed in only a small proportion of cases of 'sudden death'.

Two modifications were made to the concept of registering *all* cases. First, registration was restricted to patients under the age of 70. Second, available medical staff resources were not sufficient to cover home visits to the patients of all general practitioners in Edinburgh. Accordingly a sampling scheme was devised in which 180 of the 260 general practitioners in the city were asked to take part (171 in fact agreed to do so). However, *all* sudden deaths and *all* hospital admissions were included.

A system of checking was devised to ensure that the highest possible proportion of cases were recorded. Each month a newsletter about the study was sent to all practitioners in order to keep the study fresh in their minds, and comments were made in it about cases found in the various checks but not notified.

The data collected about each patient fell under four headings:

1. Diagnostic information sufficient to classify the case as one of 'definite infarction', 'probable infarction', 'ischaemia' (coronary insufficiency), 'insufficient information' or 'any other condition'.
2. Clinical information sufficient to classify the severity of the attack under four main grades.
3. Information about the timing of events following the occurrence of symptoms.
4. Simple demographic and social data.

A pilot study was run for three months before the main project began. Selected general practitioners who were known to be keen, knowledgeable and cooperative were invited to take part in it. When the sampling scheme for the main study was drawn up, these same practitioners formed one of four strata (the other three were based on practice size). In the final results, the notification rate from this special group will be compared with that from all other practitioners. The comparison will form one basis for estimating how effective notification has been.

DISCUSSION

The results of this one-year Registration scheme are now being analysed. Rather than present our findings to date in tabular form, I would like to mention the areas in which our information is likely to be helpful. We are now in a position to make a fairly precise estimate of the number of acute heart attacks occurring among people under 70 years of age in Edinburgh during the study year. We know about the medical, demographic and social background of those attacked and about the way in which they were treated. We now know how many of these patients were treated at home by their general practitioner, about the severity of their illness and about its outcome. The study has illustrated the diagnostic difficulties often presented to the GP and the need he has for diagnostic aids. We have similar information about patients admitted to hospital, whether to conventional wards or to a CCU. Our detailed data about the sequence and timing of events after symptoms began enables us to discuss in concrete terms the pros and cons of establishing mobile CCU's in the City. I may say that a first look at the information on this point is not encouraging – at best, it looks as though about 30 lives *might* have been saved in a year by the lavish use of very scarce resources. However, we are now in a position to discuss rationally how resources could best be used and what steps can be taken to improve the chances of those who live long enough to allow treatment to be begun. Moreover, the facts disclosed again bring into focus the need to intervene before the acute attack occurs if any major improvement in mortality is to be achieved. One incidental value of a Register is its provision of a defined population of patients who have suffered, and survived, an acute attack. Such a population can provide samples for other studies.

This kind of study is unlikely to increase our knowledge of the underlying causes and mechanisms of IHD, but I believe it is nevertheless an important step in making sure that existing knowledge is properly applied. In every country where IHD is a major health problem, the way in which patients react to the same symptoms may differ, depending upon the cultural and social milieu and the way in which health services are organised. The findings of a Registration study in Edinburgh cannot be generalised to other places – they may apply to similar cities in Scotland but they will certainly not apply in other parts of Scotland. They will certainly be very different in Holland or in the United States. Similar studies are therefore needed in different countries and in different areas of the same country and the European Region of the World Health Organization is now actively encouraging these developments. One incidental advantage of mounting such an investigation is the bringing together of epidemiologists and clinicians; their experience of working together on a Registration Scheme may lead to other fruitful collaboration.

My plea, then, is that epidemiological studies in IHD should not be limited to fundamental investigations of aetiology but should include action studies locally which will provide the essential information for the rational application of existing knowledge in the treatment of this condition. Cardiological skills must be used for the benefit of all those who need them in a community and cannot simply be limited to self selected patients. Cardiological resources can best be mobilised for the benefit of the whole community by the joint action of clinicians and epidemiologists.

ACKNOWLEDGMENTS:
My colleagues in the Edinburgh Community Study are Dr. A. Armstrong, Professor K. W. Donald, Dr. D. G. Julian and Dr. M. F. Oliver of the Department of Medicine, and Dr. E. B. A. W. Duncan, Dr. P. M. Fulton and Mr. W. Lutz of the Department of Social Medicine. The study is financed by the Ministry of Health and the Scottish Home and Health Department.

DISCUSSION

Erkelens: How many cardiologists have been necessary to make this program possible in the hospital?

Morrison: The cardiologists in one of the hospitals form part of an advisory steering committee, but in the actual team carrying out the study we had one general physician with cardiological training who spent half of his time on this study and one junior doctor who was full-time.

METHODOLOGY OF EPIDEMIOLOGICAL SURVEYS

G. ROSE

The application of epidemiological methods to the study of chronic diseases is now so widespread that it is hard to believe that the expansion of the subject really only began about twenty years ago. In that period it has proved to be one of the chief growing points in the whole of medicine. Perhaps its greatest successes have been in the cardiovascular field: most of what we know about the aetiology of coronary heart disease (CHD) has been derived from epidemiology.

It is now widely recognised that the control of cardiovascular diseases depends primarily on prevention. Just as treatment represents the practical outcome of clinical research, so prevention represents the practical application of epidemiology. It is therefore likely that the importance of the subject will be as great in the future as it has been hitherto.

In the past there has been an unfortunate separation of epidemiology from clinical medicine. Happily there are signs that the estrangement is ending. The two approaches are complementary rather than opposed, and co-operation can bring great benefits to both sides. However, it is a mistake to blur the distinctions. To speak of 'clinical epidemiology' is to obscure the fact that the two approaches are fundamentally different. The clinical researcher studies disease in patients, whereas the epidemiologist by definition studies a representative sample of a defined population.

FUNCTIONS OF EPIDEMIOLOGY IN THE STUDY OF CARDIOVASCULAR DISEASES

Hospital admission data for CHD (fig. 1) show that the case-load for men reaches a peak in middle life, with smaller numbers of patients among the elderly (1). This is a useful thing to know. Unfortunately it has led many clinicians (including writers of well-known textbooks) to suppose that the *incidence* reaches a peak in middle life and then declines. But the definition of incidence is

$$\text{Incidence} = \frac{\text{Number of new cases occurring in a period}}{\text{Number of persons at risk} \times \text{length of period}} \times 100$$

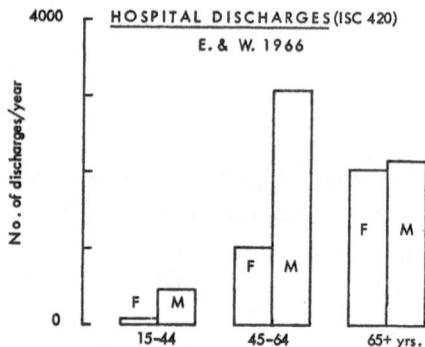

Fig. 1. Numbers of admissions for CHD (ISC 420) to hospitals in England and Wales in 1966, by age and sex.

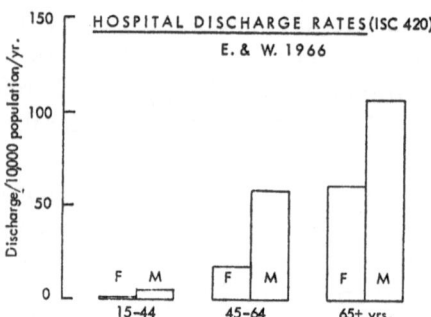

Fig. 2. Admission rates for CHD (ISC 420) to hospitals in England and Wales in 1966, by age and sex.

For its calculation we need to be able to relate the number of cases to the numbers at risk in the general population. When this is done, a very different age-trend emerges (fig. 2). Figure 1 is clinical; it presents an interesting but incomplete picture. Figure 2 is epidemiological, and provides both an actual measure of the risk to the individual, and a truer idea of the age-trend. The incidence of a disease can only be measured by epidemiology.

Clinical research permits us to describe the personal characteristics of patients – for example, the smoking habits of cases of myocardial infarction (fig. 3: data from our own department). But such information by itself does not tell us anything about differences in smoking habit between cases of myocardial infarction and the general population in which they occurred. The risk of CHD in relation to smoking habit can only be measured by a survey. The results (2) may then be presented in terms either of relative risk (fig. 4) or of the absolute risk (fig. 5).

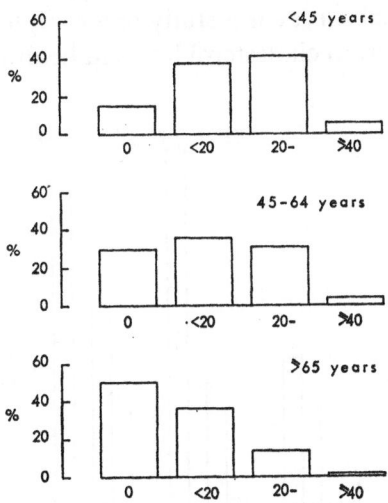

Fig. 3. Cigarette smoking habits of men admitted to hospital with myocardial infarction.

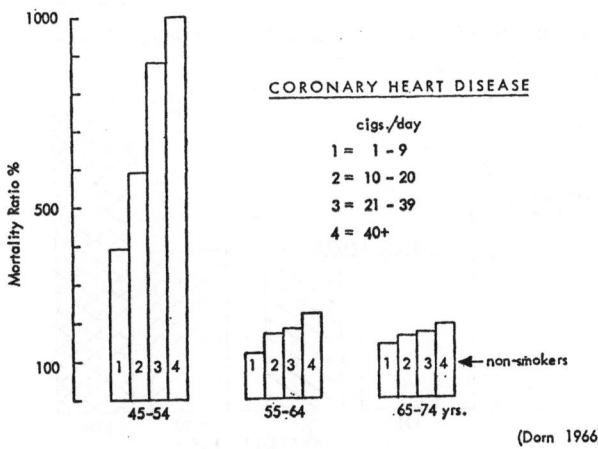

Fig. 4. Relative risk of dying of CHD among males according to cigarette consumption, by age.

Each is perfectly valid, although in this case they provide very different pictures of the relation of risk to age.

Epidemiological research can further permit us – provided that the studies are large enough – to examine the effect of combinations of risk factors. These may be very striking, as for instance when we see the combined effect of cigarette smoking and hypertension on the risk of CHD (fig. 6, taken from data of Doyle et al. (3)).

An epidemiological survey is a study of a sample of a defined population. A survey of serum cholesterol levels in healthy laboratory staff is

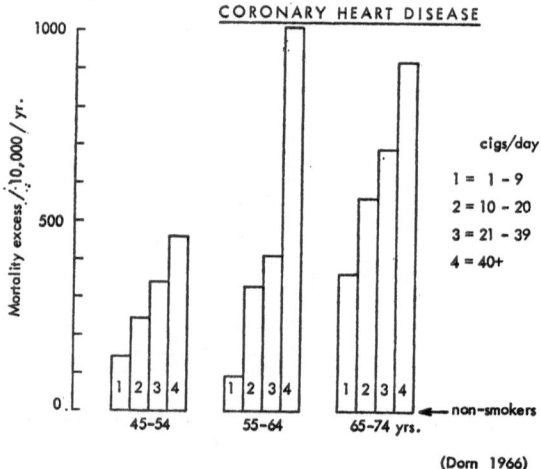

Fig. 5. Actual mortality rates from CHD among males according to cigarette smoking, by age.

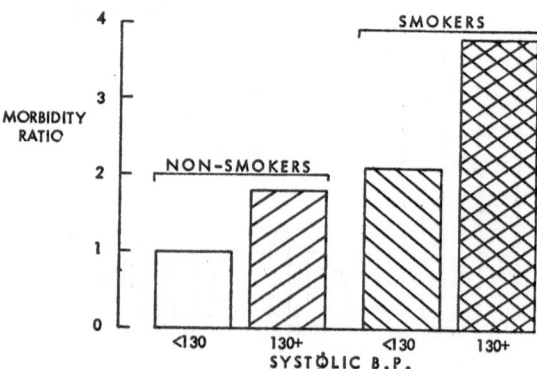

Fig. 6. Mortality ratios for CHD in the Framingham and Albany studies, related to cigarette smoking and to elevated blood pressure.

not epidemiological, because no-one can say what population the volunteers are supposed to represent. In epidemiology there must always be a list ('census') of the individuals or groups from which the sample is to be taken, and the sample itself must be statistically chosen so as to be representative of its parent population. The value of this approach is that it permits generalisations: for example, if the mean serum cholesterol level in a random sample were found to be 200 mg %, then we could know that this would be an unbiased estimate of the level in the population as a whole.

OBSERVATIONAL SURVEYS

These may be of two types. In the first ('cross-sectional' or 'prevalence' survey) the sample is examined once only, and this permits us to make statements about the state of the population only at a particular point in time. In the second type ('prospective' or 'incidence' survey), the sample is later re-examined on one or more occasions: this allows us to estimate the frequency of changes in the status of individuals (incidence, recovery and mortality rates).

Cross-sectional surveys have proved successful in identifying all the main risk factors in CHD. They also permit comparisons of the frequency of disease in different populations. For example, in a recent co-operative study sponsored by WHO European Office (4) we studied the prevalence of CHD in middle-aged clerical workers in various European cities. Figure 7 provides an example of the remarkably uniform pattern that emerged.

The same survey also illustrated a need that is fundamental in all

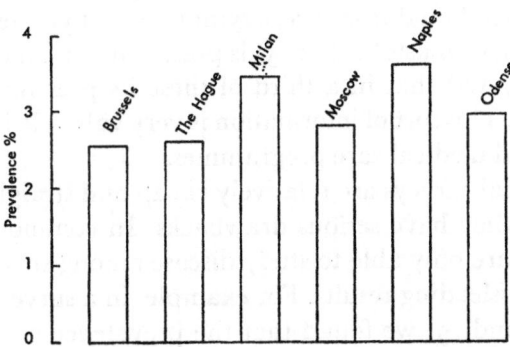

Fig. 7. Prevalence (age-adjusted) of ischaemic-type s-t depressions in men aged 40-59 in various European cities.

epidemiological work, namely, the standardisation and validation of methods. In clinical medicine it would not be particularly serious if doctors in different countries varied in some of their criteria for ECG interpretation; but the same lack of uniformity could be disastrous in a study whose aim was to compare the prevalence of disease in different countries. In this WHO enquiry we first compared prevalence using ECG reports provided by the individual teams of investigators in each country. Fortunately we then recognised that there was some doubt about the comparability of these reports, and so all the records were re-coded by a single group, using highly standardised techniques. The outcome is shown in table 1, which shows that a comparison based on the local reports would indeed have been totally misleading.

Table 1. Results of using (a) local, and (b) central coding of ECGs as the basis for comparing the prevalence of s-t depressions in surveys in various european cities

| | Prevalence % (and Rank) | |
	(a) Local coding	(b) Central coding
Brussels	9.2 (1)	2.5 (6)
The Hague	6.1 (2)	2.6 (5)
Odense	5.1 (3)	2.9 (3)
Moscow	3.5 (4)	2.8 (4)
Naples	2.4 (5)	3.6 (1)
Milan	2.2 (6)	3.4 (2)

Prevalence surveys also serve to identify the total amount of disease in a community. In a current survey of middle-aged male civil servants in London, we have found that severe symptomless hypertension (systolic pressure $\geqslant 200$, or diastolic $\geqslant 115$) is present in a total of about 26 per thousand men, and that in a third of these its presence was not previously known. This sort of information is very valuable in the planning of screening and medical care programmes.

Cross-sectional surveys are relatively cheap and straightforward, but unfortunately they have serious drawbacks. In common with clinical research, they are only able to study disease among survivors, and this can produce misleading results. For example, in a survey of diabetes in Bedford, England (5) we found that the prevalence of ischaemic-type s-t depressions was higher in women than in men (Table 2); yet it is clear from prospective studies that the incidence of ischaemia is actually much higher in men. Possibly sex differences in mortality account for this paradox.

Table 2. Prevalence of ischaemic-type s-T depression in men and women

Age	Prevalence %	
	M	F
<50	7	9
50—	7	25
60—	17	30
>70	31	40

(Bedford Diabetes Survey 1965)

It is also only by a prospective survey that we can measure the natural history of disease. This may yield information very different from what we should have been led to expect by cross-sectional surveys or by clinical experience. For example, repeated annual examinations of the same sample of men revealed that the prevalence of angina was approximately 4% in each individual year (6); but most of the men who were positive in one year were negative in the other years, so that each year the total of 4% was made up of substantially different subjects. Thus the longer the period of surveillance, the higher became the

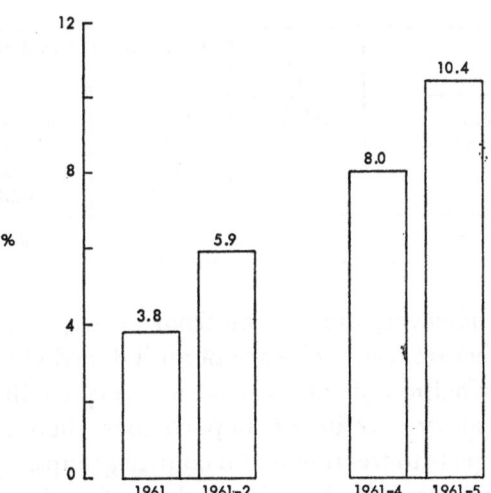

Fig. 8. Contrast between 'point prevalence' of angina (based on single examination) and 'period prevalence' (based on successively longer periods of surveillance) in a cohort of 1136 men aged 35-59 years.

proportion of men who were angina-positive at some point within it. In technical terms, the 'period prevalence' over four years was more than three times the 'point prevalence' in one year (Figure 8). A single examination grossly underestimated the total frequency of the condition.

EXPERIMENTAL EPIDEMIOLOGY

Observational epidemiology may demonstrate an association between some environmental factor, or a habit, and the occurrence of disease. For example, in our study of civil servants in London (7), we observed a strong association between the duration of the walk to work each morning and the prevalence of ischaemic-type ECG findings.

Such an association may be either causal or coincidental. The first thing is to see whether it can be accounted for in terms of other factors that are already known to be important. In this case the search has so far been essentially negative, with the exception of a small association with overweight (table 3). The second step should be to test whether the association is consistent in further studies in different populations.

Table 3. Relation between duration of walk to work and mean levels of blood pressure. Serum cholesterol. Blood sugar (2 hours after 50 g of glucose) and relative weight, in 9778 civil servants (males aged 40-64, excluding messengers and men with dyspnoea or angina of effort)

| | Duration (min) of walk to work | | | |
	0	1-9	10-19	> 20
Systolic blood pressure	135.5	134.1	134.8	134.5
Serum cholesterol (mg %)	204.0	201.6	205.2	204.0
Blood sugar (mg %)	76.4	76.8	77.0	76.7
Relative weight	1.019	0.997	0.994	0.990
Number of men	389	1185	4073	3301

The final test, however, must come from an experiment which will examine the effect on CHD incidence of an induced change in physical activity. The principles of such a trial are very similar to those of a controlled laboratory experiment; in particular, there must be random allocation of subjects to treatment and control groups.

The past twenty years in the epidemiology of cardiovascular diseases have been devoted largely to observational studies. These have been highly productive of valuable information on frequency, (data obtained from 8959 British civil servants aged 40-59; excluding men with exertional dyspnoea or angina, and messengers) distribution and natural history. They have also developed a rather large number of aetiological hypotheses. So that we may test the truth of these hypotheses and learn what their value may be in prevention, it is to be hoped that we are now entering a period in epidemiology when experiment will take its place alongside observation.

REFERENCES

1. Registrar-General *Hospital In-patient Enquiry for England & Wales for 1966*, London, Her Majesty's Stationery Office (1966).
2. Dorn, H. *National Cancer Institute Monograph* 19 (U.S. Public Health Service), 1 (1966).
3. Doyle, J. T., T. R. Dawber, W. B. Kannel, S. H. Kinch, and H. A. Kahn, *J. Amer. med. Ass.* 190, 886 (1964).
4. Rose, G., M. Ahmeteli, L. Checcacci, F. Fidanza, I. Glazunov, J. de Haas, P. Horstmann, M. D. Kornitzer, C. Meloni, A. Menotti, D. van der Sande, M. K. de Soto-Hartgrink, Z. Pisa, and B. Thomsen, *Bull. Wld Hlth Org.* 38, 885.
5. Keen, H., G. Rose, D. A. Pyke, D. Boyns, C. Chlouverakis and S. Mistry, *Lancet.* 2, 505 (1965).
6. Rose, G. *Brit. J. prev. soc. Med.* 22, 12 (1968).
7. Reid, D. D., P. J. S. Hamilton, J. Jarrett, H. Keen and G. Rose, – in preparation.

EPIDEMIOLOGY OF ISCHAEMIC HEART
DISEASE IN FINLAND

M. J. KARVONEN

I. MORTALITY

1. 1. International Comparisons

My country, Finland, has been selected to present some of the problems which are to be faced, when ischaemic heart disease (IHD) is approached as a public health problem. For this choice there is at least one very good reason: IHD is more common in Finland than in any other European country. The mortality of middle aged Finnish men from cardiovascular disease (CVD) in general and from IHD in particular has been among the highest in the world.

This position Finland has shared with the United States, Great Britain, Australia, New Zealand and Canada. It is notable that IHD mortality of working-age men in Finland is about twice as high as in its Scandinavian neighbour countries, Sweden, Norway and Denmark. The high Finnish mortality stood in obvious contrast to the often expressed view that IHD was an unavoidable concomitant of the western civilization. The Finns have always been the poorest member of the Nordic family; still they had the largest share of this 'disease of civilization'.

1. 2. Mortality within Finland

Also within Finland there are regional differences in the recorded IHD mortality (fig. 1). The poorest eastern part of the country has the highest load of IHD, while the most well-to-do southwestern part comes closest to the Scandinavian figures.

While the death is a clearly definable occurrence, its cause may often be subject to different opinions. Geographic comparisons of total mortality may be relied upon, but when dealing with its subgroups, diagnostic accuracy and differences in coding practices may cause errors and bias. However, in special situations much interesting information may be derived from a close scructiny of the mortality. Varpela (1) subjected the cardiovascular (cv) mortality of those dying in Helsinki to a analysis according to their place of birth. Men who had migrated from various parts of the country to the capital, had a

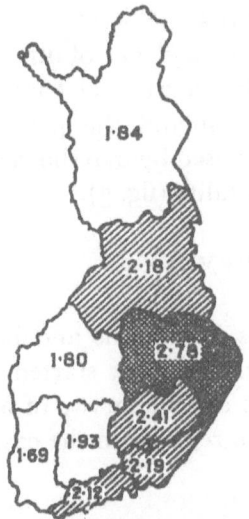

Fig. 1. Mortality of men aged 30-59 to arteriosclerotic heart disease (International List, Sixth Revision, nos. 420-422) in Finland, 1953 (Keys, Karvonen & Fidanza 1958).

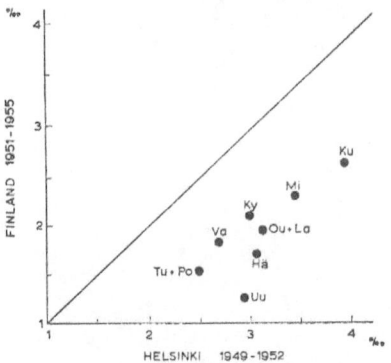

Fig. 2. Mortality of men aged 30-59 to arteriosclerotic heart disease in Helsinki, according to the place of birth (1949-52), and in the corresponding home counties (1951-1955). Age standardized figures. Hä = Häme, Ku = Kuopio, Ky = Kymi, Mi = Mikkeli, Ou + La = Oulu & Lapland, Tu + Po = Turku & Pori, Uu = Uusimaa, Va = Vaasa (Varpela 1960).

higher cv mortality than those who had stayed at home. An interesting observation was that those who had come from the regions with high cv mortality, also in Helsinki had higher mortality than those coming from the low cv regions (fig. 2). There was no tendency to a levelling off of the regional difference.

2. DISABILITY STATISTICS

Statistics on prevalence or incidence of IHD are not generally available from standard sources. However, social insurance may provide some useful figures. Thus in Finland the percentage of those receiving pension for disability as caused by CVD showed a rather similar regional distribution as the cv mortality (fig. 3).

3. CROSS-SECTIONAL SURVEYS

3. 1. Prevalence of IHD

These statistics served as a stimulus and background for a series of more direct epidemiological studies started in 1956, and still continuing. In 1956, we made a field survey of a sample of the clinically healthy population in two regions, in the east and in the southwest, in

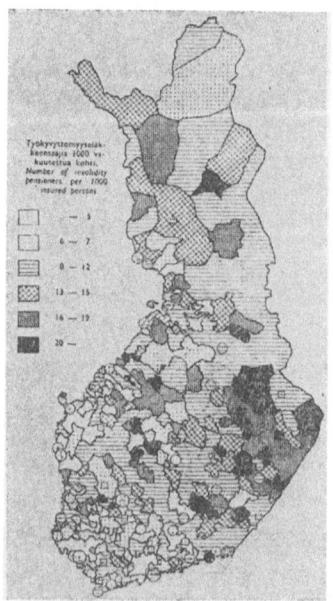

Fig. 3. Disability due to cardiovascular disease in Finland, 1955 (Kansaneläkelaitos 1956).

order to obtain a picture of such relevant factors as serum cholesterol, blood pressure, smoking habits, diet etc. (2, 3, 4, 5). The experiences obtained in the 1956 study were drawn upon for a new study in 1959, in which all men from 40 to 59 years of age in two rural areas were included. The participation rate was 99.3% in the east and 97.0% in the west. The initial population, 1677 men, has been followed since then. A 5-year re-examination was made in 1964, and a 10-year re-examination is due in 1969. The Finnish study is linked to a collaborative family of studies in six other countries, which comprises 18 cohorts, altogether some 12000 men, all examined using standardized methods (6).

The most substantial epidemiological evidence for IHD among the living is supplied by electrocardiography (ECG). The prevalence of ECG signs ascribable to IHD was slightly higher in the east than in the west, but the difference hardly reached statistical significance. On the other hand, angina pectoris was diagnosed significantly more often in the east, in 5.1%, than in the west where its prevalence was less than a third, 1.4%. Several explanations may be suggested for the discrepancy between prevalence of ECG signs and of angina. The men in the east, e.g., may be exposed to hard physical work in very cold weather, which elicits angina, while those in the west live in a less harsh climate and are economically more secure to avoid such precipitating conditions. There may also be substantial differences in the emotional set-up and sensitivity between the Finnish east and west.

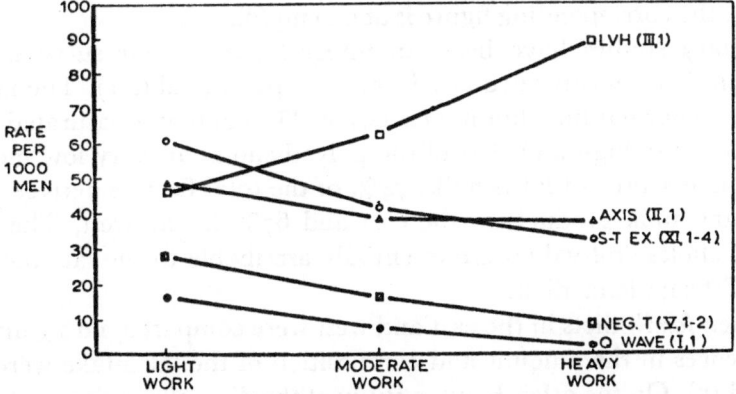

Fig. 4. Relationship of electrocardiographic findings to physical activity of occupation in men aged 40-59. LVH = left ventricular hypertrophy, Axis = left axis deviation, S-T EX. = S-T depression after exercise, NEG. T = negative T wave, Q wave = Q or QS pattern of old infarct (Keys et al. 1967).

When the men in the international collaborative study were divided into subgroups following a number of criteria, such as skinfold thickness, relative body weight, blood pressure, serum cholesterol, smoking habits and occupational physical activity, an impressive accumulation of ECG signs of IHD was observed in men with sedentary occupations (fig. 4), (6).

As a group, the east Finns do more physical work than most other European populations, and should therefore be relatively free from IHD. However, the prevalence of IHD is very high among the sedentary and semisedentary east Finns. ECG signs associated with an old infarct (Q and QRS; Minnesota Code 1, 1-3) occurred in 0.8% among 380 men engaged in heavy work, and five times more often, in 3.9% among men in less strenuous occupations (7). It is, of course, to be expected that men who have had a myocardial infarct try to earn their living in lighter occupations.

3. 2. Risk factors
3. 2. 1. Serum cholesterol
Current research has demonstrated a number of factors associated with an increased risk of the clinical manifestations of IHD. In several longitudinal studies, serum cholesterol has come out as the most potent predictor of IHD. The Finns have a cholesterol which matches their high mortality from IHD. In men at the age of 50 years, the mean in the east was appr. 270 mg/dl, and in the west 260 mg/dl. These are among the highest population averages recorded anywhere. In the United States, the corresponding figure is at 240 mg/dl.

Dietary studies have been an integral part of our surveys. The Finnish diet appears adequate in most respects (Table 1). The fat intake is somewhat high but not excessive. The content of saturated fatty acids is quite high and that of the polyethenoid fats very low indeed. The main source of fat is milk: 74% of the total fat was derived from milk and milk products in the east and 67% in the west. The high serum cholesterol values are essentially ascribable to the fat composition of the national diets.

When *family* diets in the east and west were compared, no significant differences in the amount and composition of the fat intake were observed (5). On the other hand, a study of the diets of *men* demonstrated a significantly higher contribution of fat to total calories in the east, and a greater intake of saturated fats. Evidently the men in the east chose more fatty foods from the family diet than the other members do.

3. 2. 2. Blood pressure

As a risk factor, blood pressure has been found to come close to choles-terol in predictive power. The west Finns do not differ much from other nations in blood pressure, but, the east Finns have definitely high blood pressures. In the east, the median rises from 141/87 mm hg at age 40-44 to 153/90 mm hg at 55-59; in the west the corresponding figures are 133/80 and 143/82 mm hg. However, the blood pressure measurement should never be taken as something absolute. In addition to technical errors, it is affected also by such subtle factors as by the physician-patient interaction. The east-west difference may also in-clude such hidden sources of bias.

3. 2. 3. Smoking

The Finns are a nation of cigarette smokers. Although the total con-sumption of tobacco per person is of the same magnitude as in the Scandinavian countries, a much greater share of it is smoked as cigarettes. (8).

In the east, smoking is more common than in the west. The propor-tion of smokers in our 1959 series was 68.5% in the east and 57.2% in the west. Heavy smoking (20 or more cigarettes daily) was also more prevalent in the east, where 31.4% of the men belonged to this cate-gory, as against 14.8% in the west.

3. 2. 4. Physical activity

Sedentary life habits and/or poor physical fitness have come out as risk factors of IHD in some studies. Our investigation was, in fact, stimulated by the puzzling accumulation of recorded IHD in such parts of Finland, where forest work, physically a most heavy occupation, is a source of living for many men. A part of the riddle was cleared by the observa-tion that even in the east, the ECG signs of IHD were to be found mainly among the sedentary men, much less among those physically active (7). It is worth also noting that forest work is not carried out all the year round. Many small farmers work hard on their farms for a few weeks in the spring and during the summer, and in the forest during one to two winter months, while the rest of the year are relatively slack periods. Thus, the east and west may differ in peak work rates, but in the mean energy expenditure there is not much difference, as shown e.g. by the caloric value of the food intake by the men (table 1).

Table 1. Daily intake of calories and nutrients by rural men in west and east Finland, 1959 (9).

	West	East	P
Food energy, kcal	3760	3805	..
Protein, g	114	120	..
Fat, g	148	166	..
Fat, % of calories	35.4	39.2	0.01
Fatty acids, g			
Saturated	18.8	22.1	0.02
Monoene	11.5	12.1	..
Linoleic	2.3	2.1	..
Other polyethenoid	0.9	0.8	..
Carbohydrate, g	509	479	..
Calcium, mg	1760	1865	..
Iron, mg	19	19	..
Iodine, mg	98	73	0.001
Vitamin A, I.U.	4630	5750	..
Thiamine, mg	2.3	2.1	..
Riboflavin, mg	3.4	3.8	..
Nicotinamide, mg	18	17	..
Ascorbic acid, mg	105	102	..

3. 2. 5. Obesity

Marked obesity also enhances the risk of IHD. On an average, however, the rural Finns are thin. The thickness of the subcutaneous fat, as measured with a skinfold caliber, stands markedly on the low side in international comparisons, and slightly lower in the east than in the west.

3. 2. 6. Water hardness and minerals

In some countries, regional variations in the hardness of the drinking water appear to be reflected in the incidence of IHD, in the sense that soft water and hard arteries go together. Also in Finland, this general tendency seems to prevail. Recently, several characteristics of the drinking water of 21 Finnish cities and towns were correlated to the prevalence of pensioned disability due to CVD (11). Significant negative correlations were obtained for conductivity, and for the calcium, chloride, bromine and iodine content. The correlation was most marked for iodine ($r = -0,62$); when the content of iodine was below 2 or 3 µg/l, the prevalence of CVD seamed to increase steeply.

The supply of iodine is in Finland somewhat low, less than the accepted minimum recommendation of 100 µg per day. Moreover, it is lower in the east than in the west (Table 1). In medico-legal autopsies in Helsinki, the degree of coronary atherosclerosis was positively correlated to the size of the thyroid (12). Among a population with critical iodine intake, thyroid enlargement is generally compensatory due to lack of iodine. Both these studies thus lend support to the hypothesis that lack of iodine contributes to the epidemic of IHD, particularly in east Finland.

4. LONGITUDINAL STUDIES
4.1. Mortality
A follow-up of the cohorts of the international collaborative study provides data on the mortality of thoroughly examined men, with a standard evaluation of the cause of death. Table 2 shows the 5-year mortality from IHD in the cohorts. The marked differences shown in the national vital statistics are essentially confirmed by these results.

Table 2. 5-year mortality from IHD in cohorts of men of 40-59 years on entering the study. The number of expected deaths is based on the IHD mortality of white males in the United States in 1962 (10).

Cohort	Observed	Expected	o/E
US Railroad	63	59.7	1.06
East Finland	17	17.7	0.96
West Finland	7	20.5	0.34
Slavonia	4	17.9	0.22
Rural Greece	3	27.7	0.11
Rural Japan	2	23.9	0.08
Dalmatia	0	18.0	0.00

4.2. Incidence
In a longitudinal study, various criteria for new IHD may be used. In countries with much IHD, it is reasonable to assume that the majority of otherwise unexplained sudden deaths are manifestations of IHD. New myocardial infarcts (Minnesota Code I, 1-3) are another rather valid indicator of the incidence. Table 3 shows the 5-year incidence of new infarcts and of sudden deaths in men previously free of ECG signs of IHD in the Finnish cohorts. The total incidence was practically identical in the east and west, while there were more sudden deaths in the east, and more survivors of myocardial infarct in the west (13).

Table 3. 5-year incidence of new myocardial infarcts (Minnesota Code I, 1-3) and of sudden deaths in the Finnish cohorts of healthy men of 40-59 years on entering the study (13).

	Number		Annual incidence/1000	
	West	East	West	East
Initially free of				
ECG signs of IHD	809	763	.	.
Myocardial infarct	23	14	5.7	3.7
Sudden death	6	14	1.5	3.7
Total infarcts				
and sudden deaths	29	28	7.2	7.3

4. 3. Prognosis

Differences in mortality from IHD may be due to different incidence, different survival of the illness, or both. Table 4 shows the 8-year mortality of three categories of men, those previously free of ECG signs of IHD, those with myocardial infarction and these with other signs of IHD (13). Obviously the men in the east stand their IHD poorer than those in the west. We do not know, whether this difference in prognosis is due to any of the known risk factors, or possibly to some other, hitherto unknown, factor.

Table 4. 8-year mortality in the Finnish cohorts of men of 40-59 years on entering the study. ECG characterization refers to the Minnesota Code (13).

Initial ECG	Initial number		Annual mortality/1000	
	West	East	West	East
No signs of IHD	809	763	11.0	13.3
IHD, no infarct (IV 1-3; VI 1,2,4; VII 1,2,4; VIII 3)	33	34	26.5	62.5
Myocardial infarct (I 1-3)	15	18	41.7	62.5
Total	857	815	12.1	16.4

5. EXPERIMENTAL EPIDEMIOLOGY

5. 1. Diet

The aim is to prevent. After risk factors have been demonstrated it is logical to ask, whether a manipulation of a risk factor will also cause a corresponding change in the sickness experience. Among the risk factors of IHD, serum cholesterol alone places the majority of middle aged Finns in a high risk group. It was therefore appropriate to select serum cholesterol as the first risk factor to be changed.

A dietary study is in progress since 1958 in two mental hospitals (14). In one of them, the milk fat in the typical Finnish house diet was replaced by soybean oil, 'soft' margarine and an emulsion of soybean oil in skimmed milk. After six years, the experimental and control diets were exchanged between the hospitals. In the hospital with the experimental diet, the serum cholesterol level during the first six years was on an average 217 mg/dl, while in the control hospital it stayed at the typical 'Finnish' level of 268 mg/dl. The fatty acid composition of the subcutaneous fat also became quite different in the two hospitals. The dietary change in the experimental hospital was evidently also able to prevent IHD: the annual incidence of new manifestations of IHD in men was significantly lower with the experimental diet, less than half of that in the control hospital.

5. 2. Exercise

Men may also be able to change their habitual physical activity. In order to find out, whether this is practically feasible, an experimental and a control group were recruited from the clientele of an annual comprehensive health examination offered to executives (15).

The experimental group of initially 89 men takes part three times a week in a regular fitness programme, while their matched controls have agreed not to change their exercise habits. After three months, the physical fitness of the experimental subjects had clearly improved, while none of the other studied risk factors had shown any change. The study is to continue for eighteen months.

The experimental group has adhered to its schedule with a devotion which gives promise for planning a larger scale study of prevention.

6. CONCLUSIONS

The starting points of the reported series of studies were the high cv mortality in Finland, particularly among the middle aged men, and the regional differences within Finland, with the east exceeding by some 60% the west in mortality. International cohort studies have confirmed the existence of marked differences in mortality and proved that the high Finnish figures are due to IHD. Between east and west of Finland, different statistics give somewhat discrepant figures. On one hand, the cv sickness experience, as indicated either by the disability or by angina, gives an even more marked gradient between east and west than the mortality, while, on the other hand, the prevalence of old infarcts in a cross-sectional study is only some 16% higher in the east than in the west. The discrepancy between the prevalence and mortality disappears with the observation tha prognosis of IHD in the east is poorer than in the west. The marked regional difference in the cv sickness experience remains without an obvious explanation, perhaps ascribable also to social and economic differences.

In searching for a cause of the Finnish epidemic of IHD, the high mean serum cholesterol level of the Finns appears impressive. However, the regional difference in cholesterol is small and only some 10% extra IHD in the east should be expected on account of it. High blood pressure seems to add to the handicaps in the east.

Cigarette smoking may contribute to the difference between Finland and its Scandinavian neighbours, but certainly does not explain the difference in IHD between the Finns and the Japanese, who smoke even more than the Finns. On the other hand, east and west Finland differ in smoking relatively more than they do in the other known risk factor, and cigarette smoking might well be a major determinant of the regional difference. The soft drinking water in the east, and the deficient intake of iodine, may contribute to it. Whatever the cause of the regional differences, it is not essentially affected by migration to a common environment. Heredity, early environment or life habits acquired before migration, evidently offer the possible mechanism, which, however, do not operate over the serum cholesterol level, after the men have moved to a common environment (3). Within each region, the habitual physical activity is the most potent discriminator of the prevalence of IHD.

While the role of each risk factor deserves further elucidation, it has been demonstrated that the Finnish epidemic of IHD can be effectively prevented by a change of one risk factor only, by the dietary manipulation of the serum cholesterol. It remains for further studies to show, whether corresponding effects are to be attained through experimental changes in other risk factors. Prevention on a nation-wide scale is a challenge for the public health authorities.

REFERENCES

1. Varpela, E., *Nord. Med.* 63, 127 (1960).
2. Karvonen, M. J., E. Orma, A. Keys, F. Fidanza, & J. Brozek, *Lancet* I, 492 (1959).
3. Keys, A., M. J. Karvonen & F. Fidanza, *Lancet* II, 175 (1958).

4. Rautaharju, P. M., M. J. Karvonen & A. Keys *J. chron. Dis.* 13, 426 (1961).
5. Roine, P., M. Pekkarinen, M. J. Karvonen & J. Kihlberg, *Lancet* II, 173 (1958).
6. Keys, A., C. Aravanis, H. W. Blackburn, F. S. P. van Buchem, R. Buzina, B. S. Djordjević, A. S. Dontas, F. Fidanza, M. J. Karvonen, N. Kimura, D. Lekos, M. Monti, V. Puddu & H. L. Taylor, *Acta med. scand.* Suppl. 460 (1967).
7. Karvonen, M. J., P. M. Rautaharju, E. Orma, S. Punsar & J. Takkunen, *J. Occup. Med.* 3, 49 (1961).
8. Pedersen, E., K. Magnus, T. Mork, A. Hougen, E. Bjelke, M. Hakama & E. Saxen, *Acta pathol. microbiol. scand.* Suppl. 199 (1969).
9. Roine, P., M. Pekkarinen & M. J. Karvonen, In: *Dietary Studies and Epidemiology of Heart Diseases*, ed. by Den Hartog, C., R. Buzina, F. Fidanza, A. Keys & P. Roine, p. 29. The Hague.
10. Keys, A., C. Aravanis, H. Blackburn, R. Buzina, M. J. Karvonen, N. Kimura & H. L. Taylor, Paper presented at the Fifth International Congress of Hygiene and Preventive Medicine, Rome, Italy 8-12 October. (1968).
11. Häsänen, E., *Suomen Lääkärilehti* 24, 757 (1969).
12. Uotila, U., J. Raekallio & W. Ehrnrooth, *Lancet* II, 171 (1958).
13. Punsar, S., M. J. Karvonen & K. Pyörälä, *Scand. J. clin. Lab. Invest.* 23, Suppl. 108, 52 (1969).
14. Turpeinen, O., M. Miettinen, M. J. Karvonen, P. Roine, M. Pekkarinen, E. J. Lehtosuo & P. Alivirta, *Am. J. Clin. Nutr.* 21, 255 (1968).
15. Teräslinna, P., T. Partanen, K. Pyörälä, S. Punsar, R. Kärävä & P. Oja, *Work Environment Health* (1969). To be published.

REGIONAL DIFFERENCES IN PREVALENCE, INCIDENCE AND MORTALITY FROM ATHEROSCLEROTIC CORONARY HEART DISEASE

J. STAMLER, ROSE STAMLER, R. B. SHEKELLE

HISTORICAL BACKGROUND

There is no doubt that marked regional differences exist in the occurrence of atherosclerotic disease. Medical research has been accumulating data on this phenomenon for several decades. It is by no means a *de novo* discovery stemming from the post-World War II surge of research on this problem. Valuable reviews of the earlier literature, published in the 1930s, remain worthy of study (1-6). At this Boerhaave Course, it is appropriate to refer specifically to researches in the Dutch East Indies by European investigators:

'Dutch East Indies: the diet of the natives consists chiefly of cereals. Blood cholesterol is low but rises in those who adopt European dietary habits (de Langen). The blood pressure of the natives is low: arteriosclerosis 'at least in its pronounced form' is rare (Sitsen). Angina pectoris is uncommon (Wenckebach.)' (6)

The references to De Langen, Sitsen and Wenckebach are to works published during the years 1921-3 (7-9). These are only three among more than two score references on the subject of regional differences, noted in the literature by the cited reviewers thirty-five years ago.

RECENT FINDINGS

Since World War II, the expanded research effort on atherosclerosis has included systematic investigation of the matter of regional differences. Several methods have been utilized. All of them have confirmed the existence of marked regional differences in occurrence of atherosclerotic coronary heart disease (CHD).

84

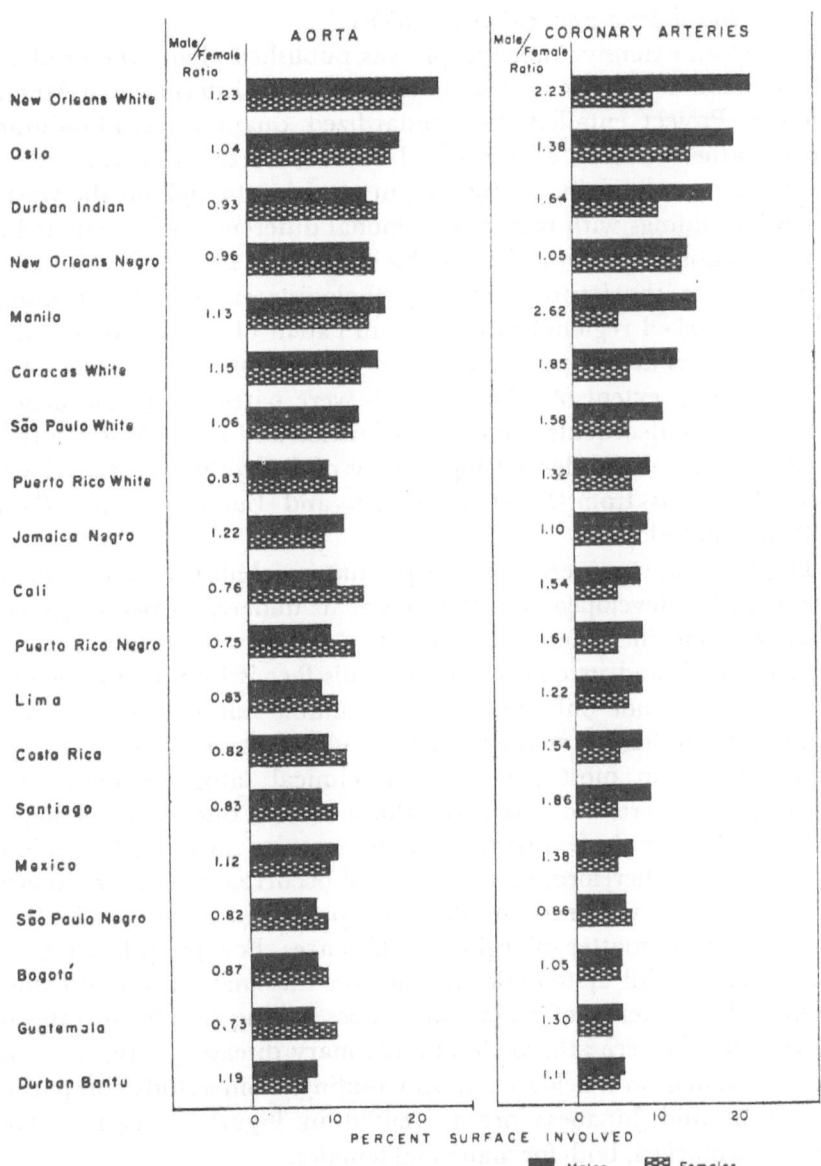

Fig. 1. Extent of aorta and coronary atherosclerosis at autopsy (10).

Findings from international pathologic studies

Recently an extensive monograph was published giving the results of one of the most comprehensive studies (10). This International Athero-sclerosis Project entailed the standardized, quantitative, blind grad-ing for atherosclerosis of aorta and coronary arteries of over 21,000 persons age 10-69 dying in 1960-65 in 15 cities throughout the world. Essential findings with respect to regional differences are presented in figure 1. As is evident, the data of this systematic, massive investigation fully confirm the impressions of pathologists early in the century. Clearly, marked regional differences in extent of aorta and coronary atherosclerosis at autopsy were present in persons dying in the 1960s. Differences in extent of atherosclerosis were particularly conspicuous between male decedents from cities of Africa and Latin America (i.e., from economically underdeveloped areas of the world), compared with male decedents from North American and European cities (New Orleans and Oslo).

The contemporary epidemic of premature clinical coronary heart disease in the developed countries has as its underlying pathology not atherosclerosis in general, but rather – quite specifically – *severe* atherosclerosis and its complications. This fact is by now thoroughly documented – not only by autopsy studies, but by the extensive findings of coronary arteriography in living human beings (11, 12). Undoubtedly, in most persons with clinical CHD, the underlying pathology is severe and extensive atherosclerotic disease, involving at least one, frequently two or three main coronary arteries. Exceptions are very rare. Therefore, data on rates of occurrence of *severe* athero-sclerotic coronary disease in different populations are particularly relevant for the matter of regional differences. Few published reports are available with systematic findings on this matter. Those extant confirm the existence of major differences among peoples in rates of occurrence of severe atherosclerotic coronary disease (cf. ref. 10, and the quotation from it below). Autopsy findings from a study comparing Americans and Japanese are presented in Figure 2 (13-15). The contrast is marked, both for males and females.

(As is evident in both figures 1 and 2, males – at least white males – from the more prosperous countries manifested considerably more ex-tensive atherosclerosis of the coronary arteries than females, whereas the sex differential tended to be slight or non-existent for populations from the less developed countries.)

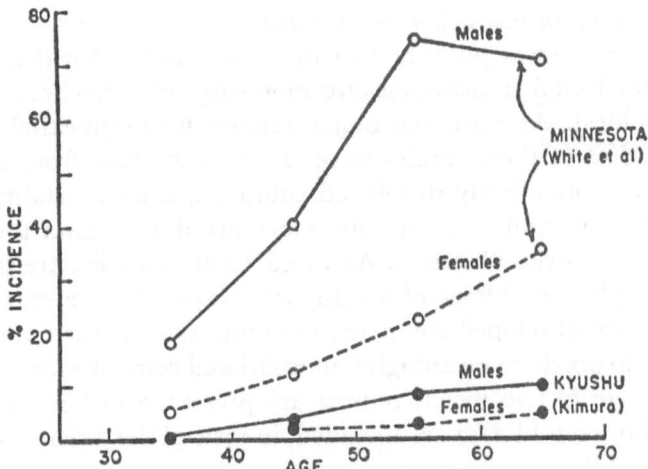

Fig. 2. Incidence of high grade coronary sclerosis in consecutive autopsies, U.S. vs. Japan (13-15).

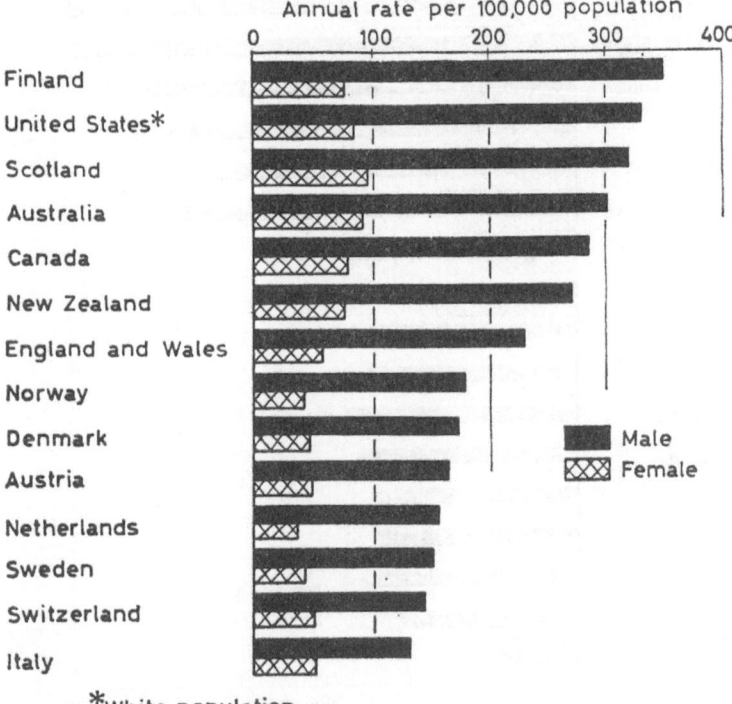

Fig. 3. Age-adjusted death rates (ages 25-64) for arteriosclerotic and degenerative heart disease, by sex, in 14 countries (20).

Findings from international vital statistics studies

Several papers were published in the 1950s and 1960s dealing with international vital statistics on CHD mortality (cf. references 16-18 for bibliographies). At least five major reports have appeared recently (19-23). Most of these studies have dealt with data from a limited number of economically developed countries, since mortality data – particularly age-and cause-specific mortality data – from the under-developed countries of Africa, Asia and Latin America are generally deficient. While problems also exist with respect to comparability of data from the developed countries, the limitations of the data are not so gross as to preclude meaningful international comparisons.

Findings from two recent reports are presented in figures 3 and 4 (20, 23). Both sets of data are included, in view of the differences in age

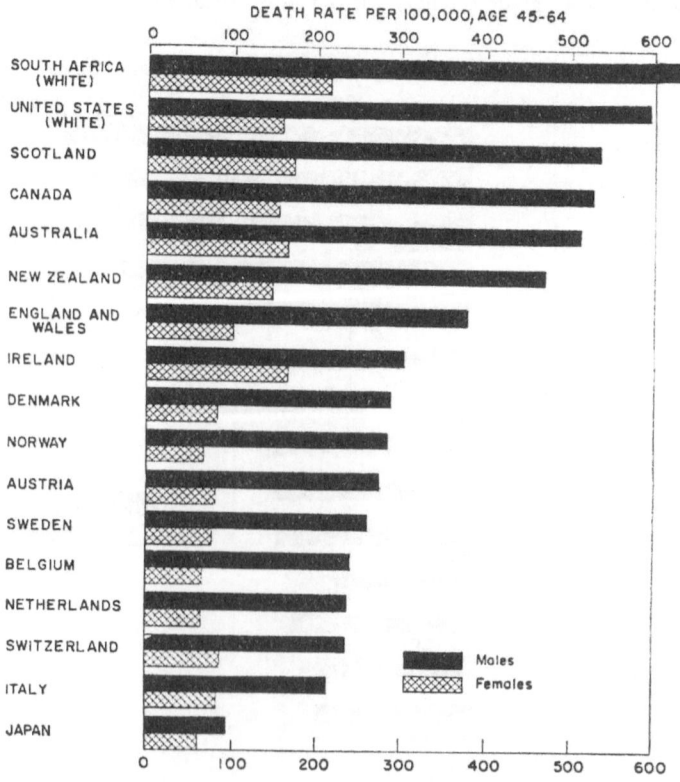

Fig. 4. Age-adjusted death rates of males and females aged 45-64, for arteriosclerotic and degenerative heart disease, in 17 countries, 1960 (23).

span and countries represented. Figure 3 includes the data for Finland, comprehensively discussed in the preceding paper of this Course. In both lists, obviously, the United States is second from the top in mortality rates for premature atherosclerotic heart disease. It seems that we Americans are adhering to the familiar slogan of a well-known u.s. car rental company: 'We 're number Two – and trying harder!' Be that as it may, these international mortality data – even though encompassing only limited numbers of the developed countries – indicate the presence of sizeable regional differences in CHD death rates for middle-aged persons, especially males.

Clearly, the United States is vast in geographic size and population, equalling or exceeding several of the foregoing countries combined. It is not surprising therefore – particularly in the light of the differences reported from East and West Finland – that sizeable differences exist among the major regions and the fifty states of the u.s.a. in mortality rates for premature CHD. For the states, these differences were almost 100 per cent in 1959-61 for white males and females age 45-64. Even greater differences were recorded for non-whites (principally Negroes) (fig. 5) (23).

Data are also available on the time trend of CHD mortality rates for the different countries (19-23). Findings for 17 countries, comparing 1960 with 1950, are presented in figure 6 (23). It is evident that for most countries CHD mortality rates for middle-aged men rose over the decade from 1950 to 1960. For several countries e.g. – Norway, Netherlands, Denmark, Australia – the increase was marked, 30 per cent or more. (The trend for rates for females was not as consistent.) Evidently the crest of the worldwide CHD epidemic has not yet been reached. The continuing increase in rates threatens – as the World Health Organization Executive Board recently noted (24) – to lead to the greatest epidemic disease problem mankind has ever faced.

The comprehensive vital statistics tabulations for twenty-two countries recently published by the World Health Organization underscore the scope of the problem arising from the raging CHD epidemic (21). Table 1 has been abstracted from that publication. It ranks the twenty-two countries from high to low, based on 1964 mortality rates from all causes of death for men age 45-54. Table 2 gives the ranking of these 22 countries for mortality rates from CHD and all cardiovascular diseases (CVD). Two facts stand out clearly: First, sizeable differences exist among these twenty-two countries – almost all of them economically developed countries – in total mortality rates for middle-aged men. Thus, Finland – at the top of the list – has a rate more than double that of Sweden, with the lowest rate. The mean rate for the three countries at the top of the list (Finland, u.s.a. Scotland) is almost double that of the mean rate for the countries at the bottom (Israel, Norway, Sweden) (1,006 vs. 553 per 100,000). Second, to a considerable degree the differences in rates for all causes are due to differences in rates for

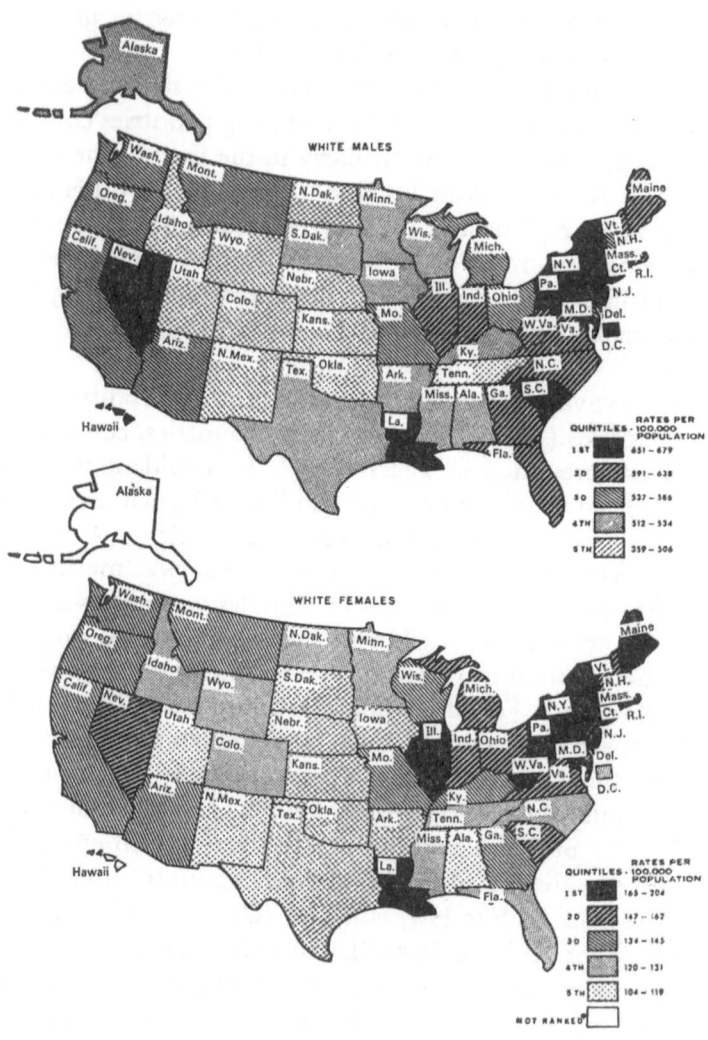

coronary and cardiovascular diseases. Thus, the mean CHD mortality rate for the three countries with the highest mortality rates from all causes is 385/100,000. The mean CHD mortality rate for the three countries with the lowest mortality rates from all causes is 167/100,000. A mean reduction in CHD mortality rate for Finland, U.S.A. and Scotland to this level of 167 would effect a reduction in mortality from all causes of 21.7 per cent (from 1,006 to 788 per 100,000). A corresponding

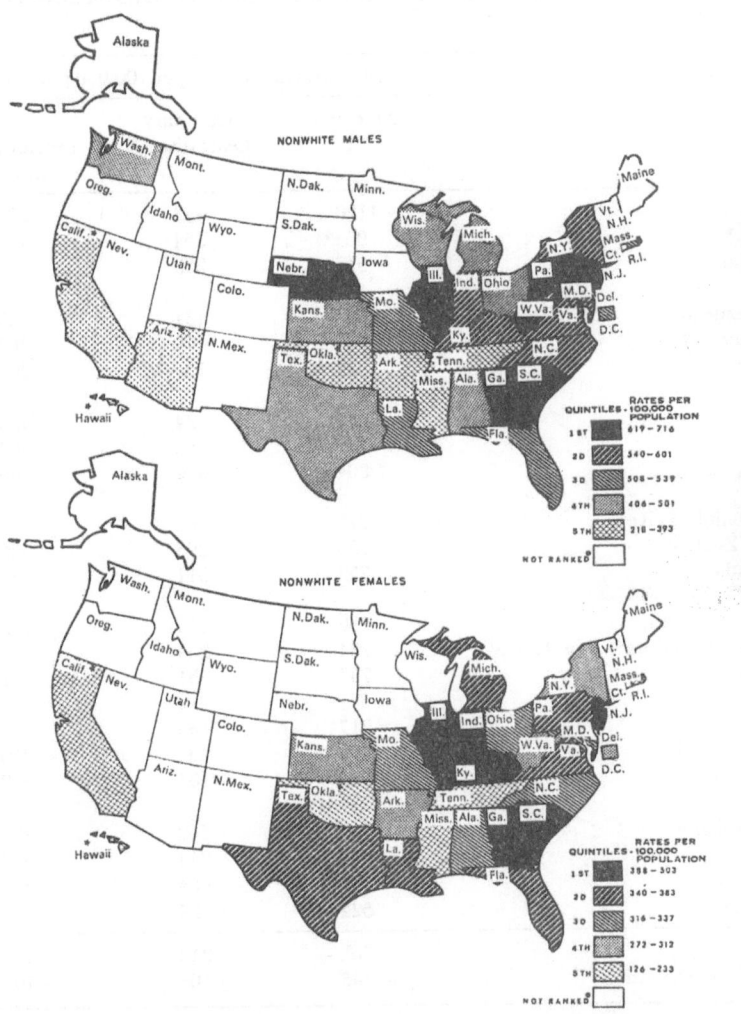

Fig. 5. Quintile ranking of age-adjusted death rate for coronary heart disease at ages 45-64 by State: 1959-61. The left figure is for whites, the right is for nonwhites (23).

reduction in mortality from all cardiovascular diseases would decrease mortality from all causes by 26.8 per cent (from 1,006 to 736 per 100,000). These achievements would lower the mean mortality rate from all causes for the three highest countries to approximately the median rate for the 22 countries (755 per 100,000 for all causes).

A similar improvement would result if the three countries with the highest mortality rates from all causes were to succeed in reducing

Table 1. 1964 Mortality rates for 22 countries ranked by mortality rates for all causes, males, age 45-54

Country	1964 Mortality rates per 100,000 population		
	All causes	Coronary heart disease	All cardiovascular diseases
Finland	1120	442	579
U.S.A.*	964*	354*	477*
Scotland	933	359	463
Venezuela	897	131	235
France	863	74	202
Austria	823	159	263
Australia	821	324	425
Belgium	820	159	302
No. Ireland	804	324	465
German Fed. Rep.	772	182	275
New Zealand	758	293	386
Canada	752	311	385
Czechoslovakia	738	151	263
United Kingdom – Eng. & Wales	734	254	341
Japan	733	51	251
Italy	717	133	239
Switzerland	658	134	210
Denmark	613	181	248
Netherlands	582	162	222
Israel	572	214	302
Norway	566	164	218
Sweden	522	124	189
Mean	762	212	315
Standard Deviation	± 145	±103	±109

* For white males only, mortality rates are: All causes = 900, CHD = 355, CV = 450.

their mean CHD and CVR mortality rates to the median levels for the 22 countries (172 and 269 per 100,000 respectively).

Mortality rates and rankings for women are presented in tables 3 and 4 respectively (21). The findings are essentially similar.

For the countries at the two poles of the distribution, therefore, two opposite – but obviously complementary – challenges exist: For the countries with the high rates, the problem is: What can they do to emulate the countries with the low rates, i.e. what can they do to achieve a sizeable reduction in mortality rates from coronary disease,

Table 2. Ranking of 1964 mortality rates for specified causes, males age 45-54, 22 countries – Primary ranking based on rates for all causes

Country	Rank order – High to low		
	All causes	Coronary heart disease	All cardiovascular diseases
Finland	1	1	1
U.S.A. *	2*	3*	2*
Scotland	3	2	4
Venezuela	4	19	17
France	5	21	21
Austria	6	14	12
Australia	7	5	5
Belgium	8	15	9
No. Ireland	9	4	3
German Fed. Rep.	10	10	11
New Zealand	11	7	6
Canada	12	6	7
Czechoslovakia	13	16	13
United Kingdom – Eng. & Wales	14	8	8
Japan	15	22	14
Italy	16	18	16
Switzerland	17	17	20
Denmark	18	11	15
Netherlands	19	13	18
Israel	20	9	10
Norway	21	12	19
Sweden	22	20	22

* If only white males are included, rank is: All causes = 3, CHD = 3, CV = 4.

cardiovascular diseases and all causes? On the other hand, for the presently favored countries with low rates, the problem is: What can they do to avoid following in the footsteps of the countries with high rates, with development of mounting mortality from coronary disease and cardiovascular diseases in general? The seriousness of this problem is underscored by statistics from Norway, for example, with a more than

Table 3. 1964 Mortality rates for 22 countries ranked by mortality rates for all causes, females, age 45-54

Country	1964 Mortality rates per 100,000 population		
	All causes	Coronary heart disease	All cardiovascular diseases
Venezuela	706	56	151
Scotland	547	86	198
U.S.A.*	523	82	183
No. Ireland	509	74	189
Australia	478	76	175
Japan	472	33	161
Israel	461	72	157
Austria	457	38	105
New Zealand	449	63	156
German Fed. Rep.	446	49	103
Belgium	446	38	116
Czechoslovakia	442	29	131
Finland	441	62	175
United Kingdom – Eng. & Wales	438	42	131
France	434	14	93
Canada	408	59	128
Italy	403	36	125
Denmark	400	29	86
Sweden	355	26	79
Switzerland	351	29	76
Netherlands	342	22	65
Norway	294	26	77
Mean	446	47	130
Standard Deviation	± 84	± 22	± 41

* For white females only, mortality rates are: All causes = 460, CHD = 71, CV = 143.

90% increase in CHD mortality rate for middle-aged males over the decade 1950 to 1960 (fig. 6).

One of the further consequences of the mounting epidemic of premature CHD is its impact on life expectancy of middle-aged persons. This is well illustrated by data of table 5, for the United States (25, 26). Despite the tremendous advances in medical science and public health since 1900, life expectancy for middle-aged men in the United States today is only a few years greater than it was at the turn of the

Table 4. Ranking of 1964 mortality rates for specified causes, females age 45-54, 22 countries – Primary ranking based on rates for all causes

Country	Rank order – High to low		
	All causes	Coronary heart disease	All cardiovascular diseases
Venezuela	1	9	9
Scotland	2	1	1
U.S.A.*	3*	2*	3*
No. Ireland	4	4	2
Australia	5	3	4
Japan	6	15	6
Israel	7	5	7
Austria	8	13	15
New Zealand	9	6	8
German Red. Reg.	10	10	16
Belgium	11	12	14
Czechoslovakia	12	16	10
Finland	13	7	5
United Kingdom – Eng. & Wales	14	11	11
France	15	22	17
Canada	16	8	12
Italy	17	14	13
Denmark	18	17	18
Sweden	19	19	19
Switzerland	20	18	21
Netherlands	21	21	22
Norway	22	22	20

* If only white females are included, rank is: All causes = 7, CHD = 5, CV = 9.

century. The paucity of the achievement is particularly conspicuous for white males.

This situation prevails despite the tremendous reduction in mortality of adults from tuberculosis and lobar pneumonia, for example, major causes of death in 1900. The decisive factor responsible for this is, of course, the increase – particularly for males – in premature mortality from CHD and atherosclerosis in other vascular beds. Clearly, for the developed countries there can be no major further advance in life expectancy without control of the CHD epidemic.

Findings from living population studies
Data from living population studies are consistent with those of autopsy and vital statistics analyses in demonstrating large regional differences

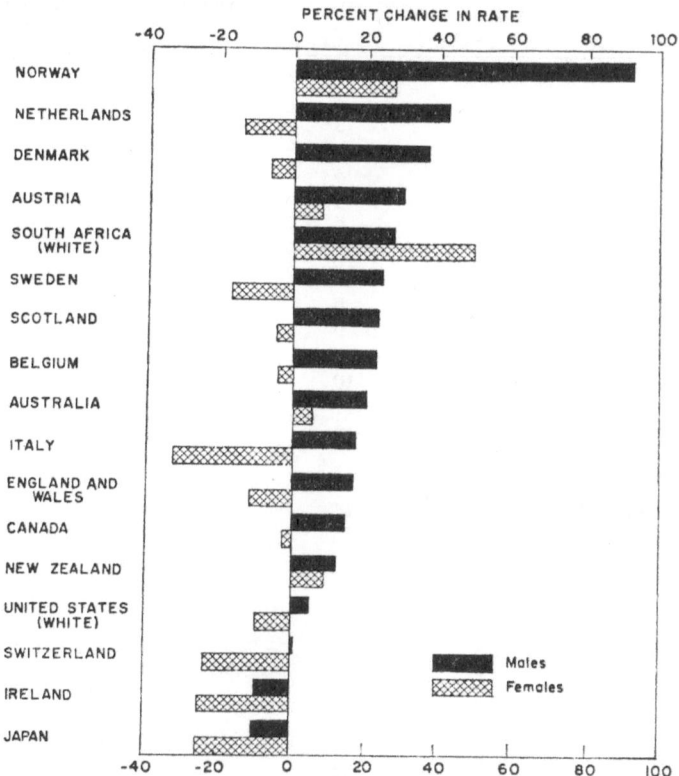

Fig. 6. Percentage changes from 1950 to 1960 in age-adjusted death rates of males and females, 45-64, for arteriosclerotic and degenerative heart disease: 17 countries, 1960 (23).

in occurrence of atherosclerotic CHD. Practically all the findings on prevalence and incidence have been collected in studies since World War II (see references 16-18, 27, 28 for reviews and bibliographies). The most comprehensive of these studies is a prospective international cooperative endeavor involving 18 population samples in seven countries (Finland, Greece, Italy, Japan, Netherlands, United States and Yugoslavia). About 12,000 men originally age 40-59 are being followed. Prevalence findings were recently reported in a major monograph (29). In addition, a preliminary presentation was made of five year incidence data before the 1969 meeting of the Council on Epidemiology, American Heart Association (30).

On initial examination, marked differences in CHD prevalence were recorded among the populations of middle-aged men from these seven countries (29, 30). Consistent with the findings from international autopsy and vital statistics studies, low rates were observed for populations from Greece, Italy, Japan and Yugoslavia, with high rates for population samples from East Finland and the United States. (The populations from West Finland and Holland were intermediate.) The

Table 5. Average number of years of life remaining at age 20, 40 and 65, United States, by sex and color, 1900-02 and 1967 (25, 26)

Age 20			
	Average number of years of life remaining		increase: vs. 1900-02
Sex-color	1900-02	1967	Years
White Male	42.2	50.2	8.0
White Female	43.8	56.9	13.1
Nonwhite Male	35.1	44.8	9.7
Nonwhite Female	36.9	51.3	14.4
Age 40			
White Male	27.7	31.8	4.1
White Female	29.2	37.8	8.6
Nonwhite Male	23.1	28.3	5.2
Nonwhite Female	24.4	33.4	9.0
Age 65			
White Male	11.5	13.0	1.5
White Female	12.2	16.5	4.3
Nonwhite Male	10.4	12.7	2.3
Nonwhite Female	11.4	15.8	4.4

highest prevalence rate (56.6 per 1,000, recorded for the men from East Finland) was about forty times greater than the lowest (1.4 per 1,000, for the Dalmatian men). For the four best cohorts, numbering almost 2,600 men, the prevalence rate for CHD of all types was 4.8 per thousand (2.9 for 'hard' infarct, 1.2 for angina pectoris, 0.7 for other CHD). For the four worst cohorts, numbering slightly more than 5,000 men, the prevalence rate for CHD of all types was more than seven times higher, 36.7 per thousand (17.5 for 'hard' infarct, 9.9 for angina pectoris, 9.3 for other CHD).

The preliminary report on five year incidence data presented findings completely consistent with the prevalence data. In fact, the correlation coefficient between prevalence and incidence data was .97. The highest five year incidence rate was recorded for men from East Finland (in excess of 120 per 1,000); the second highest was for men from the U.S.A. In contrast, incidence rates were well under 20 per 1,000 for the populations from Dalmatia, Crete and Japan.

The overall conclusion is self-evident from all the sets of data: Large regional differences exist in prevalence, incidence and mortality rates from premature atherosclerotic coronary heart disease.

FACTORS POSSIBLY RESPONSIBLE FOR REGIONAL DIFFERENCES IN OCCURRENCE OF CHD

Race, ethnic origin, geography, climate

Regional differences in occurrence of atherosclerotic CHD cannot be attributed to differences in race, ethnic origin, geography or climate. The evidence on this matter is extensive (1-6, 16-18, 27, 28). In fact, some of the investigations done during the early decades of this century yielded valuable information on this matter (1-6).

Four types of data are now available demonstrating that race, ethnic origin, geography and climate are inconsequential in accounting for regional differences in occurrence of atherosclerotic CHD (see refs. 16-18, 27, 28 for bibliographies). First, there are the contrasting findings recorded for different social classes within the same country. Data of this type are available from several countries in economically less developed regions of the world. In these countries, the small strata of the affluent upper classes have adopted living patterns quite similar to those prevailing in the developed countries. In contrast to the underprivileged masses in these countries, the well-to-do manifest rates of occurrence of premature atherosclerotic CHD approaching those of the developed countries. Obviously, these differences in occurrence of CHD have become manifest despite similarities among the different social strata in racial and ethnic background, and in geographic and climatic exposure – q.e.d., these factors cannot be etiologically very relevant per se.

Another set of data – on the effects of migration – has produced complementary findings, and therefore reinforces the foregoing conclusion, at least with respect to racial-ethnic background and its insignificance etiologically. Studies along these lines have included comparisons of Japanese in Japan, Hawaii and the United States; Italians in Italy and the United States; Irish in Ireland and the United States; and immigrants to Israel – recent vs. long-term – from underprivileged Jewish communities in Asia and Africa. The findings consistently indicate that changes in socioeconomic aspects of the mode of life consequent upon immigration are associated with increases in occurrence rates of CHD in all racial-ethnic groups studied.

The findings on time-trends of atherosclerotic disease in several European countries after World War I and during World War II are a third source of data on this matter. Again, marked socioeconomic changes in mode of life, resulting from the exigencies of war, were associated with sizeable declines in occurrence of atherosclerotic disease.

Finally, the sizeable increase since World War II of mortality rates for premature CHD in several European countries, (e.g., cf. fig. 6) lend further substantial support to the conclusion that neither racial-ethnic genetic factors nor aspects of the physical environment are key determinants of regional differences in occurrence of CHD, since obviously neither of these sets of factors have undergone significant changes in the last one or two decades.

Aspects of mode of life related to socioeconomic development – national income
As already noted in earlier sections of this presentation, occurrence rates of atherosclerotic disease are much lower in populations from the underdeveloped countries of Africa, Asia and Latin America, compared with the developed countries of the British Commonwealth, Europe and North America. Obviously, per capita income varies markedly among nations, in relation to level of economic development. Data on the relationship between per capita national income and mortality rates from coronary disease and all cardiovascular

diseases have recently been presented by the World Health Organization (22). Representative findings for CHD for men age 55-59 are presented in figure 7. They encompass 1964 data for 37 countries. Highly significant relationships are demonstrated, with high order correlation coefficients.

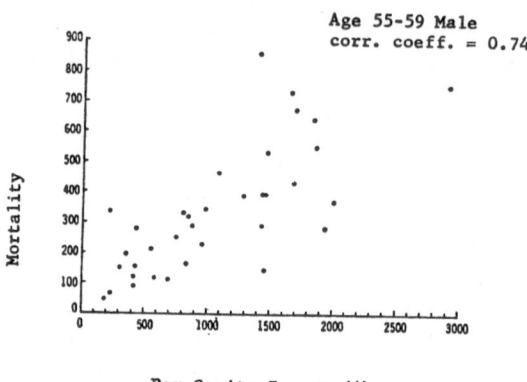

Per Capita Income ($)

Fig. 7. Relation between death rate per 100,000 population, from arteriosclerotic and degenerative heart disease (B 26) and per capita national income in 1964 (22). Countries included: Taiwan, Philippines, Mauritius, Nicaragua, Hong Kong, Portugal, Chile, Mexico, Bulgaria, Panama, Greece, Poland, Japan, Venezuela, Yugoslavia, Hungary, Czechoslovakia, Italy, Puerto Rico, Austria, Israel, Netherlands, Finland, Belgium, England, No. Ireland, Norway, France, Denmark, Germany, Iceland, Australia, New Zealand, Canada, Switzerland, Sweden, United States.

Of the 22 developed countries dealt with in detail in the recent WHO special report on CV and CHD mortality (21), national income data for 1963-5 were available for all but Czechoslovakia, Ireland and Scotland. Table 6 presents data on the correlations between income and mortality. The correlation coefficients (r) for males – .444 and .515 for the 45-54 and 55-64 age groups respectively – reach approximately the .05 level of significance. The r values are small and insignificant for females.

Although these findings are valuable, they are limited by the fact that the independent variable – per capita national income – is not explicit per se in describing mode of life. Therefore, to evaluate whether specific socioeconomic factors are responsible for regional differences in occurrence rates of atherosclerotic CHD, it is essential to go beyond per capita national income, and examine concrete aspects of the mode of life influenced by income.

Table 6. Relationships between per capita national income from coronary heart disease, and mortality rates by age and sex, 1964 – 19 countries[4]

Age-sex group	1964 CHD Mortality rate per 100,000	Correlation coefficient – per capita national Income and CHD mortality rate
45-54 Male	202 ± 101	.444[44]
45-54 Female	45 ± 20	.259
55-64 Male	570 ± 252	.515*
55-64 Female	188 ± 79	.365

[4] Mean per capita national income for the 19 countries was $ 1,373. ± $ 503. in 1963-5.
[44] P slightly greater than .05.
* P less than .05, slightly greater than .02.

Aspects of mode of life related to socioeconomic development – nutrition
As is well known, a vast literature – clinico-pathologic, epidemiologic and animal-experimental – exists on the relationship between nutrition and atherosclerosis. A comprehensive review of this subject is beyond the scope of this presentation (see refs. 16-18, 27, 28, as well as other papers in the present volume).

Here it is relevant to focus on the extensive data indicating that regional differences in nutrition account significantly for regional differences in occurrence rates of atherosclerotic CHD. The evidence on this matter is indeed massive. Here again, investigations early in the century pointed the way to conclusions firmly established only by the systematic research since World War II. Thus, one of the major reviews in the 1930s arrived at the following generalization, based on an analysis of 28 papers then in the literature, including findings from clinical and pathological studies in China, East Africa, Egypt, India, Malaya, Austria, Germany, the United States and elsewhere:

'. . .in no race for which a high cholesterol intake (in the form of eggs, butter and milk) and fat intake are recorded is atherosclerosis absent. . . Where a high protein diet is consumed, which naturally contains small quantities of cholesterol, but where the neutral fat intake is low, atherosclerosis is not prevalent.'(5)

In the last 25 years, numerous population surveys in many countries have yielded data reinforcing the same basic conclusion: Significant atherosclerosis is rare in peoples whose diet over the life span is predominantly vegetarian and low in calories, total lipids, saturated lipids and cholesterol. It is rare clinically and morphologically, in both males and females, particularly as premature and as severe disease – in marked contrast to the patterns prevailing in the developed countries, particularly those with habitual diets high in calories, total fat, saturated fat and cholesterol. Since several monographs contain comprehensive reviews and bibliographies covering all but the latest reports (16-18, 27, 28), it is appropriate here merely to present key recent findings in summary form.

As indicated earlier in this paper, the International Atherosclerosis Project represents the most comprehensive and systematic study of postmortem findings on aorta and coronary atherosclerosis in different populations (10). Its final report includes a valuable chapter on the relationship of nutrition to the disease. A highly significant correlation was found between intake of fat and severe atherosclerosis at autopsy:

'As many populations as the data permitted were ranked in order of percentage calories from fat, percentage of total fat of animal origin, consumption of sucrose. . . The rank order correlation coefficient of this ranking with that for the reference rank based on advanced athero-sclerotic lesions gave a highly significant r_s of 0.755 with percentage of calories from fat. . . The rank correlations of atherosclerosis reference rank with the other dietary variables were small and without signifi-cance. A strong positive correlation of animal protein consumption with reference rank was observed because this dietary variable closely paralleled the fat calories; it was not considered etiologically important because of the strong supporting evidence for a primary role of fat, rather than protein, in determining. . . severity of atherosclerosis, and incidence of CHD. Egg consumption generally paralleled protein and fat intake, but the data were too fragmentary for reliable ranking.' (31)

Prevalence and incidence data from the prospective study of 12,000 middle-aged men in seven countries lead to the same conclusion (29, 30). Amount and type of lipid habitually eaten – especially saturated fat, and inevitably cholesterol – varied markedly among the population samples studied. Thus, in Kyushu, Japan, total fat con-stituted 9 per cent of calories, saturated fat (SF) 3 per cent, polyunsatu-rated fat (PF) 3 per cent. In several of the European communities– e.g. the Greek islands of Corfu and Crete; Velika Krsna and Dalmatia, Yugoslavia; Montegiorgio and Crevalcore, Italy – saturated fat intake was also low (7-10% of calories); PF intake was never high (3-7%).

(For some of these Southern Europe populations consuming considerable olive oil, total fat made up as much as 40 per cent of calories, but SF intake was still low, as was PF intake, since olive oil is composed largely of mono-unsaturated oleic acid.) In contrast, analyses of the diets ingested by the men under study in Finland, the Netherlands and the U.S.A. revealed high saturated fat intakes, in the range 17-22 per cent of calories (total fat 35-40%, PF 3-5%). Men from East Finland exhibited the highest levels of SF ingestion – 22 per cent of total calories. Saturated fat intakes and five year incidence rates of CHD for these population samples showed a high order positive correlation that was statistically significant (30).

Use has also been made of data from United Nations Organizations (the Food and Agriculture Organization and the World Health Organization) to analyze relationships between nutrient patterns and mortality rates of different countries. Findings from such an analysis are presented in tables 7-10. The mortality data are for 1964 (21). Nutrient data were calculated from national food balance sheets, available from the Food and Agriculture Organization for 20 of the 22 countries listed in table 1 (all except Czechslovakia and Scotland) (32). A mean of three time periods – 1954-6, 1957-9 and 1960-2 – was calculated for each nutrient for each country. This was deliberately done, in accordance with the concept that long-term dietary pattern influences the occurrence of atherosclerotic disease.

As is evident from the data of table 9, statistically significant high order correlations are present between CHD mortality rates for men age 45-54 and several nutrients – total calories, total protein, sucrose, total fat, saturated fat, monounsaturated fat and cholesterol. As table 10 further shows, dichomotization of the 20 countries – using as the independent variable first dietary cholesterol and then saturated fat respectively – also reveals a positive relationship between each and CHD mortality rate for males age 45-54. With this split based on the mean for all 20 countries, the resultant two groups had significantly different average levels of nutrient intake and CHD mortality. The highest mortality ratio, 1.91, was obtained with saturated fat intake (expressed in grams per person per day) as the independent variable. These findings are generally consistent with those reported by three earlier post-World War II investigations (17, 33-35).

It is of course a truism of the scientific method that statistically significant correlations between variables do not necessarily indicate

Table 7. Mean daily apparent nutrient intake in grams – 20 countries, 1954-1962*

Country	Mean daily apparent nutrient intake									
	Calories	Protein g	Animal protein g	Carbohy-drate g	Sucrose g	Total fat g	Sat. fat g	Monoun-sat** Fat g	Poly. fat g	Choles-terol mg
Finland	3,092	96	55	423	102	114	55	44	12	400
U.S.A.	3,070	105	70	357	110	135	52	57	21	605
Scotland	—	No data available								
Venezuela⁴	2,087	62	24	344	89	52	18	17	15	143
France⁴	2,955	95	52	390	80	112	45	40	22	410
Austria	2,915	83	42	410	89	104	43	39	18	353
Australia	3,156	109	73	397	137	125	58	50	12	582
Belgium	2,957	87	47	378	80	123	49	46	23	495
Ireland	3,482	109	60	478	118	126	57	46	18	576
German Fed. Rep.	2,902	85	46	369	76	123	47	42	30	412
New Zealand	3,416	117	82	400	118	151	75	58	12	741
Canada	3,046	101	70	362	117	132	56	56	15	572
Czechoslovakia	No data available									
U.K. – Eng. & Wales	3,223	102	66	409	128	130	55	54	16	547
Japan	2,170	67	20	425	37	17	5	5	6	151
Italy	2,644	76	25	417	51	72	24	35	11	235
Switzerland	3,107	92	53	410	106	124	50	43	26	428
Denmark	3,359	99	60	402	126	152	59	57	31	495
Netherlands	2,861	73	41	367	111	123	47	41	30	331
Israel	2,803	81	34	428	75	81	27	35	17	328
Norway	2,964	84	53	358	103	131	50	59	20	355
Sweden	2,962	90	57	360	110	130	53	51	21	478
Mean	2,959	91	52	394	98	113	46	44	19	432
Std. Deviation	±350	±15	±18	±33	±26	±33	±16	±14	±7	±154

* Data calculated from Food Balance Sheets of the Food and Agriculture Organization; unless otherwise specified, data are the means for three time periods – 1954-6, 1957-9, 1960-2.

⁴ Mean of latter two time periods; no data available for 1954-6.

** Oleic acid.

Table 8. Mean daily apparent nutrient intake as per cent of total calories – 20 countries, 1954-62*

| Country | Calories | Protein | Mean daily apparent nutrient intake as per cent of total calories | | | | | | |
			Animal protein	Carbohydrate	Sucrose	Total fat	Sat. fat	Monoun-sat.	Poly. fat
Finland	3,092	12	7	55	13	33	16	13	4
U.S.A.	3,070	14	9	47	14	40	15	17	6
Scotland	No data available								
Venezuela	2,087	12	4	66	17	22	8	7	7
France	2,955	13	7	53	11	34	14	12	7
Austria	2,915	11	6	56	12	32	13	12	6
Australia	3,156	14	9	50	17	36	17	14	3
Belgium	2,957	12	6	51	11	37	15	14	7
Ireland	3,482	12	7	55	13	33	15	12	5
German Fed. Rep.	2,902	12	6	51	10	38	14	13	9
New Zealand	3,416	14	9	47	14	40	20	15	2
Canada	3,046	13	9	48	15	39	17	17	4
Czechoslovakia	No data available								
U.K. – Eng. & Wales	3,223	13	8	51	16	36	15	15	5
Japan	2,170	12	4	78	7	7	2	2	2
Italy	2,644	12	4	63	8	24	8	12	4
Switzerland	3,107	12	7	53	14	36	15	12	7
Denmark	3,359	12	7	48	15	41	16	15	8
Netherlands	2,861	10	5	51	16	39	15	13	9
Israel	2,803	12	5	61	11	26	9	11	5
Norway	2,964	11	7	48	14	40	15	18	6
Sweden	2,962	12	8	49	15	39	16	15	6
Mean	2,959	12.4	6.7	54.1	13.2	33.6	13.8	13.0	5.6
Std. Deviation	±350	±1.1	±1.7	±7.7	±2.8	±8.3	±4.1	±3.6	±2.0

* See footnotes of Table 7.

cause-and-effect relationships. As the foregoing quotation from the report of the International Atherosclerosis Project infers, it is essential to utilize the totality of data available from all methodologies – clinico-pathologic, animal-experimental, epidemiologic – in evaluating the meaning of these several statistically significant correlations between nutrient patterns and mortality rates. In such an assessment, it is illuminating to keep in mind the effect of economic development and increased per capita income on nutrition patterns. Traditionally, from the time man ceased to be a food gatherer and became a food producer (particularly, as in the majority of societies, a farmer rather than a herdsman), from ancient times right down to the present – and inevitably from an economic standpoint – inexpensive high-starch grains and tubers (breads, cereals, rice, potatoes, etc.) have constituted the 'staff of life', supplying 60 to 88 per cent of daily calories. The essence of the economics of this phenomenon is summarized in figures 8-11 (32).

In the poorest nations, with the lowest per capita national income

Table 9. Correlations of nutrients and mortality rates, 20 countries. males 45-54, 1964[A]

Nutrients	Mortality		
	All causes	CHD	CV
Calories, daily total	—.021	.570***	.437*
Protein, g daily	.206	.675***	.605***
Protein, % of calories	.397	.527**	.594***
Animal protein, g daily	.112	.650***	.512**
Animal protein, % of calories	.129	.604***	.481*
Carbohydrate, g daily	.087	.191	.325
Carbohydrate, % of calories	.086	—.429	—.204
Sucrose, g daily	—.026	.579***	.376
Sucrose, % of calories	—.046	.372	.161
Total fat, g daily	—.093	.463*	.255
Total fat, % of calories	—.111	.391	.156
Saturated fat, g daily	.046	.580***	.409
Saturated fat, % of calories	.045	.546***	.350
Monounsaturated fat, g daily	—.114	.518**	.302
Monounsaturated fat, % of calories	—.112	.470*	.238
Polyunsat. fat, g daily	—.336	—.213	—.369
Polyunsat. fat, % of calories	—.203	—.340	—.456*
Cholesterol, mg daily	.093	.617***	.517**

*p = .05   **p = .02   ***p = .01 or less

[A] As indicated in Tables 7 and 8, of the 22 countries listed in Table 1, no nutrient data were available for Czechoslovakia and Scotland.

Table 10. Relationship between national apparent nutrient intake and 1964 mortality rates for coronary heart disease, men age 45-54 – 20 countries

Nutrient	Mean level of nutrient intake		1964 Mean CHD mortality rate/100,000		Mortality ratio
	Countries below mean for all 20	Countries above mean for all 20	Countries above mean nutrient intake for all 20	Countries below mean nutrient intake for all 20	
Saturated fat – g/person/ day	54.5	27.0	242.8*	127.0**	1.91
Saturated fat – % of total calories	15.7	8.0	231.5ᴅ	137.6ᴅᴅ	1.68
Cholesterol – mg/person/ day	572.3	322.4	257.3+	167.8++	1.53

* Australia, Belgium, Canada, Denmark, Finland, German Fed. Rep., Ireland, Netherlands, New Zealand, Norway, Sweden, Switzerland, United Kingdom (Eng., Wales), U.S.A.
** Austria, France, Israel, Italy, Japan, Venezuela.
ᴅ Australia, Belgium, Canada, Denmark, Finland, France, German Fed. Rep., Ireland, Netherlands, New Zealand, Norway, Sweden, Switzerland, United Kingdom, U.S.A.
ᴅᴅ Austria, Israel, Italy, Japan, Venezuela.
+ Australia, Belgium, Canada, Denmark, Ireland, New Zealand, Sweden, United Kingdom, U.S.A.
++ Austria, Finland, France, German Fed. Rep., Israel, Italy, Japan, Netherlands, Norway, Switzerland, Venezuela.

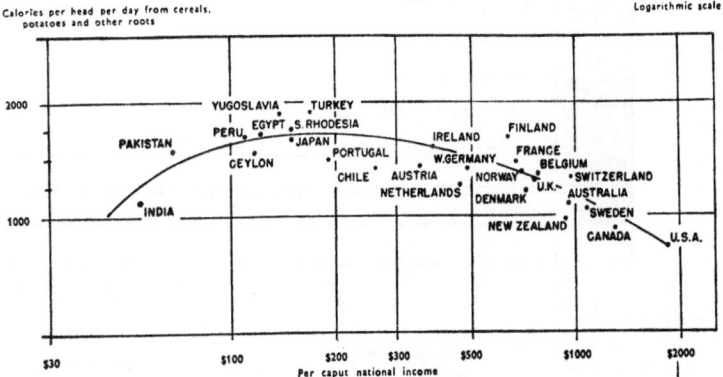

Fig. 8. Per capita consumption of cereals and roots in relation to per capita national income (32).

(e.g. India and Pakistan), cereals are the main staple, but they are in short supply, so that too little is available to assure a reasonable per capita calorie intake. Almost none can be spared for fodder for animals (fig. 10).

With slightly greater per capita national income, consumption of cereals tends to become greater, as exemplified by data for countries with per capita national incomes of $100-$200 per year (fig. 8). In

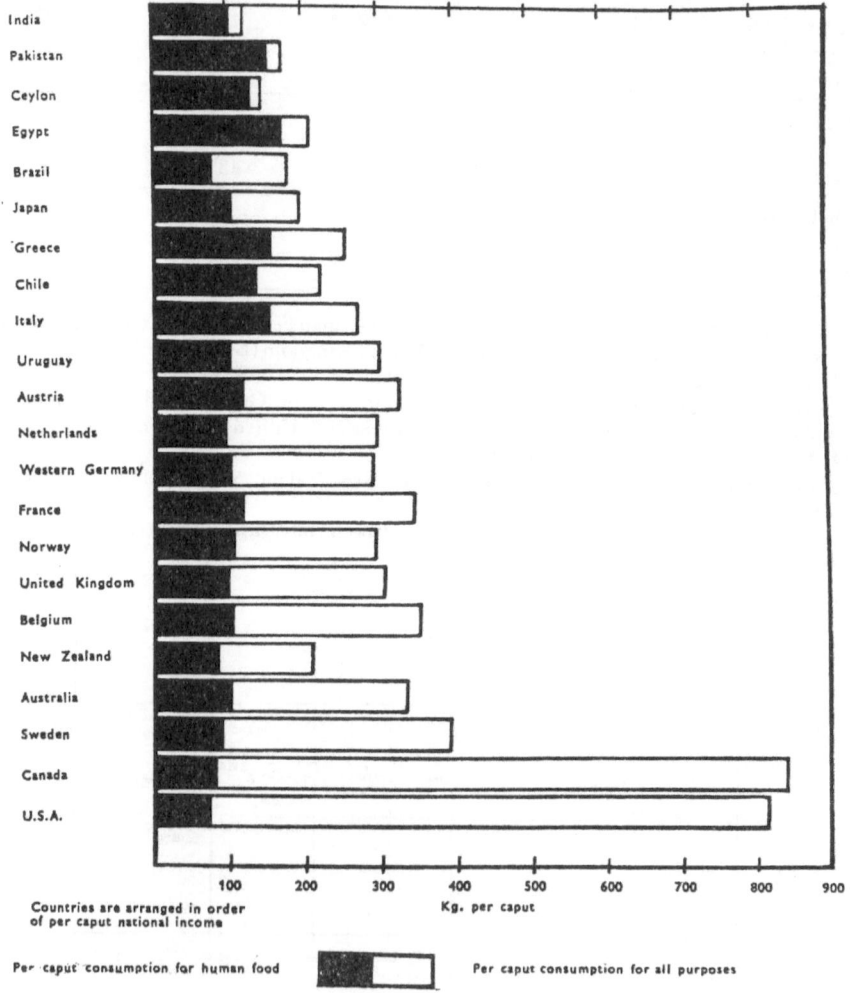

Fig. 9. Per capita supply of cereals for all purposes (including livestock feeding) and for direct human consumption (32).

addition, it becomes possible to make significant amounts of grain available for livestock feeding, i.e. for conversion of grain to meat and dairy products for human consumption (fig. 9). Among the developed countries, with high per capita national incomes, cereals cease to be the 'staff of life'. They no longer supply a majority of calories. For the most advanced countries intake of cereals is lower than in the poorest countries. For the United States, for example, apparent consumption of grain products – about 295 pounds per person per year in 1909 – has

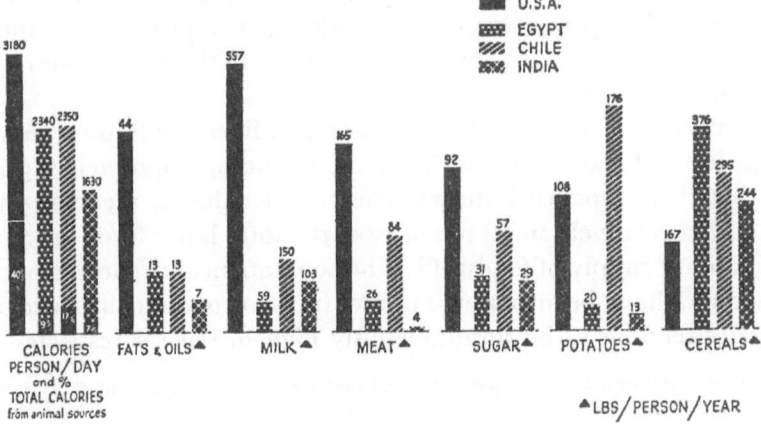

Fig. 10. Diet in more developed and less developed countries, 1950 (32).

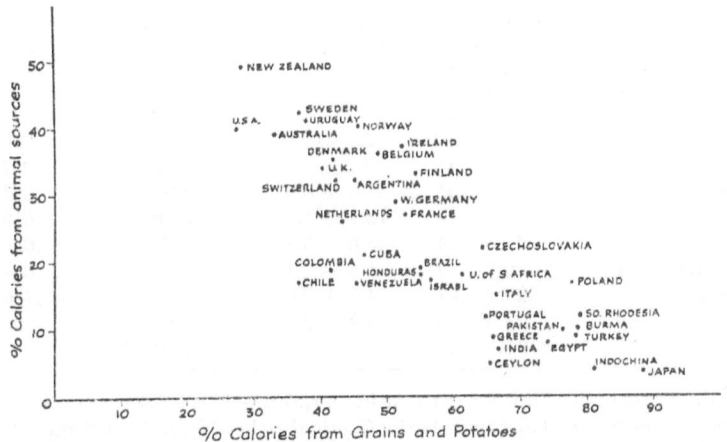

Fig. 11. Percent calories from animal sources and from grains and potatoes, in different countries (32).

been about 165 pounds in recent years. The corresponding figures for potatoes are about 202 pounds in 1909, about 103 pounds in recent years (17, 36, 37). While human consumption of cereals is low in these affluent countries, total supply for all purposes is high; a high proportion is utilized for livestock feeding. This is the phenomenon known to us in the United States as the 'corn-hog' economy. One of its important aspects is that grazing of livestock, particularly cattle, is supplemented by feeding of high-energy feeds in confined pens, to accomplish optimal fattening quickly and efficiently, prior to slaughter. The result is the highly 'marbled' prime and choice grade meats typically consumed in large quantities, especially by the populations of the United States and Canada.

This pattern of foodstuff consumption and livestock feeding requires a high level of economic development, including high-yield agriculture, based on modern industry, chemical fertilizers, mechanization, etc., with a relatively small minority of the total labor force producing an abundant supply of foodstuffs. The consequences of these economic phenomena have been patterns of diet in the economically developed countries tending to be simultaneously high in several respects – i.e.

Table 11. Relationship between per capita annual income[Δ] and apparent daily nutrient intake – Simple correlation coefficients – 19 countries

Nutrient	Mean and standard deviation[ΔΔ]		Coefficient of correlation with income	
	Nutrients in absolute units[ΔΔΔ]	Nutrients as % of calories	Nutrients in absolute units[ΔΔΔ]	Nutrients as % of calories
Total calories/day	2,931 ± 337	—	.626***	—
Total protein	90 ± 14	12.3 ± 1.0	.702***	.516**
Animal protein	52 ± 18	6.7 ± 1.7	.748***	.814
Total fat	112 ± 34	33.6 ± 8.6	.709***	.694***
Saturated fat	46 ± 16	13.7 ± 4.2	.663***	.658***
Oleic acid	44 ± 14	13.0 ± 3.7	.718***	.685***
Polyunsaturated fat	19 ± 7	5.6 ± 2.1	.317	.091
Carbohydrate	390 ± 27	54.0 ± 8.0	—.374	—.730***
Sucrose	97 ± 26	13.2 ± 2.9	.592***	.397
Cholesterol	424 ± 154	—	.753***	—

[Δ] Mean and standard deviation for 19 countries: $ 1,373. ± 503. Of 22 countries in Table 1, no data on both income and diet available for Czechoslovakia, No. Ireland, Scotland.
** P = .02.
*** P < .01.
ᵥ [ΔΔ] g/person/day, except for calories and cholesterol; cholesterol in mg/person/day.

total calories, total protein, animal protein, total fat, animal fat, saturated fat, cholesterol – in marked contrast to the situation in underdeveloped countries (tables 7, 8, 10-12).

Economic development and high per capita income also lead away
from a 'natural' subsistence economy, and to widespread availability
of money for purchase of foods in the open market. A further major
consequence of this is a high intake of sugar (tables 7, 8, 10-12), an
item available only by purchase in almost all countries, except for a
few major sugar producers (17, 18, 32, 38). Per capita sugar consumption in the United States, for example, has in recent decades fluctuated
around 100 pounds per person per year, whereas it was about 8 pounds
in 1820, 30 in 1860 (17).

In general, with few exceptions (see below), the masses in most underdeveloped countries, with low per capita incomes and subsistence
livelihoods from agriculture in 'natural' economies, consume sugar in

Table 12. Interrelationships among nutrients – Simple correlation coefficients – 20 countries

Nutrient pairs	Correlation coefficient	
	Absolute amount[4]	% of calories
Total calories, Total protein	.893***	.436*
Total calories, Animal protein	.815***	.757***
Total calories, Saturated fat	.918***	.851***
Total calories, Monounsaturated fat	.857***	.725***
Total calories, Sucrose	.733***	.341
Total calories, Cholesterol	.875***	—
Total calories, Polyunsaturated fat	.302	—.008
Total calories, Carbohydrate	.291	—.794***
Total protein, Saturated fat	.859***	.306
Total protein, Sucrose	.710***	.137
Total protein, Cholesterol	.950***	.675***
Total protein, Animal protein	.920***	.632***
Total protein, Polyunsaturated fat	—.003	—.503**
Total protein, Carbohydrate	.235	—.214
Saturated fat, Monounsaturated fat	.904***	.836***
Saturated fat, Cholesterol	.902***	.850***
Saturated fat, Sucrose	.823***	.596***
Saturated fat, Polyunsaturated fat	.322	.134
Saturated fat, Carbohydrate	—.039	—.944***

[4] g person/day for all nutrients except calories and cholesterol; mg/person/day for cholesterol.
*p slightly greater than .05.
**p < .02
***p < .01

modest amounts. In contrast, the populations of the developed countries, with relatively high per capita incomes and food supplies chiefly
purchased in the market, consume large quantities of sugar.

The foregoing basic economic facts serve to clarify the findings
summarized in table 9, particularly the significant correlations between several nutrients and mortality rates for premature CHD. Clearly,
circumstances of economic development make it inevitable that levels
of intake of several key nutrients are highly intercorrelated – particularly total calories, total protein, animal protein, total fat, animal fat,
saturated fat, cholesterol and sucrose. Since intakes of all of these tend
to increase with economic development and rise in per capita income,
it is to be anticipated that each and every one of these nutrients would
correlate with mortality rates for CHD – if these rates are in any basic
way related to per capita income and patterns of nutrition.

The question therefore becomes: Which, if any, of the statistical
correlations between levels of nutrient intake and CHD death rates
reflect cause-and-effect relationships? These data pose this question
but cannot answer it. The answer must be sought from other available
evidence.

As the foregoing quotation from the International Atherosclerosis
Project notes, extensive data indicate that the correlations between intakes of protein (total, animal) and CHD mortality rates do not indicate
cause-and-effect relationships. Extensive data are also available from
hundreds of studies, using a diversity of research methodologies
(clinico-pathologic, animal-experimental, epidemiologic) indicating
that the correlations between lipid intakes (saturated fat, cholesterol)
and mortality rates are indeed highly indicative of cause-and-effect
relationships. (As already noted, the vast amount of evidence on these
matters is summarized, reviewed and documented bibliographically
in references 16-18, 27 and 28.) It is valid at the present time to conclude that – at a high level of probability – a cause-and-effect relationship has been demonstrated between dietary lipid (specifically,
saturated fat and cholesterol) and widespread, premature CHD, even
though substantial direct proof from definitive, large-scale, longterm
mass field trials is still to be obtained. This conclusion is almost certainly valid since: data on the epidemiologic associations are available
from many sources, the associations persist when confounding variables
are taken into account, are strong and consistent (so-called 'exceptions' do not invalidate this estimate), are in harmony with findings

from other research methods (i.e., animal experimentation and clinico-pathologic investigation), are coherent in terms of reasonable pathogenetic mechanisms relating apparent causes and the disease (see below), and all alternative hypotheses purporting to account for the nutritional aspects of the etiology of premature atherosclerotic disease (e.g. the polyunsaturated fat deficiency and the high sucrose hypotheses) are invalidated by the totality of the data (17, 18, 27, 28, 38, 40, 41). This conclusion of course, does not mean that dietary lipid composition is the sole cause of the current epidemic of premature, severe atherosclerotic disease (see below). It does mean that habitual high intake of saturated fat and cholesterol is a key, primary, indispensable etiologic factor in the epidemic.

Evidence is also available indicating that the correlation between total calorie intake and CHD mortality rate (table 9) is meaningful, in a limited adjuvant fashion, in terms of cause-and-effect relationships (see below).

Recently, a few investigators have emphasized the positive correlation between sucrose intake and CHD mortality rate. Of course, insofar as sucrose ingestion may be a major factor accounting for level of total calorie intake, this particular foodstuff may be regarded as playing a role, non-specifically. However, the proponents of the sucrose hypothesis do not emphasize this aspect of the matter, but rather invoke for sucrose a major, primary and specific role in atherogenesis (42-44). This issue has been reviewed at length elsewhere, and its detailed examination is beyond the scope of this presentation (18, 38). Suffice it to note here that at least three major sets of evidence render the hypothesis untenable that sucrose is a prime and decisive factor influencing atherogenesis. The first is the failure of the International Atherosclerosis Project to find a significant correlation between sucrose intake and advanced atherosclerosis at autopsy (see quotation above and ref. 31).

The second set of data bringing the sugar hypothesis into question relates to the underdeveloped nations of the world, and the comparative findings on the major sugar producers, e.g., Columbia, Cuba, Venezuela. Their populations in the mass – in marked contrast to those of other underdeveloped countries, but like those of the developed countries – habitually consume large amounts of sugar. Like the masses in other underdeveloped countries, but unlike those in the developed countries, they habitually subsist on diets low in animal products (meats, dairy products). Therefore, while sugar intake is high, intakes of total calories, total fat, saturated fat and cholesterol are low. These three countries, therefore, resemble the United States and other developed countries in having high sugar intakes, e.g. 88 or more pounds per person per year (40 or more kg). But here the resemblance stops (cf. fig. 11). Thus, there is available to epidemiology an 'experiment of nature', or – more correctly – a socioeconomically induced set of differences in national nutrition patterns permitting a unique test of the sucrose hypothesis (cf. above for other such ready-made 'experiments', e.g. intra-national social class differences, changes with migration, effects of World Wars I and II, trends since World War II). If level of sugar intake is indeed a key factor in the etiology of the coronary epidemic, then the middle-aged populations of Colombia, Cuba and Venezuela should have high rates of premature CHD, as is indeed inferred by one set of papers presenting the sugar hypothesis (42, 43). Contrariwise, if sugar intake is relatively unimportant etiologically, and of minor significance compared with dietary saturated fat and cholesterol, then rates of CHD should be low. Although only limited data are available, none indicate the existence of an epidemic of premature CHD in the middle-aged populations of these countries (cf. fig. 1 and tables 1-4) (10, 21). The proponents of the sugar hypothesis have failed to address themselves to these data and their implications (44).

A third and even more telling critique of the sugar hypothesis arises from animal-experimental data (1, 16-18). It is indeed a cardinal fact of more than a half century of animal-experimental research that high sugar intake is totally incapable of inducing atherosclerotic lesions in the arteries of any animal species, in marked contrast to the positive results emanating from feeding of diets supplemented with fats and cholesterol. To the authors' knowledge, the proponents of the sugar hypothesis have also failed to acknowledge this fact, and its meaning for their view (44).

Finally, the sugar hypothesis has been promulgated based on the reported finding in one study that levels of dietary sucrose were higher in patients with occlusive atherosclerotic disease than in controls (43). The inadequacies of this report have been discussed previously (18, 43). It is now evident that other investigations have not substantiated the observation (45, 46). This then is still further reason to doubt the validity of the sugar hypothesis.

In summary, there is no substantial basis for the hypothesis that the statistical association between sucrose ingestion and CHD mortality rates (cf. table 9) reflects a cause-and-effect relationship, i.e. sucrose – in contrast to saturated fat and cholesterol – is not a key, essential, primary nutritional factor in the etiology of premature severe atherosclerotic disease. However, this does not mean that high levels of sucrose intake are without relationship to the current CHD epidemic in the developed countries. It remains possible that high sugar intake acts as a secondary contributing cause, e.g. via its role in contributing to chronic caloric imbalance. Unquestionably, chronic caloric excess and resultant obesity add significantly to risk of both hypertension and hyperlipidemia (particularly hypertriglyceridemia), and possibly to risk of maturity-onset diabetes as well (18, 41). Thus, insofar as high sucrose intake contributes to the development of obesity as a mass social phenomena in affluent countries, it may be significantly related to high prevalence rates of key coronary risk factors, and thereby may be a contributing cause of the current CHD epidemic. Moreover, in populations also ingesting diets high in saturated fat and cholesterol, high intake of sugar may be an adjuvant cause of hyperlipidemia even in the absence of caloric excess. Although evidence on this matter is scanty and contradictory, this possibility cannot be entirely ruled out at present (47, 48).

Based on these considerations, a possible minor role of high sugar ingestion as a presumptive secondary and contributory etiologic factor becomes reasonable at this time as a working hypothesis. However, it is reasonable only on this basis, within the context of a multifactor concept of etiology, and the recognition of the primary, essential and decisive role of dietary lipid (saturated fat and cholesterol) in the epidemic.

One of the most important research advances since World War II is the delineation of the chief probable *mechanism of the etiologic effect of dietary lipid on atherogenesis.* This has been the demonstration that populations differing in habitual intake of saturated fat and cholesterol also differ markedly in serum cholesterol-lipid-lipoprotein levels. To appreciate the significance of this contribution, it is worthwhile to turn to a classic of medicine, the great work by Peters and Van Slyke 'Quantitative Clinical Chemistry' (49). The second edition of this invaluable work draws the conclusion in virtually categoric terms that diet composition does not influence the serum cholesterol of man. At the time that monograph was written, in the middle 1940s, it was taken for granted that the rise in serum cholesterol recorded in populations of the developed countries was an inevitable and invariate physiologic response, completely endogenous in origin and not amenable to environmental influence. As is evident from Figure 12, this is not the case. The slope of serum cholesterol with age varies markedly among different populations, depending upon habitual diet and habitual serum cholesterol level. The differences among populations in this regard are not related to their different ethnic and racial backgrounds. This is clear from such comparisons as those of Neapolitan working men and bankers in Italy, and Neapolitans in Boston (fig. 12) (50, 51).

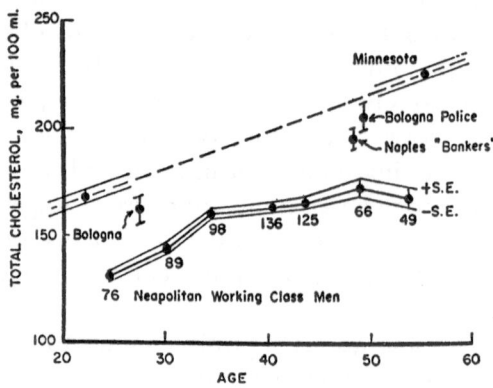

Fig. 12. Field studies in Italy, 1954 (50, 51).

This conclusion is based on many such research studies, another one of which is illustrated by figure 13 (52). For further documentation, the reader is referred to comprehensive monographs summarizing the findings and their sources (16-18, 27, 28).

The conclusions from the epidemiological data are fully supported by massive animal experimental evidence. And, by way of negative collaborative evidence, research on both animal and man indicates that other components of diet – e.g. protein, carbohydrate, sugar – are not capable of markedly influencing serum lipid levels of the population.

In summary, the two-way correlation indicated by the early research work, prior to World War II, has been broadened and extended to a three-way correlation – among habitual diet (particularly habitual saturated fat and cholesterol intake), levels of serum cholesterol – lipid-lipoprotein and occurrence rates of premature severe atherosclerotic coronary disease. The pathogenetic mechanism of the biologic action of the key environmental etiological agent – nutrition – has been delineated.

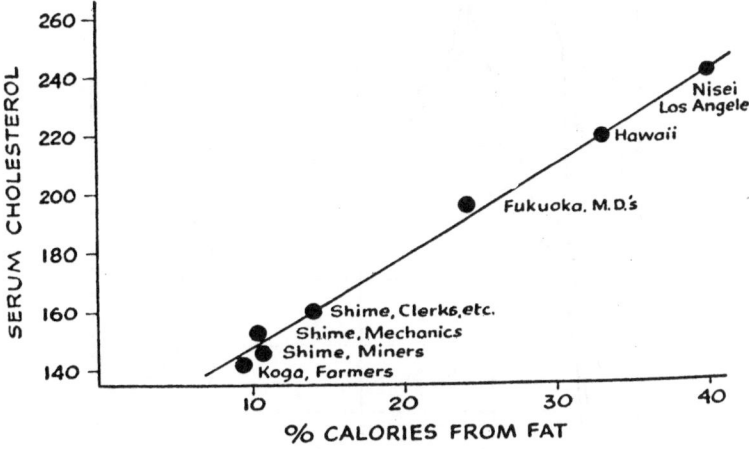

Fig. 13. Diet and cholesterolemia in 284 clinically healthy Japanese men age 40-49, in seven groups (52).

Aspects of mode of life related to socioeconomic development – cigarette smoking
Of course, it is generally known today that other aspects of Man's contemporary behavior in the developed countries interact synergistically with habitual diet in producing the current epidemic of premature atherosclerotic disease. Here it is appropriate to note that this habit of cigarette smoking is a relatively recent acquisition. Although tobacco has been widely used since introduced by Sir Walter Raleigh in the seventeenth century, mass cigarette consumption is a recent twentieth century phenomenon, dating from World War I. The data for the United States are typical in this regard (fig. 14) (53). A decisive prerequisite for mass adoption of cigarette smoking was a cheap package of a commercially produced cigarettes. This became possible with the development of machines for mass mechanized production of cigarettes, late in the nineteenth century. The circumstances of World War I and the immediate post-war period led to a wide spread shift of tobacco usage in this form, by men, and the adoption of the cigarette smoking habit by women.

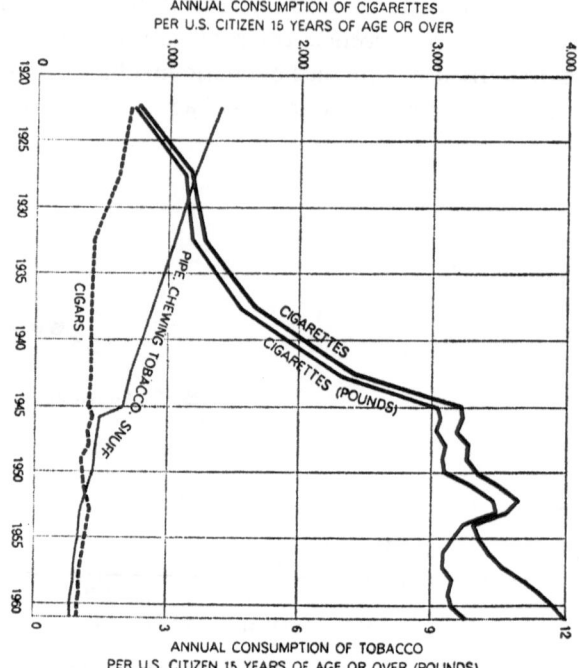

ANNUAL CONSUMPTION OF CIGARETTES
PER U.S. CITIZEN 15 YEARS OF AGE OR OVER

ANNUAL CONSUMPTION OF TOBACCO
PER U.S. CITIZEN 15 YEARS OF AGE OR OVER (POUNDS)

Fig. 14. Changes in tobacco use in the United States produced a five-fold rise in cigarette consumption between the early 1920's and 1961, and a drop of nearly 70 per cent of all other tobacco products (53).

Despite the relatively low cost of a package of cigarettes, it remains true that even for the developed countries, consumption of cigarettes is related to per capita income. Among the 22 developed countries under discussion throughout this paper, data on mean annual cigarette consumption were available for 17. The correlation coefficient between per capita income and cigarette consumption for these 17 countries is .507, with a p value < .05.

For these 17 countries, the correlation coefficient between annual cigarette consumption per capita and CHD mortality rate for men age 45-54 was .648 for the year 1964. For women, age 45-54, it was .782. The higher correlation coefficients for women, compared with men, merit attention, particularly since this is the only set of correlations differing between the sexes in this direction.

When the 17 countries were dichotomized into low and high groups, using the mean annual cigarette consumption per capita for all 17 as the cutting point, the two groups were found to differ markedly in mean average cigarette consumption and CHD mortality rate (table 13).

Further support for the conclusion that cigarette smoking is contributing significantly to the current coronary epidemic has recent been forthcoming from a study in the United States. This investigation demonstrated highly significant correlation between age-adjusted death rate for coronary heart disease and per capita consumption in 44 American states (fig. 15) (54). This relationship was further shown to be independent of degree of urbanization.

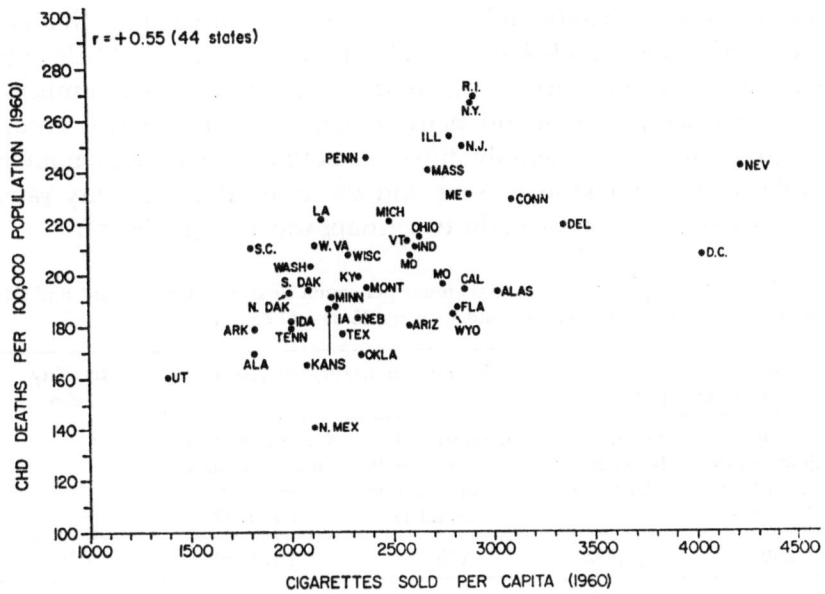

Fig. 15. Relationship between age-adjusted death rate for coronary heart disease and per capita cigarette consumption in 44 states in 1960 (54).

Aspects of mode-of-life related to socioeconomic development – physical inactivity – sedentary living habit
Considerable evidence (albeit contradictory to a degree) is available implicating habitual lack of exercise as another contributory cause of the epidemic of premature coronary disease. Status of populations in this regard is not readily assessed. In an effort to explore whether differences among countries in habitual physical activity may be

related to the differences among them in CHD mortality rates, several socioeconomic indices were examined, since they may be regarded as possibly reflecting sedentary living habits. These included number of motor vehicles, radios, television sets, telephones and newspapers per capita, proportion of the population urbanized, per capita energy consumption, et al. Simple correlation coefficients between these variables and CHD mortality rates for men age 45-64 in 1964 are presented in table 14. The statistically most significant correlation coefficient was between number of motor vehicles in use per thousand persons and CHD mortality rates. In contrast to earlier reports, no statistically significant correlation was observed between number of television sets per capita and CHD mortality. Based on these findings, the countries were divided into two groups, those above and below the mean for the 20 countries for which data were available on number of motor vehicles per thousand persons. Once again, the two groups were found to be considerably different, both for the average number of vehicles per thousand persons and the respective mortality rates. The mortality ratio between the two groups was 1.41 (table 15).

Table 13. Relationship between national annual per capita cigarette consumption* and 1964 mortality rates for coronary heart disease, men age 45-54 – 17 countries[4]

Mean annual cigarette consumption per capita		1964 CHD mortality rate/100,000		Mortality ratio
6 countries above mean for all 17[4]	11 countries below mean for all 17	Countries above mean cigarette consumption for all 17	Countries below mean cigarette consumption for all 17	
3,307	1,592	276.8**	184.6***	1.50

* Per Capita for all persons 15 years and over, 1961-63 data.
[4] No data available on cigarette consumption for Czechoslovakia, Ireland, Israel, Scotland, Venezuela. Mean for 17 countries is 2,200 annually, per capita.
** Australia, Canada, New Zealand, Switzerland, United Kingdom, U.S.A.
*** Austria, Belgium, Denmark, Finland, France, German Fed. Rep., Italy, Japan, Netherlands, Norway, Sweden.

Aspects of mode-of-life related to socioeconomic development – combined effect of several variables

When the indices discussed above are found together, the contrast between the extreme groups – i.e. those high on both variables vs. those lower on both – is generally more marked than when only one variable

Table 14. Correlations of indirect indices of sedentary living and mortality rates, 19 countries, males 45-54, 1964

Indices	CHD Mortality
Motor vehicles/1000 persons	.511*
Radios/100 persons	.419
TV sets/100 persons	.368
Telephones/100 persons	.371
Energy consumption – short tons, per capita	.440
Percent of population urban	.037
National income, per capita	.444

*p = .02

Table 15. Relationship between number of motor vehicles in use[4] and 1964 mortality rates for coronary heart disease, men age 45-54 – 20 countries

Mean no. of motor vehicles per 1,000 persons[4]		1964 CHD mortality rate/100,000		Mortality ratio
9 countries above mean for all 20	11 countries below mean for all 20	Countries above mean number of vehicles for all 20	Countries below mean number of vehicles for all 20	
285.0	112.2	247.8*	175.5**	1.41

* Australia, Canada, Denmark, France, Ireland, New Zealand, Sweden, United Kingdom, U.S.A.
** Austria, Belgium, Finland, German Fed. Rep., Israel, Italy, Japan, Netherlands, Norway, Switzerland, Venezuela.
[4] No data on moter vehicles available for Czechoslovakia or Scotland; mean for 20 countries is 190.0 vehicles in use per 1,000 persons.

is considered. Thus, when cigarette consumption was considered by itself, the CHD mortality ratio of the higher vs. lower groups was 1.50 (table 13). When apparent saturated fat consumption is the second variable, the mortality ratio for the extreme groups (both high vs. both low) is 2.196 (Table 16).

Similarly, the combined variables of motor vehicle use and saturated fat intake have a CHD mortality ratio for the 'both high vs. both lower' groups of 1.96 (table 17). The high vs. low comparison for motor vehicles alone yielded a mortality ratio of 1.41 (table 15).

Saturated fat intake as a single variable does show a mortality ratio between the high vs. lower groups as large as when other variables are added. However, the absolute CHD rate for groups with an additional

Table 16. Apparent intake of saturated fat, consumption of cigarettes and 1964 mortality rates for coronary heart disease, men 45-54 – 17 countries[Δ]

Apparent daily intake of saturated fat	CHD mortality rate per 100,000	
	Cigarette consumption above mean of 2,200	Cigarette consumption below mean of 2,200
Above mean of 48.4 g	278.5*	214.0**
Below mean of 48.4 g	—	126.8***

Mortality Ratio: 278.5/126.8 = 2.196
[Δ] Data were lacking for one or both variables for five countries – Czechoslovakia, Ireland, Israel, Scotland, Venezuela.
* Australia, Canada, New Zealand, Switzerland, United Kingdom, U.S.A.
** Belgium, Denmark, Finland, Norway, Sweden.
*** Austria, France, German Fed. Rep., Italy, Japan, Netherlands.

Table 17. Apparent intake of saturated fat, use of motor vehicles, and 1964 mortality rates for coronary heart disease, men 45-54 – 20 countries

Apparent daily intake of saturated Fat	CHD mortality rate per 100/1000	
	Motor vehicles in use above mean of 190 per 1,000 persons	Motor vehicles in use below mean of 190 per 1,000 persons
Above mean of 46.2 g*	269.5**	207.1***
Below mean of 46.2 g	74[Δ]	137.6[ΔΔ]

Ratio of both factors high to neither high (269.5/137.6) = 1.958
* Mean of 20 countries for which there is both dietary data and data on use of motor vehicles.
** Australia, Canada, Denmark, Ireland, New Zealand, Sweden, United Kingdom, U.S.A.
*** Belgium, Finland, German Fed., Rep., Netherlands, Norway, Switzerland.
[Δ] France.
[ΔΔ] Austria, Israel, Italy, Japan, Venezuela.

variable high is somewhat greater than for the group with saturated fat as the single high variable measured (278.5 per 100,000 when combined with cigarette consumption, 269.5 when together with motor vehicle use, 242.8 for saturated fat as the single variable) (tables 10, 16 and 17).

Table 18 describes the effect on CHD mortality rates of having none, 1, 2 or 3 of these variables high. While the rate does not increase step-wise, the contrast is marked between the group with all three high and that with none high (305.4/100,000 vs. 137.4, for a mortality ratio of 2.222).

Table 18. Saturated fat intake, cigarette consumption, motor vehicles in use, and 1964 CHD mortality rates, men 45-54 – 17 countries

Number of factors high*	Countries	CHD mortality/100,000
None	Austria, German Fed. Rep., Italy, Japan, Netherlands	137.4
1	Belgium, Denmark, Finland, France, Norway	236.8
2	Sweden, Switzerland	129.0
All 3	Australia, Canada, New Zealand, United Kingdom, U.S.A.	305.4

Mortality ratio for 3 factors above mean vs. 3 factors below mean = 2.222
* 'High' is defined as above the mean for all 17 countries:
 Mean apparent saturated fat intake – 48.4 g/day/person
 Mean per capita annual cigarette consumption – 2,200
 Mean number of motor vehicles in use – 204.3 per 1,000 persons

SUMMARY

The major methods of comparing impact of coronary heart disease on different populations yield similar findings. Regional differences are marked, whether the data examined are from international pathological studies, comparison of mortality rates or studies of living populations. The latter, for example, yield differences in prevalence of coronary heart disease as great as 40 times when comparing rates for East Finland and Dalmatia.

In certain areas of the world, essentially the more economically developed countries, premature coronary heart disease is already a major epidemic. Time trend studies indicate both an increase in CHD in these countries and beginning of change in less developed countries that are on the road to greater economic development.

If CHD mortality rates in countries with the highest rates (such as the U.S.A., Finland, United Kingdom) could be reduced to those prevailing in the countries not afflicted with this epidemic, the saving in human life would be enormous. Therefore, understanding the causes of the differential in CHD prevalence and mortality is critically important to these countries. Moreover, if the less developed countries are to avoid the increase in deaths from coronary heart disease that thus far has always accompanied economic growth, pinpointing causes is equally important to them.

Racial, ethnic, geographic or climatic factors as possible causes can be eliminated by data coming from time trend studies, migration statistics on prevalence and mortality, as well as study of class differences in CHD rates within single countries.

The high order correlation between CHD mortality and national income provides an important etiologic clue. While higher income itself cannot explain the higher mortality, it is, at least until now, accompanied by a mode of life whose characteristics can be etiologically connected to excess CHD mortality.

Chief among these characteristics are a nutrition pattern high in total calories, total fat, saturated fat and dietary cholesterol. In addition, heavy cigarette smoking and sedentary living habits are important features of this mode-of-life.

The international comparative data pinpoint intake of saturated fat as the major dietary factor accounting for differences in CHD mortality among the 22 countries surveyed. Although other nutrients are often found in association with high saturated fat intake (protein, sucrose) the data do not justify attributing an independent causal role to them.

When such factors as atherogenic dietary patterns, cigarette smoking and sedentary living habits are present together, CHD mortality rates are increased even further.

Knowledge shed by such international comparisons dealing with the etiology of coronary heart disease could help lower the coronary and overall mortality to the lower level still prevalent in the less developed countries. If applied, it could also prevent this epidemic from becoming an inevitable concomitant of the economic development taking place in the countries who have thus far escaped the epidemic.

ACKNOWLEDGEMENTS

It is a pleasure to acknowledge the cooperation and support of Eric Oldberg, M. D., President, Chicago Board of Health and Chairman, Chicago Health Research Foundation. It is also gratifying to pay tribute to my colleagues for their help with the nutrition work –

particularly Louise Mojonnier, Ph. D., and Dorothy Moss, M. S.

The research of our group presented in this paper was made possible by grants from the American Heart Association, Chicago Heart Association, Corn Products Institute of Nutrition, National Dairy Council, National Heart Institute, National Institutes of Health, United States Public Health Service (HE 04197 and HE 09426) and Wesson Fund for Medical Research.

REFERENCES

1. Cowdry, E. V., Ed., *Arteriosclerosis*, Macmillan Company, New York, NY, (1933).
2. Sydenstricker, E., Statistical Study of Arteriosclerosis, in Cowdry, E.V., Ed., *Arteriosclerosis*, Macmillan Company, New York, NY, 131 (1933).
3. Stocks, P., Race and Climate as Possible Factors, in Cowdry, E.V., Ed., *Arteriosclerosis*, Macmillan Company, New York, NY, 195 (1933).
4. Weiss, S. and G. R. Minot, Nutrition in Relation to Arteriosclerosis, in Cowdry, E.V., Ed., *Arteriosclerosis*, Macmillan Company, New York, NY, 233 (1933).
5. Rosenthal, S. R., Studies in Atherosclerosis: Chemical, Experimental and Morphologic. *Arch. Path.*, 18, 473, 660 and 827 (1934).
6. Raab, W., Diet, Hormones and Arteriosclerosis – *Data and References from the Older European and Oriental Literature*. Assembled and Published by the Author.
7. de Langen, C. D., [Arteriosclerosis and Lipid Metabolism.] *Nederl. Tijdschr. Geneesk.*, 92, 1811 (1948).
8. Sitsen, A. E. [About the Influence of Race in Pathology.] *Virchow's Archiv.*, 245, 281 (1923).
9. Wenckebach, K. F., Personal Communication to Dr. W. Raab; see ref. 23 of bibliography in ref. 6 above.
10. McGill, H. C., Jr., Ed., *Geographic Pathology of Atherosclerosis*, William and Wilkins, Baltimore, Md., 1968.
11. Katz, L. N., J. Stamler, and R. Pick, *Nutrition and Atherosclerosis*, Lea and Febiger, Philadelphia, Pa., 45, 1958. (cf. also references 290-292, 294-300 of bibliography of this monograph.)
12. Proudfit, W. L., E. K. Shirey, W. C. Sheldon and F. M. Sones Jr., Certain Clinical Characteristics Correlated with Extent of Obstructive Lesions Demonstrated by Selective Cine-Coronary Arteriography. *Circulation*, 38, 947 (1968).
13. Kimura, N. Analysis of 10,000 Postmortem Examinations in Japan, in: Keys, A. and P. D. White, Eds., *World Trends in Cardiology*, I. Cardiovascular Epidemiology, Hoeber-Harper, New York, NY, 159,(1956).
14. White, N. K., J. E. Edwards and T. J. Dry, The Relationship of the Degree of Coronary Atherosclerosis with Age, in: *Men. Circulation*, 1,645 (1950).
15. Reproduced from: Katz, L. N., J. Stamler, and R. Pick, *Nutrition and Atherosclerosis*, Lea and Febiger, Philadelphia, Pa., 26 (1958).
16. Katz, L. N. and J. Stamler, *Experimental Atherosclerosis*, Charles C. Thomas, Springfield, Ill., (1953).
17. Katz, L. N., J. Stamler and R. Pick, *Nutrition and Atherosclerosis*, Lea and Febiger, Philadelphia, Pa., (1958).
18. Stamler, J. *Lectures on Preventive Cardiology*, Grune and Stratton, New York, NY, (1967).
19. Epstein, F. H., Coronary Heart Disease at Younger Ages: Epidemiology. *Proceedings*

of the V World Congress of Cardiology, Oct. 30 – Nov. 5, 1966, Acta Cardiologica, Brussels, Belgium, 345 (1966).

20. Epstein, F. H. and D. E. Krueger, The Changing Incidence of Coronary Heart Disease, in: Morgan Jones, A., Ed., *Modern Trends in Cardiology* 2, Butterworths, London, 17 (1969).

21. Mortality Statistics, Cardiovascular Diseases, Annual Statistics 1955-1964 by Sex and Age. *Epidemiological and Vital Statistics Report*, World Health Organization, 20, 539 (1967).

22. *Programme Review, Cardiovascular Diseases*, Prepared for the Executive Board, World Health Organization, Geneva, Switzerland, January 1969.

23. Moriyama, I. M., J. Stamler, and D. E. Krueger, *The Major Cardiovascular Diseases – An Epidemiologic Analysis*, American Public Health Association, New York, NY, in press.

24. Executive Board, World Health Organization. *Mankind's Greatest Epidemic: Heart Disease*. Resolution and Press Release, Division of Public Information, World Health Organization, Geneva, Switzerland, Feb. 1969.

25. U.S. Bureau of the Census. *Statistical Abstract of the United States, 1963*. (84th edition). Washington, DC, 61 (1963).

26. *Vital Statistics of the United States, 1967*, Vol. II, Section 5, Life Tables. U.S. Department of Health, Education, and Welfare Public Health Service, Washington, DC, (1969).

27. Keys, A., The Role of the Diet in Human Atherosclerosis and Its Complications, in: Sandler, M. and G. H. Bourne, Eds., *Atherosclerosis and Its Origin*, Academic Press, New York NY, 263 (1963).

28. Keys, A. Dietary Factors in Arteriosclerosis, in: Blumenthal, H. T., Ed., *Cowdry's Arteriosclerosis*, Charles C. Thomas, Springfield, Ill., 675 (1967).

29. Keys, A., C. Aravanis, H. W. Blackburn, F. S. P. van Buchem, R. Buzina, B. S. Djordjevic, A. S. Dontas, F. Fidanza, M. J. Karvonen, N. Kimura, D. Lekos, M. Monti, V. Puddu and H. L. Taylor, Epidemiological Studies Related to Coronary Heart Disease: Characteristics of Men Aged 40-59 in Seven Countries. *Acta Med. Scand*, Suppl. 460 (1966).

30. Keys, A., H. L. Taylor, and H. Blackburn, *Coronary Heart Disease-Five-Year Incidence in 12,000 Men Aged 40-59 in Seven Countries*. Paper presented at the Conference on Cardiovascular Disease Epidemiology, Council on Epidemiology, American Heart Association, March 3-4, 1969, New Orleans, La.

31. Scrimshaw, N. S. and M. A. Guzman, Diet and Atherosclerosis, in: H. C. McGill, Jr., *Geographic Pathology of Atherosclerosis*, Williams and Wilkins, Baltimore, Md., 168 (1968).

32. Food and Agriculture Organization of the United Nations. *Food Balance Sheets: 1954-56*, Rome, (1958); 1957-59, Rome, (1963); 1960-62, Rome, (1966).

33. Yerushalmy, J. and H. E. Hilleboe, Fat in the Diet and Mortality from Heart Disease – A Methodological Note. *New York State J. Med.*, 57, 2343 (1957).

34. Jolliffe, N. and M. Archer, Statistical Associations between International Coronary Heart Disease Death Rates and Certain Environmental Factors. *J. Chronic Dis.*, 9, 636 (1959).

35. Connor, W. E., Dietary Cholesterol and the Pathogenesis of Atherosclerosis. *Geriatrics*, 16, 407 (1961).

36. US Bureau of the Census. *Historical Statistics of the United States, Colonial Times to 1957*, Washington, D. C., (1960).

37. U.S. Bureau of the Census. *Statistical Abstract of the United States. 1966*. (87th edition), Washington, D. C., 86 (1966).

38. Stamler, J. Nutrition, Metabolism and Atherosclerosis – A Review of the Data and Theories, and a Discussion of Controversial Questions, in: Ingelfinger, F. J., Relman A. S. and M. Finland, Eds., *Controversy in Internal Medicine*, W. B. Saunders Co., Philadelphia, Pa., 27, 1966.

39. Katz, L. N., J. Stamler, and R. Pick, *Nutrition and Atherosclerosis*, Lea and Febiger, Philadelphia, Pa., 33 (1958).
40. Stamler, J., F. H. Epstein, J. G. Green, and A. Keys, *Mass Field Trials on the Prevention of Coronary Heart Disease*. Perspectives and Tasks. Report of an International Working Meeting, Makarska, Yugoslavia, September 19-24, 1968. Privately printed, Chicago, Ill., (1969).
41. Stamler, J., L. Mojonnier, Y. Hall, D. M. Berkson, H. A. Lindberg, D. B. Cohen, J. J. Frankel, M. B. Epstein, R. Stamler, R. B. Shekelle and R. Soyugenc, Prevention of Atherosclerotic Coronary Heart Disease by Change of Diet and Mode of Life. *Boerhaave Course on Ischaemic Heart Disease*, 1969, Leiden, the Netherlands, in press.
42. Yudkin, J. Dietary Fat and Dietary Sugar in Relation to Ischaemic Heart Disease and Diabetes. *Lancet*, 2, 4 (1964).
43. Yudkin, J. and J. Roddy, Levels of Dietary Sucrose in Patients with Occlusive Atherosclerotic Disease. *Lancet*, 2, 6 (1964).
44. Yudkin, J., Sucrose and Heart Disease. *Nutrition Today*, 4, 16 (Spring 1969).
45. Papp, O. A., L. Padilla and A. L. Johnson, Dietary Intake in Patients with and without Myocardial Infarction. *Lancet*, 2, 259 (1965).
46. Paul, O., A. MacMillan, H. McKean and H. Park, Sucrose Intake and Coronary Heart-Disease. *Lancet*, 2, 1049 (1968).
47. McGandy, R. B., D. M. Hegsted and F. J. Stare, Dietary Fats, Carbohydrates and Atherosclerotic Vascular Disease. *New Engl. J. Med.*, 277, 186 and 242 (1967).
48. Little, A. Personal Communication.
49. Peters, J. P. and D. D. Van Slyke, *Quantitative Clinical Chemistry – Interpretations*, Vol. 1, 2nd edition, Williams and Wilkins, Baltimore, Md., (1946).
50. Keys, A. Field Studies in Italy, 1954, in: Keys, A. and P. D. White, Eds., *Cardiovascular Epidemiology*, Hoeber-Harper, New York, NY, 1956.
51. Miller, D. C., M. F. Trulson, M. B. McCann, P. D. White and F. J. Stare, Diet, Blood Lipids and Health of Italian Men in Boston. *Ann. Intern. Med.*, 49, 1178 (1958).
52. Keys, A. Diet and Epidemiology of Coronary Heart Disease. *J.A.M.A.*, 164, 1912 (1957).
53. Hammond, E. C. The effects of Smoking. *Scientific Amer.*, 207, 3 (July 1962).
54. Friedman, G. D. Cigarette Smoking and Geographic Variation in Coronary Heart Disease Mortality in the United States. *J. Chronic Dis.*, 20, 770 (1967).

PANEL DISCUSSION ON EPIDEMIOLOGICAL APPROACH

MODERATOR: J. STAMLER

The first question to be put before this panel is related to the often repeated statement: that we are having an epidemic of coronary disease. Classically, the term epidemic has been used in speaking about outbreaks of infectious diseases – e.g., cholera, plague, smallpox, etc. Is it correct to talk about the current situation with regard to coronary disease as an epidemic?

Joossens: We think that one can speak about an epidemic if one is dealing with middle aged males in western countries. Signs of an epidemic disappear if you consider the middle aged females in the same countries. In the Netherlands, as professor De Haas has shown, the incidence of premature deaths is rising in males and falling in females. The same is true in England for cardiovascular mortality at the age of 50; it is rising in males and falling in females. This is also seen in Belgium. Wherever you compare the mortality of cardiovascular disease in males and females, you find that the sex ratios at a given age are increasing over a period of time.

Stamler: It may be helpful to remind ourselves of the Greek roots of the word *epidemic: demos – people* and *epi – above or among*. This literal sense of the word makes it appropriate for use to indicate any disease – infectious or non-infectious – common in the population. This meaning emphasizes the concept of widespread major disease afflicting a population. I think this was first used in that sense for coronary disease by Paul White. It seems to me to be very appropriate, especially in regard to the onslaught among young and middle-aged adults, as well as the elderly. I am pleased that the WHO Executive Board Statement last January used the term. It serves as a clarion call to action, especially prevention.

I would like to go back to the questions Dr. Joossens just raised –

touched on very little here thus far – relating to the sex differential. What lies behind it? What are the factors that account for it? As Dr. De Haas has pointed, it is unlikely that diets of men and women differ markedly in the developed countries. Does any one wish to discuss these questions, firstly the basis for the difference in rates, and secondly the basis for the continuing divergence of trend of CHD rates for males and females?

Kannel: I shall discuss this question because we at Framingham have undertaken one of the few studies which has provided longitudinal data on population that includes women. We did this because we recognized that the sex difference was one of the major factors in this disease, about as strong as any of the others. It has been noted in some of the international comparisons that in countries with a low incidence the sex ratio does not appear to be as striking as in countries with a high incidence. This suggests that in countries with a high incidence there is a male predominance which is attributable to an excess of the disease occurring in the males particularly, with the females exhibiting a relative immunity to whatever is going on. We have examined every factor that we could study and thus far we cannot explain this difference between men and women. The gap in incidence does decrease with advancing age and it appears that the immunity seen in the pre-menopausal state is lost after the menopause in women.

Groen: If one considers the differences between men and women, one can think, of course, about genetic differences in the x and y chromosomes or about hormonal differences. We should not forget to consider differences in the psycho-social worlds in which they live. The responsibilities which go with many professions and with being the provider for the home are different for the two sexes. The prescribed ways of conduct and behaviour, the codes of morals and honour are different and thereby interhuman conflicts and their ways of reacting to them. There is another major factor in western countries, namely, that one of the two sexes has recently been emancipated. The position of the woman in the western home has been on the rise while that of the male has at best remained stationary. The average western male now has sometimes conflicts that he has to cope within his family life which he did not have previously and which do not or hardly occur in so-called eastern or primitive societies.

Stamler: Stress may be in the eyes of the beholder. If we ask women, they would probably tell us that they are more stressed than men.

Joossens: The sex differential is the major factor in the epidemiology of coronary heart disease. It is up to now unexplainable as Dr. Kannel has remarked. I cannot support Dr. Groen's view. No one knows if stress is more severe in women or in men.

Stamler: There are some aspects of our knowledge that have not yet been discussed: When a population lives under socioeconomic conditions that do not lead to frequent coronary disease in middle age, little or no sex differential is present. Japan is the epitome of this situation. To me, the general inference from this – and it has the weakness of being too general – is that it requires appropriate environmental stimuli to bring out the relative susceptibility and resistance respectively of the sexes. A further, corollary conclusion is that the sex differential does not contradict the theory that the main cause of the epidemic is environmental.

Data from my earlier experience in the animal laboratory are illuminating in this regard: Neither mature hens nor roosters spontaneously develop coronary atherosclerosis. When fed an atherogenic diet containing cholesterol and fat, only the roosters develop the disease. This environmental causative agent, diet, elicits different responses in the two different biological organisms, the male and female chicken. There is a large body of evidence implicating one endogenous difference in particular – a hormone difference, i.e. normal estrogen secretion protects women premenopausally, even as it protects hens. There are data to support that from animals and from humans – e.g., data on women castrated in their 20's or 30's who become susceptible; data of the reverse sort on men castrated prior to puberty, i.e. eunuchs, whose blood lipid patterns are similar to those of women and are (according to very limited data) relatively resistant to atherosclerotic disease; etc. This is the background of the effort to assess the value of treating men with estrogen after a coronary attack, and of giving women (especially high risk women) estrogens for years and not allowing them to become hormonally postmenopausal. We do not know at present whether this is good, bad or neutral. The data on the 'pill' would suggest that there may be dangers for women, and other data suggest that there may be dangers in giving estrogens to both men and women. Hopefully the large-scale efforts of the Coronary Drug Project in the USA – involving 8,341 middle-aged men with previous MI – will clarify this matter. One other facet of this problem also merits emphasis: Very recently, and only very recently in a few countries, women have begun to achieve equality in the 'right' to smoke cigarettes. As I noted in my formal paper, this is probably very important for contemporary coronary disease in the developed countries. If this phenomenon persists, together with current dietary habits, etc., the downward trend for women may be reversed.

Joossens: I have recently presented some work linking the sex chromosomes to growth properties. Sex chromosomes are known to induce growth spurts in young persons. There is a large difference between the sexes in the levels of uric acid, hematocrit, creatinine, blood pressure and cholesterol. In males, the early growth is very rapid, while in female it is the late growth that is very rapid.

The same can be said for cardiovascular mortality. In the Netherlands considering the total cardiovascular mortality, the earlier rise is more pronounced in males than in females and the late rise is more pronounced in females than in males. The same thing can be said for Finland and Sweden.

Stamler: Dr. Hudson, we have become increasingly interested in the United States recently in the problem of apparently 'classical' symptoms of angina pectoris in some persons who lack evidence of coronary disease on angiography. While most cases correlate, there is sometimes a contradiction. Among other things, this has raised the question of small vessel disease in the coronary arteries. Would you care to comment at all on this aspect of our knowledge of coronary disease?

Hudson: This question of small coronary artery disease causing heart pain and so on has not been solved satisfactorily. I have not observed narrowing of the intramural branches of the coronary arteries in atheromatous ischaemic heart disease. This disease, in my experience, has always been in the large epicardial arteries.

Stamler: How about the disease in diabetics and hypertensives?

Hudson: Even in those, we do not see it. We do see, of course, some arteriosclerosis in these cases, but we do not see atheroma of the intramural arteries. There are, however, a few diseases like Friedreich's Ataxia, which Thomas James, now in Birmingham, has explored, where there seems to be widespread small coronary artery disease.

Stamler: That is important. You mentioned in your presentation this morning – and this is a big problem for us in epidemiology – that you are frequently presented with cases of sudden death and can do no better in terms of signs than anyone else in making a diagnosis. How would you help the epidemiologist in determining in such a circumstance whether the cause of death is coronary disease or not?

Hudson: In my experience, if a person has coronary artery disease and is found dead, then we are entitled to assume that this coronary disease has caused some focus of electrical instability in the heart leading to ventricular fibrillation and sudden death.

Stamler: Dr. Hellerstein, you seem to have a different opinion here. Would you care to make a few comments on this question?

Hellerstein: I was once a pathologist and for this reason I want to take issue here. I think that many pathologists have misled us in the past and have continued to do so. It is often an error to make a 'post hoc' type of reasoning. In Israel, Dr. Brunner and his associates, for example, studied the hearts of a group of people who met with accidental death. Many had significant coronary disease. However, there was a poor correlation between the prevalence of atherosclerosis and the clinical symptomatology. How easily their death could have been attributed to coronary disease, erroneously. I have challenged over and over again our pathologist about 'post hoc' ergo 'propter hoc' reasoning. In many instances, there has been a bullet in the head or some other lethal lesion, which if undetected, death would be erroneously ascribed to coincident 'innocent' atherosclerosis. At any given moment, many of us here, if subjected to coronary arteriography, would find that we have significant lesions because we are so highly coronary prone. The real mystery is not why we die from coronary disease but why we do not die from it.

Stamler: Dr. Hellerstein, are you not avoiding the question?! You are criticising the pathologists, but you are not saying what you would infer about these deaths. Most of them, after all, do not have a bullet in their head, even in the United States and even in Chicago!

Hellerstein: I think that it is too pat to say that death is due to coronary disease, merely because it is present.

Hudson: We can only go on the evidence, sir. People have been in consulting rooms and have been connected to electrocardiographs, being examined for ischaemic pain. The cardiologist has observed the onset of ventricular fibrillation, he has asked the patient how he is and he responds, 'I'm doing all right', yet within two minutes the patient is quite dead. There has been no sudden attack of pain or anything, but we know that they had ischaemic heart disease and a history of angina pectoris. At necropsy, all you may find in these people is severe or relatively severe coronary artery disease.

Stamler: This is a crucial question in the evaluation of all epidemiological data on coronary disease and on sudden death attributed to coronary disease.

Kannel: I suspect that a sudden death in one part of the world may not be the same thing as a sudden death in another part of the world. For example, haematuria here in Leiden is probably stone infection or tumor while in Egypt schistomosiasis would be the number one suspect. It is very possible that a sudden death in the Congo is due to myocardial endofibroelastosis. In Framingham we do not have much fibroelastosis. All I can say is that when something looks like a goat it may not be a goat, but if it begins to smell like a goat, taste like a goat and sounds like a goat you better start thinking in terms of a goat! Now, if you look at sudden deaths as they occur in the general community, you find, like in angina or myocardial infarction, that there is a marked male predominance. Looks like a goat! What kind of people develop sudden deaths? They have an excess of hypertension, of cholesterol, they are heavy cigarette smokers, they have a lot of antecedant ECG abnormalities, an excess of diabetics, obesity and they are sedentary people. Sounds like a goat! The point I am trying to make is that people with overt coronary disease and the coronary pnosie develop sudden death at a much higher rate than the general population, and we have no other explanation for the health of them.

Stamler: I agree with Dr. Kannel on this matter, and can cite a paper from the Tecumseh study in support. It will be published soon in *Circulation*. The most conspicuous fact on approximately the first 60 sudden deaths is that about 90% were previously stigmatized.

I will show a slide tomorrow of data from our Peoples Gas Company study in Chicago. I am still rather hesitant to show it because the figures are too good. In the men free of CHD at the beginning of the study, with serum cholesterol levels under 250 mg %, diastolic blood pressures under 90 mm Hg and not smoking cigarettes, there has not been one sudden death in the first ten years of the study – in marked contrast to the rates of sudden death for those with risk factors and ECG abnormalities. The pathologist, too, must use judgement. I agree with Dr. Hudson's approach to the judgement for cases seen in the developed countries. Everything in our experience in the United States indicates that in the adult population, the sudden deaths are indeed overwhelmingly coronary deaths.

Hudson: One additional point is that people with a bullet in the head may also show extensive myocardial lesions. This has not been sufficiently emphasized to those who are anxious to transplant the heart from persons who are dying of head injuries.

Stamler: This is a very important point. I have been told of a experience in the United States already, where the transplanted heart was a dying heart – dying of an unrecognized myocardial infarction.

De Haas: I would like to ask Dr. Morrison how many people had a history of angina pectoris or myocardial infarction in his series of sudden deaths? It is my recollection that it was the majority of cases.

Morrison: That is perfectly correct. I cannot give you the exact figures off-hand, but they were very much in the majority. As I have explained before, our sudden death data is poor because of the lack of autopsy data. At least, at an autopsy you can find another cause of death.

Stamler: We just analyzed that in our Gas Company study. We evaluated all sudden deaths over the first ten years, distinguishing between those with disease or without disease in the beginning and prior to death. Overall, 49% of our coronary deaths were sudden. Of the sudden deaths, approximately 50% were sudden and 'expected', in the sense that there was evidence of previous sickness, evidence of a previous acute infarct, major ECG abnormality. The other half of the sudden deaths were sudden and unexpected, in the sense that there was no previous evidence of heart disease. There were – as already noted – risk factors present, high cholesterol, etc. This is very important because the future victims of sudden and unexpected death are completely at the mercy of the disease as long as medical care is confined to treatment for those who are already clinically ill with cardiovascular disease. One quarter of the total deaths are sudden and and unexpected and they cannot be approached unless we develop treatment before illness. I think that Dr. Kannel's data are very similar in that regard.

Kannel: Ours are even blacker than that, 65% of all deaths from an initial coronary attack were sudden and unexpected.

Stamler: Dr. Morrison, could you discuss your statement: 'We should elaborate on the inability to save lives with ambulatory intensive care units.' It is a big issue in the United States as to whether every city should follow the Belfast road or not. There are sharp disagreements among us on this. I'm sure that this point is also troubling people here.

Morrison: There is not very much more that I can really say here. Dr. Oliver will present some detailed figures on Saturday on this point. The main point that we found from our study is the importance of the delay before seeking medical aid. The whole business of specially equipped ambulances, etc., begins at the moment that the patient realizes he needs aid. If there is a long delay, then, of course, it is during this period that the highest mortality occurs. On the other hand, if you try to get people to send for aid more quickly, you get into the area of dyspepsia and so on, and where are you going to stop? If people with any kind of chest pain can send for a special ambulance, I don't quite know where we would be. I believe that this is the case in Moscow, that the patient can send directly for this ambulance. I've never quite understood how they are able to cope with the load unless the Russians are very good selfdiagnosticians. We found only a relatively small number of people who might have been saved. In order to provide this service, one would need an enormous amount of resources. As far as we can see at this stage, it is simply not economic.

Stamler: Could you give us, Dr. Morrison, any information on the Edinburgh experience on the relative value of treatment in the Intensive Care Unit versus routine hospital treatment for myocardial infarction. How much do you think that the Intensive Care Units are accomplishing in terms of acute saving of life, and what evidence is there that those saved have any reasonable prognosis thereafter?

Morrison: I would not like to do this at this stage. This is the reason why we tried to get some rough measure of clinical severity at the earliest point. Of course, as soon as you establish a unit of this kind, the kind of people coming into the hospital and the stage at which they come probably alters. Any straightforward comparison of mortality before and after the installation of the unit in the hospital, or in other wards at the same time is fraught with all kinds of difficulties. There are many possible snags in a non-randomized comparison of this kind.

As far as what happens to people who are resuscitated, I think that the experience so far is good. These people do leave hospital alive, they get a follow-up at six months and they intend to follow-up at a later stage. We would like to find out in due course what happens to these people two years after leaving hospital, not only in terms of life and death but whether or not they are working and leading a normal life.

De Haas: Would Dr. Schweizer be so kind as to tell us about the survey that he has organized in Basle and why he as a clinician, has taken the initiative in organizing an epidemiological survey which as far as I know is still an exception in Western Europe?

Schweizer: In Basle a prospective epidemiological study is going on since 1959. The team of the Department of Cardiology, University Hospital for Internal Medicine joined the study in 1965. The objectives set and the methods of examination are shown in table I and II. Concerning coronary heart disease the results of the Basle Study II are not yet fully available; up to now selected questions only have been worked out. We do know the prevalence of coronary heart disease in our population of working employees (table III). We had a look at Ecg evidence for coronary heart disease in people with different arterial blood pressure (table IV and V). We investigated the frequency of angina on effort in cases with Ecg changes indicating coronary heart disease. Only 25% of those with 'positive' Ecg at rest and only 16% of those with 'positive' Ecg during and/or after effort complained of angina, indicating the low sensitivity of interrogation as a method of examination in such a study. Finally we tried to find out if A. M. Master is correct in saying that in exercise electrocardiography the Ecg can be recorded after effort only, that it is not necessary to record during effort. I can give you our answer during the round table conference to-morrow morning.

Table 1. Basle study I. 1959-1962

6470 EMPLOYEES (Pharmaceutical Industry)

OBJECTIVES SET

    Prevalence/Incidence of peripheral artery disease
    Frequency of 'risk factors'
    Sensitivity of different methods of examination

        Basle study II 1965-1968

4975 EMPLOYEES

OBJECTIVES SET

    Prevalence/Incidence of
        Peripheral artery disease
        Coronary heart disease
        Peripheral vein disease
    Correlation between diseases and signs of disease
    Frequency of 'risk factors'
    Sensitivity of different methods of examination
    Significance of signs of low specifity
    Establishment of normal values
    Functional residual capacity
    Bronchial resistance

Table 2. Basle study methods of examination

A. PERIPHERAL ARTERY DISEASE
    Standard questions about ischaemic pain
    Palpation of pulses
    Auscultation of arteries (at rest/after exercise)
    Oscillography (at rest/after exercise)
    if pos.: Aortography

B. ISCHAEMIC HEART DISEASE
    Standard questions about ischaemic pain
    Electrocardiography at rest and during/after exercise
    Chest X Ray

C. PERIPHERAL VEIN DISEASE
    Photography

D. LUNG FUNCTION
    Whole body plethysmography

Table 3. Basle Study II, ECG evidence for coronary heart disease in 4641 employees

Myocardial infarction	1.1%
St Changes (*) at rest	0.3%
St Changes (*) during/after exercise	6.3%

* St Depression more than 1 mm QX/QT Ratio more than 50%

Table 4. Basle Study II. ECG evidence for coronary heart disease in 1610 employees (age 45-64) with different arterial blood pressure

Hypotension (119.3) N 221	Normotension (141.4) N 1134	Hypertension (176.9) N 225
4.5%	6.5 %	12.6%
(10)	(72)	(32)

Table 5. Basle Study II. ECG findings in 114 employees (age 45-64) with different arterial blood pressure

	Hypotension (119.3) N 10	Normotension (141.4) N 72	Hypertension (176.9) N 32
Myocardial Infarction	10 %	18 %	21 %
St Changes At rest	0 %	5 %	15 %
St Changes During/after Exercise	90 %	77 %	64 %

Stamler: When we were talking together earlier, Dr. Schweizer, you mentioned a point repeatedly brought out by the epidemiological data, i.e. the distinction between usual observed levels for a given variable (e.g. serum cholesterol or blood pressure), what we have come to regard as normal – and the tendency to accept and be satisfied with usual levels – with the simultaneous failure to recognize optimal levels. Could you start a discussion on these points and perhaps some of the other members of the panel can join in.

Schweizer: I have some figures from our study. As doctors, we always think that normal values are good values and that normality is a good thing to have. We forget that our actual normal values are mixed figures and not the optimal ones. We took men in the age group 45-64, divided them according to their blood pressure and looked for electro-cardiographic evidence of coronary heart disease. You see that 6.5% of the normal blood pressure group (mean systolic blood pressure 141 mm Hg) has this evidence versus 12.6% of the hypertensive group (mean systolic blood pressure 176 mm Hg). The hypotensive group (mean systolic blood pressure 119 mm Hg) had a considerably lower frequency of electrocardiographic evidence (4.5%). This concerns not only the s-t segment changes of doubtful specificity but also the evidence for myocardial infarction.

Stamler: Does anyone else on the panel wish to elaborate on this point? I think that it is quite clear. I have an anecdotal experience which I find very useful, because sometimes knowledge is transmitted better by an anecdote than by a mass of statistics.

When I was at the Asian-Pacific Congress of Cardiology in 1964, one of our Japanese colleagues in giving a paper very matter-of-factly said: 'In our hypercholesterolaemic patients with serum cholesterol levels of 185 and above –' I don't know about cutting points here on the European continent, but in the United States if we define hypercholesterolaemia as 185 or above, the great majority of middle-aged adults would be designated as hypercholesterolaemic – correctly so, I venture to add!

I would like to ask Dr. Karvonen a question about the very intriguing East-West Finland comparison. Have you looked at rates for various combinations of risk factors in the two populations? Our experience in the States is that when multiple factors are present in combinations, the risk of disease is particularly marked.

Karvonen: The east Finns differ in practically everything possible to their disadvantage with the west. They smoke more, have higher serum cholesterol levels, have higher blood pressure, and a lower intake of iodine. Therefore, you are likely to get these combinations much more often.

Groen: In regard to the question of what is 'normal' serum cholesterol level, one can define this now in two ways. Either we choose as normal the level of serum cholesterol in populations where ischaemic heart disease does not occur, we will then regard that 180 mg% about the upper level of normal and the average as near to 140 mg%. One arrives at the same values when one defines as normal the level to which a man's blood cholesterol drops when he lives on a diet without saturated facts, cholesterol or sugar. Those are the three nutrients which increase the serum cholesterol; all other dietary constituents, proteins, other carbohydrates and other fats leave it unchanged. If one goes on such a diet, practically everyone's serum cholesterol will drop to below 180 mg%, at least in healthy individuals, this is why I think that we should regard this as the normal level of serum cholesterol.

Stamler: I would like to suggest that we modify what Professor Groen has said in the following ways. First, I think that total caloric balance is also important in regard to influencing the lipids, especially trig-lycerides, i.e. very low density lipoproteins (sf 20-400), which tend to rise with obesity. I also think that we must recognize the existence of persons who on a genetic basis will have aberrant lipid levels even on an optimal diet for life. I know that Professor Karvonen is aware of that. We also have to add that it is presently not entirely clear whether there is any substantial influence on serum cholesterol from sucrose in-take per se. There are disagreements on that and more work needs to be done. My impression is that the main evidence leads to a negative answer.

Groen: As far as the relationship between weight increase and total calories on the serum cholesterol is concerned, so far as I know it has never been tried on one of these diets which have been mentioned and which contain no saturated fat, no cholesterol, and no sucrose. The fact is that in the Middle East, you can have many middle aged fat women who become fat because of a combination of excessive bread intake and little exercise. These women have serum cholesterol levels in the range of 150 to 160 mg% and coronary heart disease among them is extremely rare. It is not the obesity as such, but it is the type of excess food causing the obesity that is important here.

Stamler: I think Dr. Groen is correct on the experimental evidence on that point. There is no evidence from controlled metabolic ward studies that a diet of the type he describes does lead to an increase even of the very low density lipoproteins when caloric intake is excessive.

Dr. Rose has very rightly emphasized the importance of standardization, a maximum effort at uniformity, and maximum care in the collection of data. To me this has always had important implications for clinicians for two reasons. Firstly, when they go to laboratories for cholesterol, glucose or uric acid levels, they should verify that they are going to decent reliable laboratories. Secondly, if they are to embark upon efforts to achieve prevention, they should feel that the changes being proposed are based on solid evidence, well collected and well verified by standard methods and replicated collections of data. Could you make an estimate of the solidity of the evidence with respect to the major risk factors at this juncture of our knowledge?

Rose: As epidemiologists, we are trained to be very selfcritical and as someone who works in the clinical field as well as the epidemiological I feel that this is a very helpful training but a very painful one. If you have never had your ability to measure blood pressure or to report consistently on ECG's evaluated under objective rigorous conditions, then the first time such a test is carried out and you realize how a doctor is not the reliable authorative person we imagine, this is for a time very productive of a suicidal tendency. In the same way, when we turn this skeptical attitude on the interpretation of our evidence we have to face some disheartening experiences. I'm not quite sure, Dr. Stamler, whether the full breadth of your question is really intended for me. Does it mean the evaluation of what we know about the causes of coronary disease? I take it not on that scale!

Stamler: Let me put it the way it is put to us by many physicians in the United States. Is the evidence really solid in regard to the primary risk factors and their relation to the disease? Let us consider serum cholesterol. How solid is our evidence on this risk factor, on blood pressure, on cigarette smoking?

Rose: We are certain that in all the populations that have been studied and in which coronary disease occurs cholesterol level is predictive of risk. Is it causally related? We don't know. It is a tremendous difficulty for the theory that seeks to link fat intake with coronary disease that we have in almost all studies failed within a population to show that the individuals fat intake is related either to his current cholesterol level or to his future coronary risk. That is a very big stumbling block in the theory's way. At the present we are putting that on one side and proceeding as we should to experimental studies. None of those that have been reported so far have produced more than, to my mind, suggestive evidence that dietary alteration may reduce the incidence. They have none of them been in the strictest scientific sense perfectly designed but one might say that they are encouraging. My own assessment of cholesterol is that we know it is predictive but we don't know for sure that alteration in the cholesterol level will be beneficial to the individual. You could say almost exactly the same for blood pressure. There is some hope, that within a couple of years the Veterans Administration trial on treatment of mild hypertension in the United States may perhaps turn out to give us evidence that at present we lack; namely, whether reduction in mild hypertension reduces coronary risk. This is the key question and if it is answered positively we shall be faced with a very urgent problem of implementing that knowledge.

In regard to cigarette smoking, there is again a lot of observational evidence to show that cigarette smoking is certainly predictive of risk. We are ourselves in London conducting a controlled trial in high coronary risk civil servants who smoke cigarettes. A random half are left to the care of their general practitioners as a control group, and the other random half are being persuaded very hard to give up smoking cigarettes. At present we have succeeded in convincing about 2/3 of this group to completely give up smoking cigarettes. We hope over the course of the next few years to see what influence this has on their coronary risk rate; but at the present time we cannot be certain that cigarettes are a cause, but only that they are an association. One encouraging thing that I might mention is that while coronary rates everywhere are rising or steady, British doctors are an exception. The coronary mortality in British doctors is falling and it would of course be tempting to link this to their decline in smoking rates among British doctors. As far as physical activity is concerned, as I hinted earlier, we are on much less sure ground even than these other major risk factors in attributing causality to an association.

Kannel: The question of when is an association causal is a difficult one. I sometimes think that the eminent British physician who pointed to the lack of citrus fruit as the cause of scurvy would have a difficult job today trying to convince anyone that these were causally related. They would want to know about the psychological make up of citrus fruit eating seamen as compared to non-citrus fruit eating ones etc. When is an association causal? You can never prove it is causal, even in animal experiments. All you can do at best is to show a strong association. You can talk about probability of causality. If the relationship is very strong the probability is high; namely, everybody who gets the disease has it. If it preceeds the event by some reasonable, known incubation period, it is more likely to be causal. Finally, does the relationship make sense? Can you explain it in terms of biologic phenomena? I think that blood pressure and cholesterol meet most of these criteria. The final link in the evidence that I think would convince most physicians is what Dr. Rose has alluded to: the fact that when you take it away the disease does not occur or it disappears. We are slowly gathering this final piece of evidence.

Stamler: I have been asked by the chairman to summarize this Panel Discussion. That is virtually an impossible task. The last remarks have contributed much toward a summary. I would like to take a moment to make two or three points in staccato fashion. I hope they are a reasonable substitute for a summary of what has been said here this afternoon.

First, all of us – trained in the clinical or clinical-pathologic approach to medicine – can benefit by broadening our view and recognizing a lesson from the history of medicine: scientific solutions to problems in medicine are accomplished by a variety of approaches and methods. Epidemiology is one among this constellation of approaches that medicine needs to tackle its difficult unsolved problems of today. It is one of the methods that has proved itself to be of value, not only in controlling infectious diseases and diseases of under-nutrition, but – as we have learned principally since World War II – in mastering the chronic diseases, including those relating to overnutrition, particularly coronary disease. There is no doubt that epidemiology stands on its own as one of the major methods of medicine. The issue is never whether the clinician, the animal experimentalist, or the epidemiologist is right. If their data are contradictory, there is a problem somewhere with one or the other set of data, and further probing is needed.

Secondly, I think we can agree that there is a vast amount of evidence linking multiple aspects of mode of life and the coronary epidemic. There is also abundant evidence on the pathways whereby mode of life leads to this disease, pathways relating to serum lipid levels, blood pressure levels, etc.

Thirdly, the associations between certain risk factors and this disease shown in study after study in multiple populations are indeed at this point very well documented, probably as well as anything in medicine. While direct causational implications are a matter of debate and relate to philosophic issues concerning proof, the data also afford the basis for a safe approach to treatment before illness or primary prevention. This is very important in a disease which obviously cannot be controlled without primary prevention as a major aspect of the total medical effort. Medicine, like industry, must often base itself on best judgement from available data – often at the 70% rather than the 95% probability level. Action on this basis can be proper, as long as we are sure that we do no harm with the approach we are pursuing. Since that seems to be the case, especially in regard to recommendations to the population about eating and smoking habits, it is understandable that more and more pressure is mounting for the development of a variety of action programs, to apply the knowledge already available for preventive approaches – while further work on mass field trials is proceeding. Particularly so, since this difficult work takes 10 or 15 years. This is really the challenge confronting us at the present time, I am convinced: wisely and judiciously, step by step to apply the knowledge now, while we do further research, on mechanisms and in field trials.

Hellerstein: I believe that it is essential to point out that intervention – 'action' studies may not modify the basic process of arteriosclerosis but yet conclusively modify the sequellae of atherosclerosis. Progress can be made in action studies which may not fundamentally alter the process of atherosclerosis but may decrease the sensitivity of the heart to arrhythmias, to what is called the mechanism of death.

Stamler: Dr. Snellen, would you care to close the meeting?

Snellen: I would like to thank Dr. Stamler and all the other participants of this panel for a magnificent job. I think that they conveyed a great deal of very useful information in a very short time.

CHAPTER III

DIAGNOSTIC METHODS IN ISCHAEMIC HEART DISEASE

THE CORRELATION BETWEEN CORONARY DISEASE, DEMONSTRATED BY SELECTIVE ANGIOGRAPHY, AND THE VECTORCARDIOGRAM AND ELECTROCARDIOGRAM

(WITH A NOTE ON COMPLICATIONS)

A. V. G. BRUSCHKE AND G. VAN HERPEN

A diagnosis may be regarded as a predictive statement regarding a truth, unknown as yet but which may be revealed by means of certain verification procedures. Verification procedures are methods, such as autopsy and coronary angiography, to which a high degree of reliability is assigned a priori. A diagnosis is reached by the evaluation of diagnostic parameters, sometimes a single one, generally a whole set of them. In the case of electrocardiography, for instance, a diagnosis of left ventricular hypertrophy may be made if the values of parameters such as the height of R in v_5 and the depth of s in v_1 exceed certain critical values ('criteria'). Great effort has been devoted by many workers to selecting proper parameters and determining correct criteria for the various possible diagnostic entities. For this purpose one must be able to assess diagnostic skill in a quantitative way.

In a series of cases the relations between 'prediction' and 'truth', regarding the presence of disease, can be conveniently rendered in a contingency table in which only binary (yes-or-no) statements are admitted:

PREDICTION

		yes	no
	yes	a_1	a_2
TRUTH	no	a_3	a_4

The numbers a_1 through a_4 represent the number of cases in each of the following categories: correct-positive (a_1), correct-negative (a_4), false-negative (a_2) and false-positive (a_3). Now, to express the diagnostic skill or, in other words, the discriminative ability of any diagnostic parameter or set of parameters it is necessary and sufficient to use two mutually independent figures. If the correct positive diagnoses are given as a fraction of the total number of positive cases: $\dfrac{a_1}{a_1+a_2}$,

the fraction of correct-negative diagnoses is also required: $\dfrac{a_4}{a_3+a_4}$. Alternatively, the correct-positive diagnoses may be expressed as a fraction of the total number of positive diagnoses: $\dfrac{a_1}{a_1+a_3}$, in combination with a good-negative fraction $\dfrac{a_4}{a_2+a_4}$.

Quite often this simple truth is neglected and the diagnostic performance of a given predictor is represented by one number only, e.g. the fraction of correct-positive diagnoses alone. Some examples may clarify this. It has been shown in correlation studies that in individuals in which a history of typical angina pectoris was obtained, severe coronary artery disease was present in a high proportion of cases (thus: $\dfrac{a_1}{a_1+a_3}$ was high). From this single finding several authors conclude that the history is a highly significant parameter. This conclusion is not warranted: only if, in addition, in the *absence* of typical angina pectoris the coronary arteries were generally proven to be *normal* (if $\dfrac{a_4}{a_2+a_4}$ was also high) is such a conclusion justified. It is usually easy to enhance either the fraction of correct-positive or of correct-negative diagnoses of any diagnostic parameter by shifting the criteria used for interpretation: if a Master two-step test is classified as positive when, instead of an ischemic ST depression, an isolated junction depression is observed, the number of correct-positive predictions will rise, but at the expense of the fraction of correct-negative diagnoses, as was observed in our correlation studies. Many investigators have not avoided this pitfall.

The fact that two numbers are required makes the evaluation of the performance of a predictor equivocal. However, it is possible to substitute them by a single correlation coefficient, for which purpose the 'skill score' or 'index of merit' proposed by Kuipers and Hanssen (1) is particularly convenient. The index is given by

$$I = \frac{a_1}{a_1 + a_2} + \frac{a_4}{a_3 + a_4} - 1 \, .$$

It is obvious that $0 \leq I \leq 1$. The standard deviation is given by

$$S = \sqrt{\left(\frac{1}{4 \, p \, (1-p)} - I^2 \right) / n}$$

in which $p = \dfrac{a_1 + a_2}{a_1 + a_2 + a_3 + a_4}$, and n is the total number of cases.

The standard deviation for a given number of cases is a minimum if the distribution of cases over the positive and negative groups of 'truth' is equal. One may ask whether the reduction of the diagnostic statements to an unconditional yes-or-no is not too rigorous. It is quite possible to apply 3×3, 4×4 or larger contingency matrices, but the information retained in this way is again largely lost if a single index is calculated to express the correlation. Moreover, in the clinic one is not much helped by non-committal enunciations like 'possible appendicitis', 'borderline appendicitis' or 'appendicitis not excluded'. Yes-or-no statements are required if yes-or-no decisions are to be made.

THE CORONARY ARTERIOGRAM (CAG)

From our total material of 600 patients studied by selective coronary-cine-angiography, a continuous series of 150 patients with chest pain, but without any other known cardiac disease (such as rheumatic or congenital heart disease) was selected for this study. The coronary arteriograms were graded according to the severest degree of narrowing in any of the three major branches as follows:

grade 0 – normal
grade 1 – small vessel wall irregularities up to 30% narrowing of the lumen diameter
grade 2 – 30-50% narrowing of lumen diameter
grade 3 – 50-90% narrowing

grade 4 – obstruction > 90%, but not total
grade 5 – total occlusion with collateral filling of the distal portion
grade 6 – same as grade 5 but without collaterals.

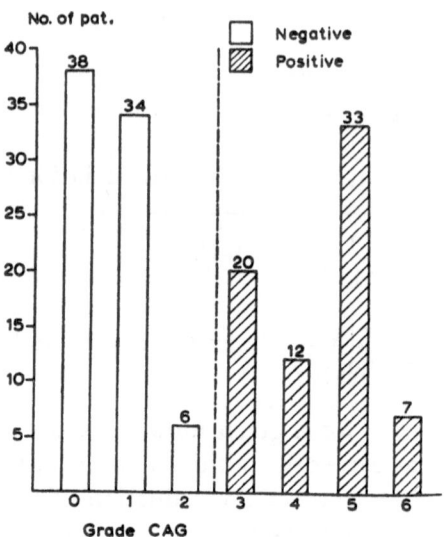

Fig. 1. Distribution of cases over the six classes of the CAG. Division into negative and positive CAG.

Figure 1 shows the distribution of cases over the 6 classes of the CAG. In order to obtain binary statements the material had to be divided into negative (normal) and positive (pathological) cases. The bisection was made between grade 2 and 3: 78 cases were classified as negative, 72 cases as positive. This provides a well balanced distribution between positive and negative cases in our material.

CORRELATION WITH THE ELECTROCARDIOGRAM (ECG)
The ECG was interpreted according to generally accepted criteria: application of more esoteric criteria led to less good results. The ECG was classified as positive if there was an infarction pattern, or a repolarization disturbance which could not be attributed to other causes (such as hypertension or digitalis effect).

Figure 2 demonstrates the correlation with the CAG. The contingency table appears to be as follows:

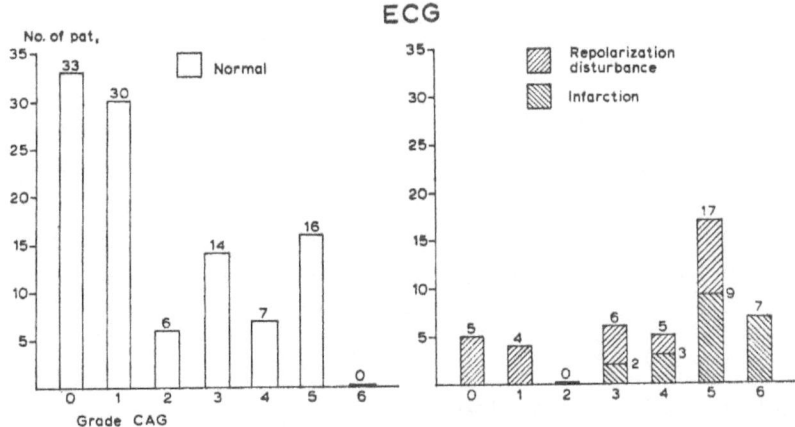

Fig. 2. Correlation between ECG and CAG. The material has been divided into cases with normal (left-hand graph) and with abnormal (right-hand graph) ECG.

	ECG	
	positive	negative
CAG positive	35	37
CAG negative	9	69

The correlation index $I = \dfrac{35}{72} + \dfrac{69}{78} = 0.37 \, (\pm \, 0.08)$.

If the cases with isolated repolarization disturbances are assigned to the normal group, I drops to 0.29.

CORRELATION WITH THE VECTORCARDIOGRAM (VCG)

In every case two lead-systems were used, namely the Burger(2) and the Frank (3) system. The three planar projections were photographed simultaneously in various enlargements (up to 1 cm = 0,14 mV). The 3 orthogonal components were recorded as well. Again, only well established criteria were used to make a diagnosis of infarction.

Figure 3 shows the correlation with the CAG. The following contingency table can be derived:

	positive	negative
positive	57	15
negative	19	59

$$I = \frac{57}{72} + \frac{59}{78} = 0.55 \, (\pm \, 0.07).$$

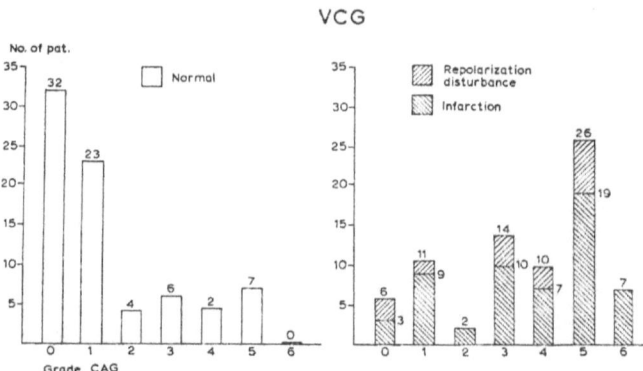

Fig. 3. Correlation between vcg and cag.

If the cases with repolarization disturbances only are considered as normal, the index becomes 0.42. Although diagnostic parameters other than ECG and VCG are outside the scope of this paper, it may be remarked that I has been calculated in the same manner for the history (I = 0.59 ± 0.07), and the serum-cholesterol (I = 0.32 ± 0.08)

DISCUSSION AND CONCLUSIONS

Coronary arteriography yields diagnostic information that cannot always be obtained by less agressive methods such as ECG and VCG. Especially the ECG suffers from a high percentage of false-negative diagnoses.

The over-all diagnostic performance of the VCG is better than that of the ECG, as is reflected in a higher correlation-index. However, the number of false-positive diagnoses is surprisingly high. Since in an asymptomatic control group the proportion of infarct diagnoses was definitely lower, it might be conjectured that the VCG reveals abnormalities which are not manifest in the CAG (such as metabolic changes, abnormalities of the micro-circulation etc.). To substantiate this concept, however, more specific diagnostic methods should be available.

The importance of accurate history-taking may again be emphasized. If the history and the VCG are both positive or both negative, one may with a high probability either predict or exclude the presence of coronary heart disease.

COMPLICATIONS
Our total material comprises 600 patients who underwent selective coronary cine-angiography according to Sones' technique (4). In order to investigate the possibility of cardiac damage caused by the procedure, serum enzyme and ECG follow-up studies were performed in approximately 200 cases, including all the patients who passed through an episode of serious arrhythmia. Apart from three cases which will be discussed in the paragraph dealing with myocardial infarction, these examinations never yielded pathological results.

The following complications were encountered:

1. Cardiac complications
a. Arrhythmias
Ventricular fibrillation occurred in 4 instances: all these patients could be defibrillated easily with direct-current counter-shock. In 3 other cases a short episode of ventricular tachycardia which terminated spontaneously was observed. Bradycardia was rather common. In 2 cases a prolonged asystole necessitated cardiac massage for less than one minute.

In all the cases which were complicated by an arrhythmia the procedure could be completed; there were no sequelae.

b. Myocardial infarction
In one case an inferior wall infarction developed, which was clearly related to the procedure. The patients' recovery was uneventful; after discharge from the hospital he went back to work normally.

An other patient with severe atherosclerotic heart disease, who had sustained the procedure well, became decompensated the day afterwards. There was a moderate elevation of the serum-enzymes. The ECG, however, remained unchanged. The patient died 5 days afterwards because of progressive cardiac failure. At autopsy signs of extensive old myocardial infarctions were found, and small foci of fresh necrosis as well. It remains doubtful whether his death should be attributed to the procedure or not.

In a third case signs and symptoms of transient cardiac ischemia were observed; the serum-enzymes were very slightly elevated, the ECG showed only slight repolarization disturbances for less than half an hour. The coronary arteriogram revealed that there had been spasm of a small branch of the left coronary artery.

2. Complications related to the arterial cut-down

Early in the series symptoms of circulatory insufficiency of the brachial artery occurred in about 4 percent. Later this complication dropped to less than 1.5 percent. Practically always the symptoms disappeared spontaneously within a few months (occasionally it took as long as 9-12 months); in only two cases was surgical intervention necessary (in both cases the result of surgery was satisfactory).

3. Cerebro-vascular complications

Two patients sustained a cerebro-vascular complication: one of them had hypertension and signs of generalized atherosclerosis, including signs of cerebro-vascular insufficiency, prior to the procedure. The recovery was reasonably good, although not complete, in both cases.

Summarizing, the major complications in this material were the following: myocardial infarction – one or two cases; transient myocardial ischemia – one case; insufficiency of the brachial artery which necessitated surgical intervention – two cases; cerebro-vascular accident – two cases.

These cases constitute 1 percent of the total material.

REFERENCES

1. Hanssen, A. W., An objective method for forecasting thunderstorms in the Netherlands. *J. Appl. Meteorology* 4, 172 (1965).
2. Burger, H. C. and J. B. van Milaan, Heart vector and leads, Part. II. *Brit. Heart J.* 9, 154 (1947).
3. Frank, E., An accurate, clinically practical system for spatial vectorcardiography. *Circulation* 13, 737 (1956).
4. Sones Jr., F. M. and E. K. Shirey, Cine coronary arteriography. *Mod. Conc. Cardiov. Dis.* 31, 735 (1962).

CORONARY ARTERIOGRAPHY. SOME ASPECTS OF CLINICAL AND ANGIOGRAPHIC CORRELATIONS

P. LICHTLEN

Coronary arteriography provides an excellent opportunity to analyse the clinical aspects of coronary artery disease (CAD) in relation to the underlying anatomical changes in a living population. In contrast to postmortem studies (1, 2, 3) it covers all phases of the disease, not only the terminal ones, allowing a better analysis of its different manifestations and its progression. Furthermore, by close analysis of the angiographic aspects considerable prognostic conclusions may be reached (4). Nevertheless, one has to realize that such correlation studies are based on a selected group of patients and by their limiting nature, are not fully representative for the living population. Finally, coronary arteriography leads to a re-evaluation of the main diagnostic methods such as history, ECG or exercise test.

PATIENTS

The analysis is based on 250 patients undergoing coronary arteriography during the last three years, 165 of them presenting an abnormal angiogram. So far more than 350 patients underwent coronary arteriography at the University Clinic, Zurich, but only the patients presenting a complete clinical record and a satisfactory angiography were included. The patients' history was assessed by at least two investigators: clinical documentation included enzyme studies, electrocardiograms, vectorcardiograms and for about half of the patients, also exercise electrocardiograms.

CORONARY ARTERIOGRAPHY

The selective technique of Sones (5) was applied for all patients. Pictures were taken in at least two positions (right and left oblique): 10 to 12 injections per patient were performed using 65% Urographin.

The last 100 of the 250 patients underwent additional left ventricular angiograms, usually in RAO position. In patients with posterolateral infarctions or occlusions of the left circumflex branch, an additional injection was performed in LAO position.

The coronary artery lesions were evaluated as follows:
– mild occlusions: the lumen being obstructed not more than 50%
– partial occlusions: obstructions of the lumen of 50 to 75%
– subtotal occlusions: obstructions of 75% or more
– total occlusions: complete interruption of the continuity of the vessel, the distal parts being either not visualized or filled through collaterals resp. anastomosis.

For statistical reasons the following branches only were included into the analysis: main right coronary artery (RCA) with its major branches (sinus node artery, marginal branches, posterior descending and right circumflex branch, av-node artery), left anterior descending branch (LAD) with major septal branches, diagonal branches (LD) and left circumflex artery (LC) (main branch, atrioventricular and posterolateral branches). The main left coronary artery was not incorporated into this analysis since its lesions were rather infrequent. Similarly,

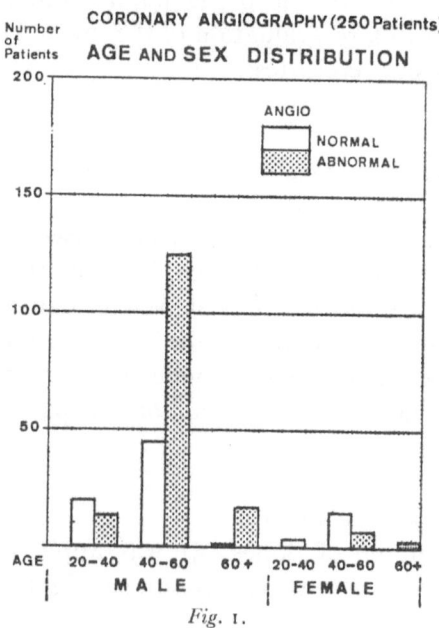

Fig. 1.

length and extension of lesions were not considered and in presence of multiple lesions on the same branch, only the most severe one was listed. A more detailed analysis of the results is given elsewhere (6, 7).

RESULTS

A. CLINICAL CORRELATION
Age and sex distribution (fig. 1)
The study includes 221 men and 29 women, the men showing abnormal angiograms in 70% versus 34% in women. 77% of the men and 76% of the women belonged to the age group of 40 to 60 years. Thus, the study reflects not only the prevalence of CAD for the middle and higher age groups, but also for the male sex.

Risk factors (fig. 2)

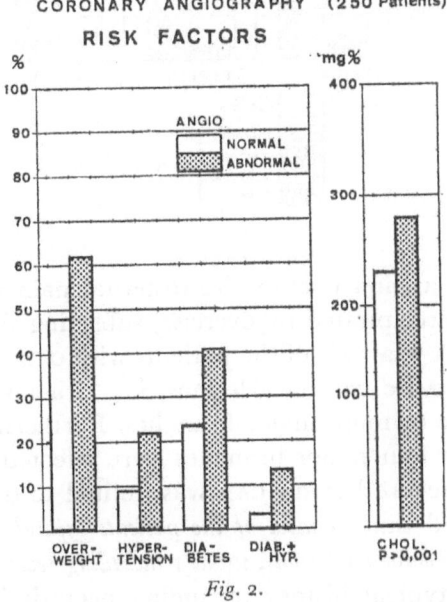

Fig. 2.

There was a clear prevalence of overweight, hypertension and diabetes (in the majority of the cases subclinical diabetes) among the patients with an abnormal angiogram. Furthermore, cholesterol levels were as a whole significantly higher in patients with CAD (p < 0,001) (231 mg% in the normal group versus 279 mg% in the CAD group).

History
a. *Angina pectoris* (*A.P.*) (fig. 3)

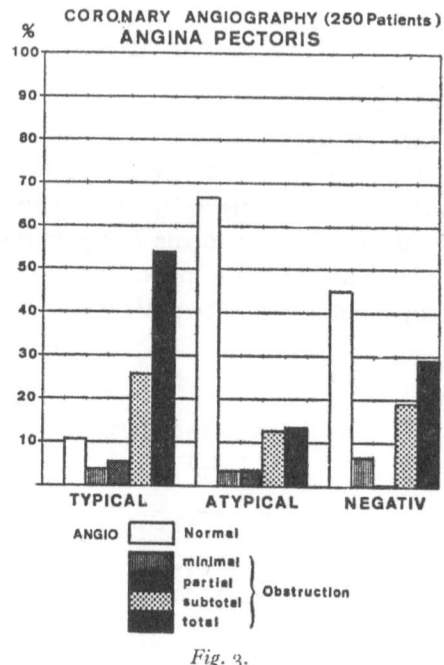

Fig. 3.

A *typical history* of angina pectoris (retrosternal pain radiating to the left arm or neck, precipitated by exercise, subsiding shortly after rest) was present in more than 2/3 of the patients with CAD. More than 70% of them showed severe coronary lesions, i.e. either total or subtotal obstructions of one or more major branches. Furthermore, in 70% of this group three or four major branches were affected; only in 7% of the patients with severe lesions, CAD was limited to one branch. It is therefore concluded that *in most of the patients typical angina pectoris is associated with severe coronary lesions, usually including several major branches.* It follows that a typical history of angina pectoris is still the most reliable clinical criterion in diagnosing CAD, provided that other heart conditions like valvular disease, obstructive or congestive cardiomyopathy, pericarditis, etc. are excluded. Thus, 8 of the 14 patients with a typical history of angina pectoris and a normal arteriogram suffered from valvular disease, 5 from cardiomyopathy, and in one patient a hiatus hernia was found.

In contrast, 66% of the patients with an *atypical history* of angina showed a normal coronary angiogram. Nevertheless, more than 20% of these patients suffered from severe coronary lesions. Therefore, in the presence of atypical chest pains, there is still considerable probability of CAD. This was also seen in patients with a *negative history* of angina in whom coronary arteriography was performed because of unclear ECG-abnormalities (unspecific changes versus ischaemia) or an equivocal history of myocardial infarction. Although free of typical symptoms, almost 50% of these patients showed severe coronary lesions, an observation which emphasizes the importance of the distinction between coronary artery disease and coronary heart disease.

b. Myocardial infarction (M.I.) (fig. 4)

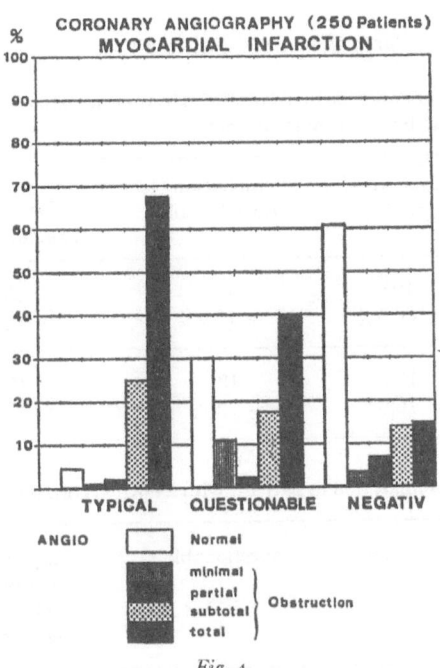

Fig. 4.

History was considered positive in the presence of classic ECG- and/or VCG-changes and typical clinical findings including positive enzyme studies. In 90% of the patients with a typical history of myocardial infarction again severe coronary lesions, i.e. either total or subtotal obstructions of one or more of the major branches were found. Like in angina pectoris, three or four major branches were affected in the majority of the cases (67,5%), although in the ECG the myocardial infarction was limited to one specific area. Isolated coronary lesions, located on one major branch only, were observed in less than 10% of these patients. In three patients a typical myocardial infarction was thought to be present at the time of hospitalization, arteriography performed three months later, however, proved negative. Retrospectively seen, acute peri-myocarditis could not be excluded in these cases.

Myocardial infarction was considered questionable if either history, ECG-changes or enzyme studies were equivocal. It was not surprising that almost 60% of these patients still showed severe coronary lesions rendering the presence of myocardial infarction retrospectively very probable.

Electrocardiogram, vectorcardiogram (Table 1)

Table 1. ECG- or VCG-diagnosis of myocardial infarction in patients with total, subtotal or partial obstructions of at least one major branch.

		Myocardial positive	infarction questionable	unspecifique ECG-changes LBBB/RBBB/LVH	Normal ECG VCG
ECG	155	103 = 66,5%	17 = 11,0%	23 = 15,0%	12 = 7,5%
VCG	148	113 = 76,5%	12 = 7,9%	18 = 12,2%	5 = 3,4%

Diagnosis of myocardial infarction in patients with a normal coronary arteriogram

		positive	questionable	unspecifique ECG/VCG-changes LBBB/RBBB/LVH	Normal ECG VCG
ECG	95	11 5 PWI 6 AWI	13	35	36
VCG	92	8 5 PWI 3 AWI	14	59	11

Considering patients with severe coronary artery disease only, i.e. partial and especially subtotal and total obstructions, the diagnosis of myocardial infarction was made from ECG in 66,5%, from VCG in 76,5%. The observation that no myocardial infarction was found in the ECG and VCG in more than 20% of these patients is in accordance with the clinical experience of underdiagnosing myocardial infarction in the conventional ECG. This is further supported by the observation of a very high incidence of ventricular abnormalities in left ventricular angiography.

With regard to the *exercise test* the yield of positive diagnosis surprisingly was not higher than from resting ECG; however, it mostly concerned another group of patients. Only those exercise test were included in which work load was sufficient and corresponded to the standardization of the double Master test in order to compare positive and negative results accurately. None of the patients was under medication at the time of the exercise test. In the presence of severe CAD, the exercise test was positive in only 66% of the patients. The conclusion has to be drawn that a negative exercise test – even in the presence of a double Master test – does not exclude CAD. The positive test, however, has to be analyzed in comparison to the patients' history. Thus, the Master test was positive in 25,7% of the patients without signs of CAD. The possible reasons for this feature are listed in table 2.

Table 2. Exercise test versus coronary arteriography. (Only those exercise tests were included, in which a double Master test was performed and any medication – except anticoagulation – was interrupted for at least two weeks prior to the test)

| | Exercise test | | |
Angiography	positive	negative	total
total or subtotal occlusion of at least one major branch	25 = 66%	12 = 34%	37
Partial obstructions	4	5	9
minimal lesions or normal	9* = 25,7%	26 = 74,3%	35

* Aortic stenosis = 2 patients, Diabetes and Hypertension = 2 patients, Diabetes alone = 1 patient, Hypertension = 1 patient, unknown = 3 patients.
For the diagnosis of a positive exercise test ST-depression of at least 1 mm had to be present in the extremity leads and of 2 mm in the precordial leads.

B. ARTERIOGRAPHY
Distribution of the coronary system (fig. 5)

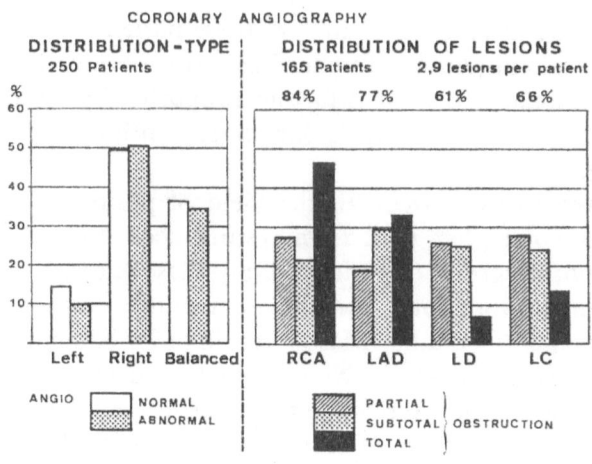

Fig. 5.

A type of right preponderance was thought to be present when the right circumflex branch extended over the crux cordis into the left atrioventricular groove. It was present in 50% of the patients. A balanced type, characterized by a joint blood supply of the crux cordis through the distal RCA and the atrioventricular branch of the left circumflex artery, was found in 35% of the patients. In contrast, a type of left preponderance where the entire crux and posterior part of the interventricular septum obtained their blood supply from the atrioventricular branch of the left circumflex artery, was seen only in about 12%. It has to be emphasized that no difference existed between normal and abnormal arteriograms with regard to the distribution of the coronary system. It might therefore be concluded that CAD is not depending on the distribution of coronary arteries whereas it may well be the case for the location and extent of a myocardial infarction as well as the development of anastomosis.

Distribution of lesions (fig. 5)
Right coronary artery and left anterior descending branch were found to be almost equally affected by CAD (84% resp. 77%) whereas lesions of the diagonal branch and the left circumflex artery were seen some-

what less frequently (61% resp. 66%). In both RCA and LAD total obstructions were prevailing, being present in 30 to 40%. The small
percentage of total occlusions of the diagonal branches has to be explained by the fact that lesions on these branches most often occurred
in association with those of the LAD, the diagonal branches, however,
originated from the main left or the proximal circumflex artery in half
of the cases.

Number of branches affected (fig. 6)

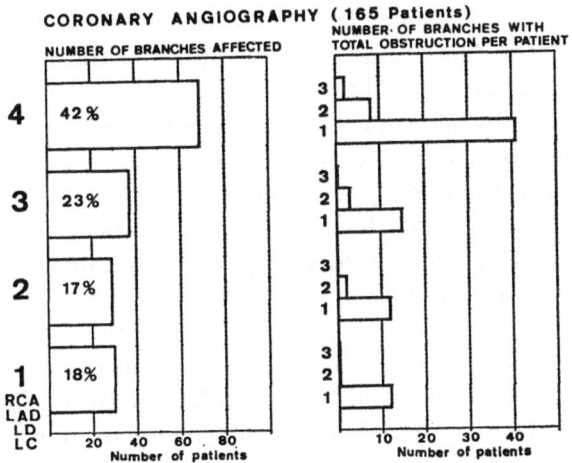

Fig. 6.

Four major branches (RCA, LAD, LD, LC) were affected in 42% of the
patients with CAD, the majority showing at least one branch completely
occluded. Total obstructions of two or even three major branches,
however, were rare; emphasizing the fact that complete occlusions of
more than one branch are probably leading to death in a relatively
short period of time. It is therefore not surprising that the 11 patients
with total occlusion of two or three major branches did not survive
angiography for more than 8 months. A similar behaviour was observed
also with regard to subtotal obstructions being simultaneously present
on three major branches in only 10% of the patients. In contrast, the
number of patients with subtotal lesions on only two branches was
significantly higher (35%). Hence, it has to be concluded that the

mortality of CAD is, as expected, in close correlation not only to the degree of severity, but even more so to the extent of coronary lesions and that reparative processes such as the development of collaterals and anastomosis are of minor importance for the long term survival. This is further supported by the fact that 80% of the patients with total obstructions presented anastomosis or collaterals. At least three major branches were affected in 23% of the patients, thus three or four major vessels were diseased in 2/3 of the patients with CAD.

It may therefore be concluded that at the time of angiography and probably also at the time of more severe clinical manifestations (myocardial infarction, angina pectoris), CAD already has a diffuse character, several branches being affected with severe lesions in at least one branch. Anastomosis (blood supply of the poststenotic area from other coronary branches) and collaterals (blood supply of the poststenotic area from the proximal part of the same vessel, bypassing the occluded segment) were seen mainly in association with total occlusions (more than 80%) and relatively seldom in the presence of subtotal obstructions (less than 20%). This emphasizes the fact that the development of anastomosis is depending on almost complete reduction of pressure and flow in the poststenotic area, creating a high pressure-gradient between the surrounding, unaffected capillaries and those of the diseased zone. The development of anastomosis and collaterals thus, has to be regarded primarily as a purely hemodynamic phenomenon and to a lesser degree dependent on additional factors such as exercise or coronary dilating drugs, although both of them may be of considerable value in further sustaining them.

Ventricular dysfunction as seen by angiography (fig. 7)
Angiographically two types of left ventricular dysfunction were observed: 1. true left ventricular aneurysms and 2. wall dyskinesia.

1. Aneurysms
Aneurysms were defined as a ventricular area without any contractions or movements during systole or diastole, protruding outside of the normal cardiac contour, often associated with 'paradox' systolic movements. They were seen mostly in the apical area of the anterior wall (19 cases); isolated aneurysms of the anterior wall, leaving the apical area intact, were found in 2 cases only. Posterior wall aneurysms were seen less frequently, usually extending from the mitral valve ring

to the midportion of the diaphragmatic part of the left ventricle.

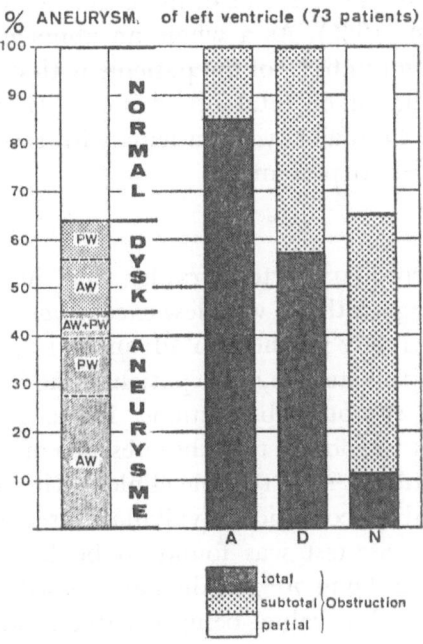

Fig. 7.

Aneurysms occurred mainly in the presence of total obstructions of a major branch; they were observed frequently in total obstructions of the LAD (20 of 24 patients), somewhat less often in those of the RCA (12 of 18 patients). In accordance with the relatively infrequent finding of two totally obstructed major branches, combinations of an anterior and a posterior wall aneurysm were rarely encountered (4 patients). Thus, whereas 28 of 38 patients with total obstruction presented a typical aneurysm (73,5%), the same abnormality was seen in only 4 of 19 patients with subtotal lesions (resp. 21%).

2. Wall dyskinesia
Alterations of the left ventricular wall, associated with impaired contractions and absence of protrusions of myocardium or any paradox movements, were defined as wall 'dyskinesia'. Their occurrence was less frequent than that of aneurysms, being present in 8 patients on the

anterior wall, in 6 cases on the posterior wall; most often they were associated with subtotal lesions. Only 10 of 57 patients presenting either subtotal or total occlusions of the LAD or RCA showed a normal left ventriculogram (16%). As a whole an abnormal left ventricular angiogram was found in 64% of the patients with CAD resp. in 84% of the cases with subtotal or total obstructions. It must therefore be concluded that in the majority of patients with severe CAD, left ventricular abnormalities are present.

DISCUSSION

The analysis of coronary arteriography and its comparison with clinical findings suggests that – with few exceptions – CAD at the time of its diagnosis, has already reached an advanced stage affecting several major branches (in this study 2,9 per patient), the lesions being severe, including total or subtotal obstructions. In accordance with other studies (8, 9, 10), it was found that the presence of a typical history of angina pectoris is still the most reliable clinical criterion of CAD, provided that other cardiac conditions (valvular disease, myopathy) are excluded. The exercise test was found to be less significant, being positive only in about 60 to 70% of the patients with CAD. Resting ECG proved to be of even less value, being positive in only about 55% of these patients. Thus, coronary arteriography represents today the most objective method in diagnosing CAD.

Nevertheless, also angiography has to be regarded with a certain caution. The possibility of a false positive angiographic diagnosis is small; but it has to be kept in mind that coronary artery disease and coronary heart disease are not identical. It is well-known that coronary lesions may exist without symptoms and in the presence of atypical chest pains, the clinical significance of angiographically demonstrated lesions may be difficult to assess.

The possibility of a false negative angiographic diagnosis in patients with typical symptoms of CAD and negative angiographic findings, is still subject of discussion. Unspecific ECG-changes resembling ischaemia or the confrontation of a positive exercise test with a normal angiogram are not infrequent. A 'false positive' exercise test may, however, result from a number of syndroms such as vegetative dystonia in younger men, orthostatic syndrom in women, rheumatic heart disease, myocardial disease or peri-myocarditis. The so-called 'small vessel disease' affecting only the branches not visualized at angiography (smaller than 0,5 mm or the av-node artery), admitted freely in the presence of these cases, has so far been lacking any anatomical corroboration (11, 12). Specific alterations of the sinus node artery or the AV-node artery, however, are well-known especially in specific vascular diseases; yet they are associated with typical ECG-changes (T-inversions) and/or arrhythmias (11).

As can be seen from this study, coronary arteriography implicates considerable prognostic values. The frequent incidence of total obstructions of one major branch in contrast to the rare occurrence of complete occlusions of several branches suggests that the multiplication of severe lesions on several branches is prognostically unfavourable, even in the presence of anastomosis. Furthermore, the extent and location of lesions seem to have an immediate impact on the outcome of the disease. In this regard it is of interest to note that in patients with both RCA and LAD involved, the pattern of a total obstruction of the RCA combined with a subtotal lesion of the LAD was seen in 52% whereas the opposite, i.e. the combination of a total obstruction of the LAD associated with a subtotal lesion of the RCA was found in only 21%. It seems therefore that total obstructions of the RCA are better tolerated than these of the LAD; further they have a more favourable prognosis once the patient has survived the critical days of infarction. This may be explained partially by the pattern of anastomosis, the poststenotic part of the occluded RCA receiving its blood supply not only from the LAD, but also from the left circumflex artery, whereas the LAD is depending on the RCA alone for further blood supply after obstruction.

SUMMARY
It may be concluded that coronary arteriography is providing a new 'inside look' into coronary artery disease, increasing our knowledge on the clinical picture of coronary heart disease considerably. It is a valuable means in assessing the diagnosis and evaluating the severity of the disease in a given patient, determining further treatment. It is an absolute necessity when considering any possibility of coronary surgery. For all these reasons coronary arteriography should be used frequently, on a much larger scale than has been the practise so far.

REFERENCES

1. Blumgart, H. L., M. J. Schlesinger and D. Davis, Studies of the relation of the clinical manifestations of angina pectoris, coronary thrombosis and myocardial infarction to the pathological findings. *Amer. Heart J.* 19,1 (1940).
2. Zoll, P. M., S. Wessler and H. L. Blumgart, Angina pectoris. A clinical and pathological correlation. *Amer. J. Med.* 11, 331 (1951).
3. Lenègre, J., J. Himbert, Critical study of the relationship between angina pectoris and coronary artherosclerosis. *Amer. Heart J.* 57, 539 (1959).
4. Ross, R. S., P. R. Lichtlen, Prognostic value of coronary arteriogram. In: *Sudden cardiac death.* Grune & Stratton, New York, (1964).
5. Sones, F. M., E. K. Shirey, Cine coronary arteriography. *Mod. Conc. Cardiovasc. Dis.* 31, 735 (1962).
6. Lichtlen, P., Zur Indikation der selektiven Koronarographie. *Schweiz. Med. Wschr.* 97, 195 (1967).
7. Lichtlen, P., P. C. Baumann and B. Preter, Zur selektiven Koronarographie. Klinisch-angiographische Analyse anhand von 250 Patienten. *Archiv f. Kreislaufforschung* 59, 287 (1969).
8. Carlsten, A., S. A. Forsberg, S. Paulin, E. Varnauskas and L. Werkö, Coronary angiography in the clinical analysis of suspected coronary disease. *Amer. J. Cardiol.* 19, 509 (1967).
9. Proudfitt, W. L., E. K. Shirey and F. M. Sones, Selective cine coronary arteriography. Correlation with clinical findings in 1000 patients. *Circ.* 33, 901 (1966).
10. Proudfitt, W. L., E. K. Shirey and F. M. Sones, Distribution of arterial lesions demonstrated by selective cine coronary arteriography. *Circ.* 36, 54 (1967).
11. James, N. T., Pathology of small coronary arteries. *Amer. J. Cardiol.* 20, 679 (1967).
12. Shirey, E. K., Correlative pathological study of the coronary microcirculation with coronary arteriography. *Circ.* 38, Suppl. 4-179 (1968).

ATRIAL PACING IN ANGINA PECTORIS

J. P. ROOS AND J. ROELANDT

Exercise is the most physiological test available in the electrocardiographic evaluation of patients with angina pectoris. However, it has several disadvantages: it cannot be used in patients with poor exercise-tolerance; comparable haemodynamic parameters are not exactly reproduced during repeated periods of exercise.

Increasing heart rate alone by means of right atrial pacing is a new technique and provides a unique opportunity for the study of rate dependent functions and responses of the heart.

It is a well-known fact that sт-segment depression may occur during tachycardia and this suggests that heart rate alone may play a significant role in uncovering subjects with coronary artery disease. It is also generally accepted that the pain of angina pectoris occurs when myocardial oxygen-requirement exceeds the capacity of the diseased coronary arteries to supply sufficient oxygenated blood. As shown by Sarnoff et al. (1) the product of heart rate and intraventricular pressure (tension time index) may be used to estimate myocardial oxygen consumption. In later studies by Sonnenblick et al. (2) it was shown that factors other than intraventricular pressure and heart rate may alter myocardial oxygen consumption. The major ones of these factors are myocardial wall-tension and the contractile state of the myocardium (LV dp/dt).

Although tension time index is only a rough indication of myocardial oxygen consumption it has some value especially in repeated investigation in the individual patient (3).

MATERIAL AND METHODS

Twelve patients aged 25 to 66 were studied. Six patients had a history of coronary artery disease; the other six were non-coronary patients. Clinical signs or symptoms of congestive heart-failure were not present in any patient.

Under local anaesthesia a Cournand needle was inserted in the brachial artery and a bipolar pacing-catheter was directed into the right atrium and positioned at the junction of the superior vena cava and right atrium under fluoroscopic control. The catheter was connected with an external battery powered pacemaker unit. Pacing was started at a rate just above the resting heart rate. Heart rates were increased gradually with increments of 10 beats/min. until angina pectoris occurred or a rate of 180/min. was reached. Each rate was maintained for 2 minutes.

In each patient the pacing procedure was repeated after 10 minutes to ascertain the reproducibility of the technique. If angina pectoris was induced it disappeared within one minute after cessation of atrial pacing. In four patients with a positive test a β-blocking agent was administered intravenously and the test was repeated after twenty minutes. Tension time index was calculated as a product of heart rate, ejection time and blood pressure. Ejection time was measured by means of an external carotid tracing. Electrocardiographic leads II, v_4 and v_6 were monitored and recorded simultaneously.

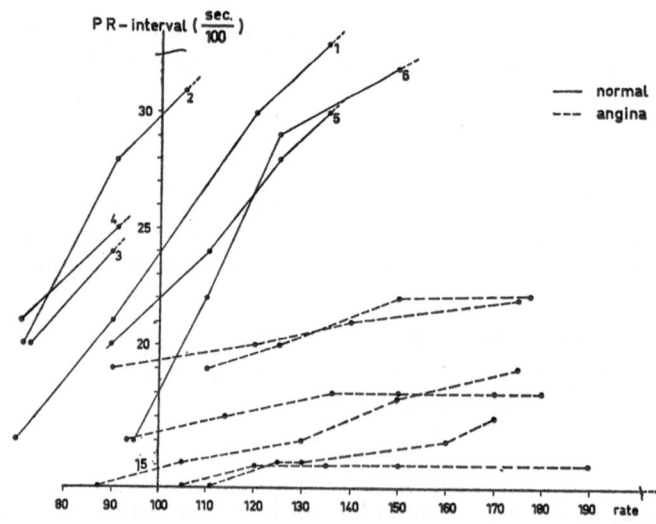

Fig. 2. In normal subjects first degree AV-block of the Wenckebach type occurred at paced heart rates between 90 and 140. Patients with coronary artery disease could be paced at a rate of 180 with a 1 to 1 ventricular response.

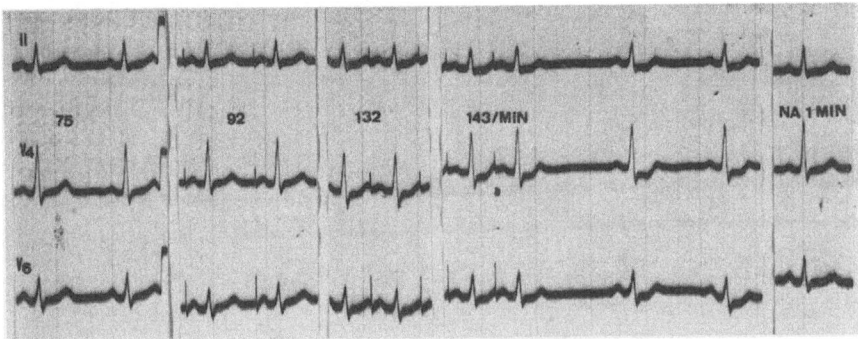

Fig. 1. Positive pacing test. Significant sᴛ-changes of myocardial ischemia in lead v₄ and v₆ are present at paced rates of 132 and 143. Recovery of sᴛ-changes within one minute after cessation of atrial pacing.

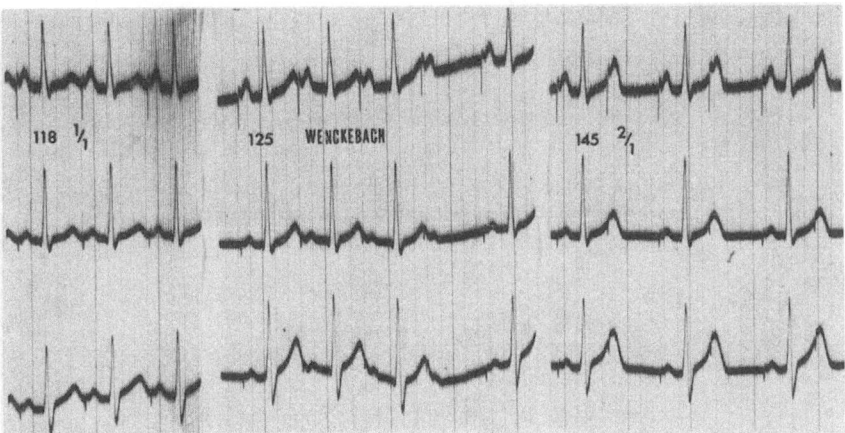

Fig. 3. First degree ᴀv-block of the Wenckebach type at a paced rate of 125 resulting in 2: 1 ᴀv-block at a paced rate of 145.

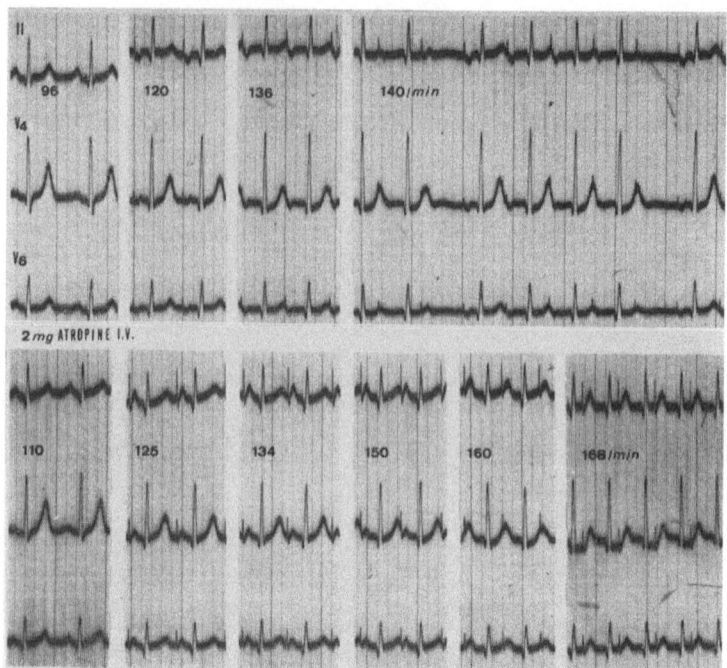

Fig. 4. First degree AV-block of the Wenckebach type at a paced heart rate of 140 (upper tracing) which disappears after administration of 2 mg atropin.

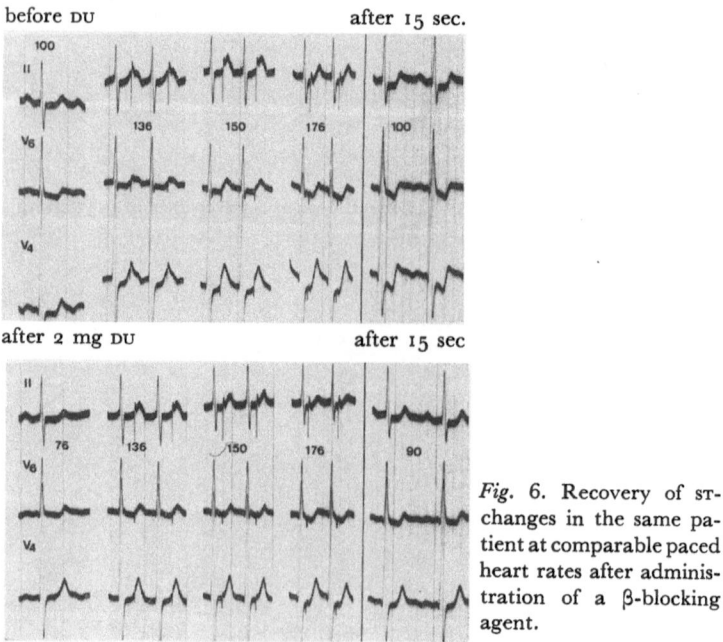

Fig. 6. Recovery of ST-changes in the same patient at comparable paced heart rates after administration of a β-blocking agent.

RESULTS

In five of six patients with a coronary artery disease the test was positive, that means that angina pectoris occurred and ST-T changes were present (fig. 1). In the remaining patients angina did not occur during atrial pacing up to a frequency of 180/min., nor did the electrocardiogram show ST-T changes.

In all patients systemic blood-pressure was not significantly changed with increased heart rates, while stroke volume reflected by ejection time diminished linearly with heart rate.

While the coronary artery patients could be paced up to rates of 170-180 with a 1 to 1 ventricular response, the non-coronary patients developed conduction disturbances at the AV-junction: an increase in rate of pacing resulted in a progressive increase in PR-interval (fig. 2) up to a point at which the refractory period of the AV-junction was reached resulting in AV-block of the Wenckebach type and 2 to 1 block (fig. 3).

This difference in response is most probably related with the blood catecholamine-level as it is shown that sympathetic stimulation results in shortening of the PR-interval at any given paced heart rate. (4).

Under the influence of atropin the normal subjects could be paced till rates of 170-180/min with a 1 to 1 ventricular response while an AV-block of the Wenckebach type occurred at paced heart rates between 90 and 140/min. before the drug was administered (fig. 4).

Atrial pacing can be used to evaluate drugs to have a beneficial effect in angina pectoris. For this purpose an investigational β-blocking agent (DU 21445, Philips Duphar) was studied in some of our patients. After administration of 2 mg DU 21445 intravenously it became evident that the heart rate was lower in the resting state than before the drug was given. When atrial pacing was started a decrease in tension time index occurred as compared without the drug at the same heart-rate (fig. 5).

The electrocardiogram before and after administration of DU 21445 shows a significant difference in the patients we investigated with this drug and reflects decreased tension time index, as compared without the drug at the same heart rate (fig. 6).

SUMMARY

Atrial pacing is a functional test which is performed at rest with a minimum of discomfort to the patient and which requires no physical action by the patient. Chest pain and electrocardiographic changes can be rapidly reversed by the cessation of pacing. In some patients AV-block of the Wenckebach type was a limiting factor for further increase of the heart rate.

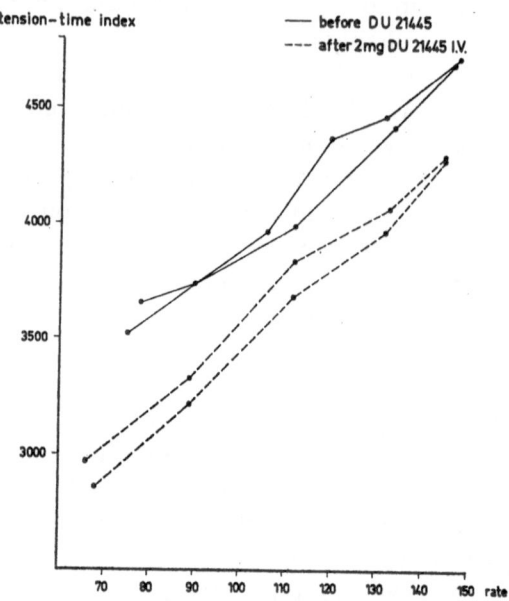

Fig. 5. Repeated pace-runs with a 10 min. interval in the same patient before and after administration of a investigational β-blocking agent (DU 21445, Philips Duphar) show a relative good reproducibility and a decrease in tension time index.

The test is relatively safe and gives reproducible results in the objective evaluation of coronary heart disease in the individual patient. The test seems useful to evaluate results of drug therapy, although the interpretation of the test can be complicated by changing factors as heart volume and the contractile state of the myocardium, which may independently alter myocardial oxygen consumption.

REFERENCES

1. Sarnoff, S. J., E. Braunwald, G. H. Welch, Jr., R. B. Case, W. H. Stainsby and R. Macruz, Hemodynamic determinents of oxygen consumption of the heart with special reference to the tension time index. *Amer. J. Physiol.* 192, 148 (1958).
2. Sonnenblick, E. H., J. Ross Jr. and E. Braunwald, Oxygen consumption of the heart: Newer concepts of its multifactorial determination. *Amer. J. Cardiol.* 22, 328 (1968).

3. Sowton G. E., R. Balcon, D. Cross and M. H. Frich, Measurement of the angina threshold using atrial pacing: New technic for the study of angina pectoris. *Cardiovasc. Res.* I, 301 (1967).
4. Granata, L., R. A. Olsson, A. Huves, D. E. Gregg, Coronary inflow and oxygen usage following cardiac sympathetic nerve stimulation in unaesthetised dogs. *Circulation Res.* 16, 114 (1965).

DETERMINATION OF MAXIMAL CONTRACTION VELOCITY AS A MEANS OF ASSESSING MYOCARDIAL CONTRACTILITY IN PATIENTS

P. G. HUGENHOLTZ

I have worked on both sides of the Atlantic Ocean and I am quite aware of how narrow it has become. Because of this and because of the similarity of our problems, I wish to inject a plan into the fighting of this epidemic. The presence of which has been signalled some years ago and the size of which, this conference now has made quite clear. I sincerely hope that we all can work together towards a solution of this problem.

Of continuing concern to the clinical cardiologist is the evaluation of myocardial muscle function apart from the performance of the ventricle as a pump. This is of particular importance when surgical intervention is considered in efforts to correct the abnormal haemodynamic load. In particular when abnormalities caused by coronary artery disease, are to be attacked, we are really asking ourselves the question: 'To what extent is muscle function as such really impaired?'

Due to the various compensations which can occur even in the presence of heart failure, moderately severe loss of myocardial muscle function may not be manifest as ventricular pump failure unless you stress the system and unless you specifically go after the function of underlying myocardium independent of the load. So far, various laboratories have used a variety of indices which were derived from routine haemodynamic measurements. Several of these have been looked at or tried out by each of us in our efforts to assess quantitatively the overall cardiac performance. The previous discussions have illustrated how difficult it is to standardize such a matter. All of us have worked with such indicators as the ventricular end-diastolic pressure, the ejection fraction, end-diastolic volume, cardiac output in response to stress or pharmacological agents etc. Some of these has been found to be really satisfactory in the assessment of inter individual differences in cardiac performance. This is very logical, because most of these indices reflect, indirectly, one more of this separate but interdependent factors. Let us look at these individually.

Firstly, the things that we really want to know is the intrinsic contractile state or those characteristics we loosely call the 'contractility' of the myocardium.

Secondly, the end-diastolic volume or the fiber length of the ventricle which with a lost of other factors determines the *pre-load* factors.

In view of the fact that the heart is a muscle with very defineable mechanical characteristics, and is not skeletal muscle, recent studies have been directed toward the analysis of ventricular performance in terms of derived muscle properties on isolated muscle strips.

If you look at the basic inter-relationship between length and tension or the force that the muscle delivers in the papillary muscle or an isolated muscle strip, all of us know that as length is increased a greater tension will be developed. (fig. 1).

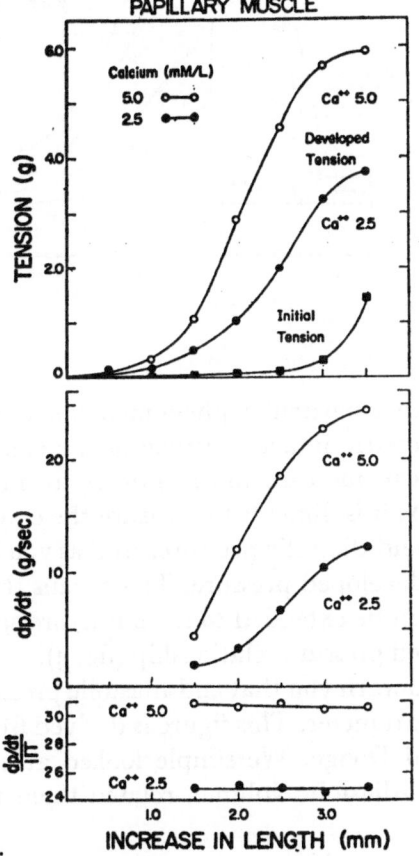

Fig. 1.

If we add different substance, in this case, Calcium, epinephrine or norepinephrine, we can get an even greater delivery of tension for a given length.

You can schematically condense a number of experiments by showing these four averaged curves. They show that as you increase the resting-length, from one to two to three to four, one gests a higher peak in the developed or delivered tension. That is only one aspect of it, i.e. the inter-relationship of length and tension (fig. 2).

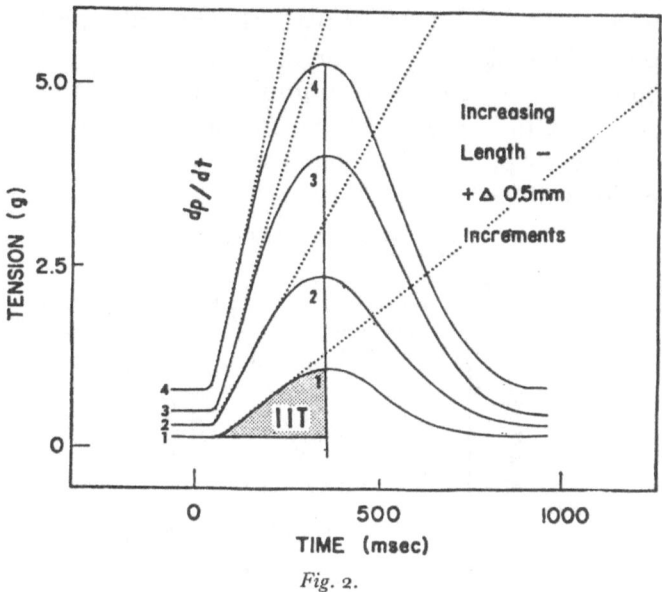

Fig. 2.

When we look at that particular phenomenon shown in the papillary muscles in the isometric intact ventricle of the experimental animal, you see that you can increase the length by an increase in LV end-diastolic volume. As it is difficult to measure the end-diastolic volume, we usually look at end-diastolic pressure. And as you load the ventricle, you get a greater developed pressure. This means that the length-tension relationship can be extended to a volume-pressure relationship or fiberlength-delivered pressure relationship (fig. 3).

Figure 4 ought to warn you that end-diastolic pressure cannot always be used as such a parameter. This figure is derived from our experience and that of Harold Dodge. We simple looked at a large number of determinations end-diastolic volume, related them to pressure in the same individual and as you can see, found no correlation at all. So, while what I have said earlier holds within a given animal, it does not hold between patients.

Sofar, I have talked about length versus tension. I now want to expand this to velocity and force. There really are three factors when we want to talk about the isolated muscle. The first one was the interrelationship of length and tension or length and developed pressure. The second one is the relationship of velocity to the force of contrac-

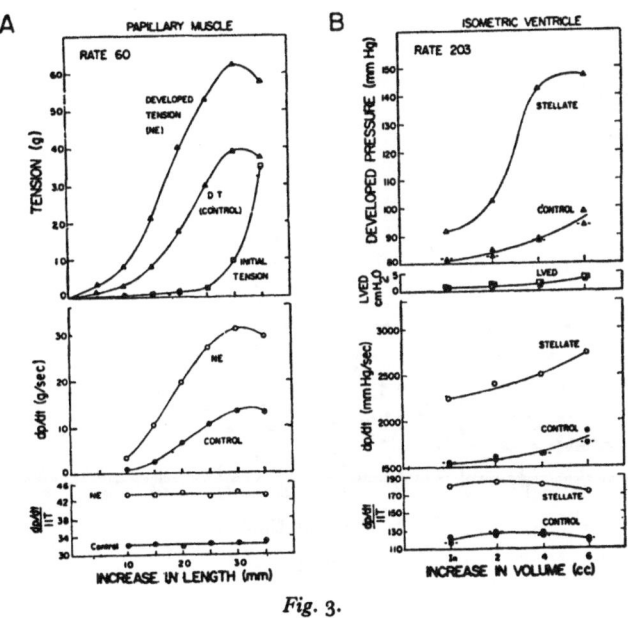

Fig. 3.

tion. As we increase the force, we will get an interaction between the velocity and the force, so that the velocity goes down. Alternatively as we decrease the force we will get an increase in velocity. If we could, in a given patient, have a number of points on force, i.e. by the system with different loads, we would get a curve which could be extrapolated to a point where it would intersect with the zero force axis. That point has been defined by Sonnenblick and co-workers as V_{max}. That is the maximum velocity, that the particular fiber of a particular pump can deliver for zero force. The thesis that I would like to explain in the next few minutes is that if we could get at a method which would give us that particular quantity, we might then obtain a really objective measurement of contractility for comparisons *between* individuals with different disorders.

We may achieve this goal by utilizing biplane angiocardiographics in the following manner. Biplane films can be quantitatively measured, from the dimensions of the heart and the wall thickness and by simultaneously recording the pressure inside the left ventricle the data can be translated through a computing process into the volume of the ventricle over a series of 3 or 4 beats and more important wall-stress.

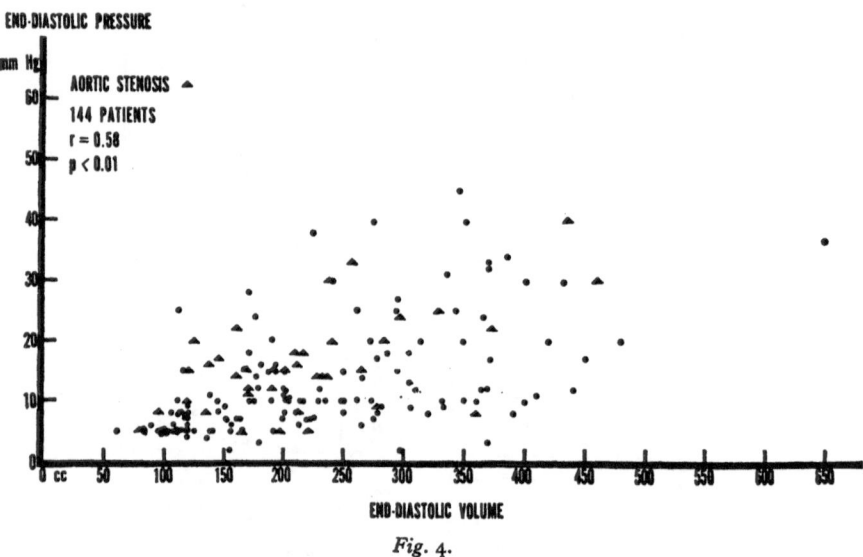

Fig. 4.

Now with wall-stress known, during the isovolumic contraction phase, we can look at the basic muscle model as proposed by A.V. Hill. Remember we were attempting to get at the quantity V_{max}. The contractile element velocity V_{CE} can be computed as the sum of the velocity of the contractile fiber V_{CF} and of the *series elastic* $V_{CE} = V_{CF} + V_{SE}$. If we have a fiber and look onto a level, we hang a load on the far arm of this lever, the muscle formation can be analyzed by 2 seperate components. The contractile element exists of the *active* part of the contraction and the passive component (a spring) the series elastic. In addition in parallel in order to hold the whole thing together, there is a parallel elastic element. Let us now see how we can get at the contractile element velocity in intact man. The contractile fiber velocity V_{CF} may be derived by using the formula: $V_{CF} = \dfrac{db/dt}{b}$ where

the b is the semi-minor radius which is determined from the angio-graphics. The series elastic SE is calculated as the change of stress in time divided by a constant stress. The latter is so far only available

from animal data. In formula $V_{SE} = \dfrac{d\sigma/dt}{k\sigma}$, where σ = stress and

k = 28. Once again, the stress we get from the angio and a good pressure measurement. By plotting V_{CE} versus stress a curve is obtained during isovolumic contraction. Extrapolation of this curve to zero load (zero stress), V_{max} is determined. We have now derived V_{max} for about 40 patients. As we look at this parameter we have wondered how good it was in terms of predicting contractility. The study is obviously still preliminary as many more cases will be needed before we know how we will use this parameter. We have found that in patients with aortic stenosis who had congestive heart failure, that there were two patients with a very poor V_{max}. The muscle even when hypothetically unloaded, had a maximum velocity of contraction which was abnormal. Both of these patients have done poorly after surgery. We also have had 3 patients who had *normal overall* cardiac function. Their cardiac output, end-diastolic pressure and volume and other parameters were normal, but their V_{max} was abnormally low. In one of these primary muscle disease developed subsequently. In two others myocarditis had been clinically present before but could not be demonstrated by conventional haemodynamic criteria. The low V_{max} did appear to indicate it. We do think that this is a way of getting at the intrinsic contractility of the muscle fiber. It is important for coronary artery disease, that if we extrapolate these data to the disease, we would then have a method which indicated the health of the cardiac muscle, without having to exercise the patient or stress him by after-loading the patient with angiotension infusions or the like. It would give us an objective measurement which we could follow and compare from patient to patient.

ROUND TABLE CONFERENCE ON DIAGNOSTIC METHODS IN ISCHAEMIC HEART DISEASE

MODERATOR: L. WERKÖ

Werkö: We are going to discuss methods used in the diagnosis of coronary heart disease. This will be divided into two parts; the first one concerned with coronary angiography and the second on methods of evaluating myocardial function or myocardial disease in ischaemic heart disease.

The first part of this round table discussion will consider the indications, complications, and usefulness of coronary angiography. Before we delve into this interesting but perhaps difficult problem, we should have a few words from those using coronary angiography as to which methods they are using. As you all are well aware of, there are several different techniques in current use, and their results, complications and indications may be different. I now ask Dr. Paulin to say a few words about the methods that he is using.

Paulin: Some years ago we developed a rather simple approach to coronary arteriography which did not involve the selective catheterization of the coronary arteries. This technique, however, requires rather advanced technical equipment which is expensive and at times difficult to operate. In other words it puts the stress on the examiner and on his equipment rather than on the patient. Therefore, we are still using this method which in the vast majority of cases gives us very satisfactory results. If it does not do so, we complete the examination with the selective techniques.

Werkö: We will now go on to the main presentations. Dr. Paulin will discuss the anatomy of the coronary arteries as seen in the angiograms and the correlation with the findings at autopsy.

Paulin: Permit me to demonstrate two specimens in which the coronary arteries of the human heart have been injected with plastic material and the organ been corroded in a subsequent acid bath. These delicate preparations which I show with the kind permission of Dr. Thomas James may serve as a base line for comparison of the findings obtainable in the living patient.

Paulin: The heart's own blood supply derives from the two main coronary arteries. The *right coronary artery* which arises from the outer wall of the right sinus of Valsalva runs in the right atrial ventricular groove in the form of a semicircle around the right heart. In more than 80% of the cases the right coronary artery reaches the crux which is the junction of the posterior atrial ventricular groove with the intraventricular and intra-atrial septum at the posterior aspect of the heart. Secondary branches arising from the right coronary artery in anterior direction are those to supply the myocardium of the free wall of the right ventricle. In about 50% of the cases this pulmonary conus branch arises separately and has its own little orifice in the right sinus of Valsalva. This relatively small 'third coronary artery' may, however, be of considerable importance in situations where disease in both the proximal coronary arteries is present, since it may provide an important pathway for collateral flow.

The *left coronary artery* arises from the left sinus of Valsalva which has an overall left posterior orientation. The length of the *left coronary main trunk* does usually not extend 40 mm before it divides into its two major branches, the anterior descending artery and the left circumflex artery.

The *anterior descending artery* represents a direct continuation of the left coronary artery main stem and runs in anterior and downward direction in the intraventricular sulcus between right and left ventricular anterior wall to terminate after curving around the apex of the heart. A varying number of relatively large side branches towards the anterior wall of the left ventricle are readily seen, whereas the corresponding branches toward the right ventricular wall are few in number and small in caliber, and therefore, barely seen angiographically. A third group of secondary branches arising from the anterior descending artery are those which run in a central direction in order to supply the interventricular septum.

The *left circumflex artery* runs in the left atrial ventricular groove in a similar fashion as the right coronary artery does on the right side. Side branches to supply the lateral wall of the left ventricle arise from it in a anterior direction. The largest of these latter branches, the branch to the obtuse margin runs at the most lateral part of the heart so that it divides the left ventricular free wall into an anterior and posterior half.

In about 30% of the cases one will find that the bifurcation of the left main coronary artery represents a trifurcation. A rather prominent branch is interposed between the anterior descending artery and the left circumflex artery and, hence, it is denoted as the *intermediate* or *diagonal branch* of the left coronary artery.

The anatomy of the coronary arteries in the human heart are submitted to a considerable amount of variations. Mention has to be made of the concept of the right or left *coronary artery preponderance* which is based upon the anatomical features of arterial supply of the posterior aspect of the heart. If the crux of the heart – the junction of the atrial ventricular and interventricular sulci – and adjacent regions are supplied by the right coronary artery, one speaks of right coronary artery preponderance, a situation found in more than 80% of normal human hearts. Unfortunately, this widely used concept is misleading since the largest blood supply to the myocardium is derived from the left coronary artery in the majority of cases.

Arterial branches to supply the atrium of the heart are relatively small. They arise from either right or left circumflex artery in a posterior direction. By far the largest and most important of these is the one to supply the sinus node located at the border between superior vena cava and right atrium. This *sinus node artery* can be demonstrated readily in vivo angiograms and has been shown to arise in 55% of the cases from the proximal portion of the right coronary artery. Another rather constant but somewhat smaller artery is the *AV-node artery* which arises from that artery which happens to supply the crux of the heart.

The supply of the interventricular septum derives mainly from the septal branches from the anterior descending artery and, therefore, belongs to left coronary artery territory. Its distal extension are linked with corresponding septal branches from the posterior interventricular artery which corresponding to the individual variation of arterial supply may arise from the right (approximately 80%) or the left circumflex artery. An interesting observation made in postmortem studies is that the septal branches tend to run in the septum close to the surface of the right ventricular cavity so that they seem to escape the intramural pressure which is generated by the myocardial contraction during systole. We may, therefore, speak of the septal branches as belonging to the epicardial or extramural arterial system of the coronary arteries.

For understandable reasons angiographic demonstration of the coronary arteries in the living patient does not give us the same opportunity for a careful and detailed inspection of the coronary arteries as compared to the situation when one is confronted with a postmortem specimen. Several factors account for this. The radiographic contrast material injected into the blood stream either close to the orifices of the coronary arteries or directly into their most proximal portions will be carried away with the existing blood flow. As shown in film series the transit time of the contrast material through the coronary circulation from the proximal aorta to the venous coronary sinus requires about 6 to 8 seconds. The phase of arterial filling, which demonstrates the most interesting part of the coronary circulation, is correspondingly shorter. Furthermore, the pulsatile pattern of flow in coronary circulation as well as spatial displacement of the coronary arteries of high rapidity during the normal heart cycle necessitates the use of technically advanced high power radiographic equipment. The three-dimensional arrangement of the coronary arterial tree requires that the contrast filled arteries are visualized in several different views. The relatively small caliber of the coronary arteries and its branches requires rather high concentration of the radiographic contrast in order to demonstrate them within the surrounding x-ray absorbing structures.

The here illustrated examples of in vivo coronary arteriograms demonstrate the feasibility of proper demonstration of the entire extramural coronary arterial tree in a technically well performed examination. This includes the demonstration of smaller arteries such as the sinus node, AV-node artery, as well as the septal branches of both anterior and posterior interventricular arteries. When compared with [the previously demonstrated] postmortem studies the impossibility to demonstrate branches of a diameter of less than 100-250 microns in diameter individually is apparent. Insight into the events in the intramurally located vascular structures is limited to the occasionally detectable defuse blush of contrast media when passing the capillary bed.

I have personally made several attempts to obtain further detailed information of the peripheral arterial tree by increasing the concentration of the contrast material. This was accomplished by selective contrast injection into a coronary artery and the use of large size radiographs of high definition. The improvement gained was surprisingly small and of no apparent practical consequence. We, therefore, concluded that it is not necessary at the present time to submit patients routinely to this more hazardous and technically more difficult examination.

The pathologic condition of greatest interest today is coronary arterosclerotic disease. Minor changes can be detected in the coronary arteriogram as slight irregularities of the artery walls, commonly located at the site of bifurcation of smaller branches. In more advanced cases one may see distinct luminal narrowings. These may be of varying degree as far as extension, caliberreduction, and multiplicity is concerned. To evaluate the hemodynamic implication of these arterial changes on the basis of their topographic appearance alone may be very difficult. Considering the different presentation of one and the same lesion in relation to the direction of the x-ray beam makes me believe that the widely used classifications of changes based on percentage caliber reduction are unreliable and do suffer from subjectivity which is inherent in most angiographic readings. I found it very useful to make a distinction between stenotic lesions which do not and which do result in any noticeable delay or weakening of contrast filling of the corresponding vascular regions distal to them. In the latter situations of obstructive changes the presence of compensating collateral circulation is very frequently seen in the angiogram. This also concerns the most advanced cases of obstructive lesions, namely when total occlusions of arteries are present.

The most frequently observed route of collateral circulation is represented by the septal arteries which usually link the anterior descending artery with the distal parts of the right coronary artery. This situation is seen in this illustrated case here which shows a short total occlusion in the proximal part of the anterior descending artery. Filling of the distally to the occlusion located artery is seen approximately 2 to 3 seconds later. In this case a confined lesion is associated with a finding of apparently uninvolved arteries in other segments.

If one confines cases with demonstrated arterial occlusions into one group a broad spectrum of more or less diffusely advanced disease can be seen. May I therefore in contrast to the proceeding case demonstrate the angiogram from a patient with the most advanced obstructive coronary artery lesions in our material. Actually all three major branches show proximally located occlusions and contrast filling of the periphery is accomplished by a network of widely branching collaterals which have replaced the normal vascular anatomy. It should be of interest to know that this patient has had a 16-year history of angina pectoris prior to the examination. When he was examined he had a large heart with signs of chronic heart failure and frequent angina pectoris. He tolerated the examination without complications and is to my knowledge still alive at the present time almost 7 years after the examination. This is to underline the unpredictability of this disease in the individual case.

With that I will finish this short introduction which was meant to show you the potentials and limitations of in vivo coronary arteriography.

Werkö: We proceed now to Dr. Lichtlen who will discuss the indications for angiocardiography and correlations of the findings with the patient's history and with other clinical findings.

Lichtlen: see original text, page 157.

Werkö: Several of the examples described have illustrated the point made by Dr. Hellerstein yesterday, that it seems to be more difficult to explain how the patient can survive than it is to explain why they die.

Dr. Bruschke will now continue the discussion of correlation of angiographic findings with clinical findings.

Bruschke: see original text, page 149.

Werkö: We could perhaps discuss some of the points that have been raised here. One of the problems that should be discussed is the correlation of the exercise-cardiogram to angio-cardiographic findings.

Bruschke: The Master two-step exercise test was routinely applied in all our cases. However, not all the patients were able to perform the test, and in addition there were cases in which the test could not be evaluated because either the patient was receiving digitalis or the pre-exercise ECG showed definite repolarization disturbances. A reliable test was obtained in 99 out of the 150 cases.

The following figure (in which the total number of patients in each category is indicated by the interrupted lines) shows the relation to the CAG:

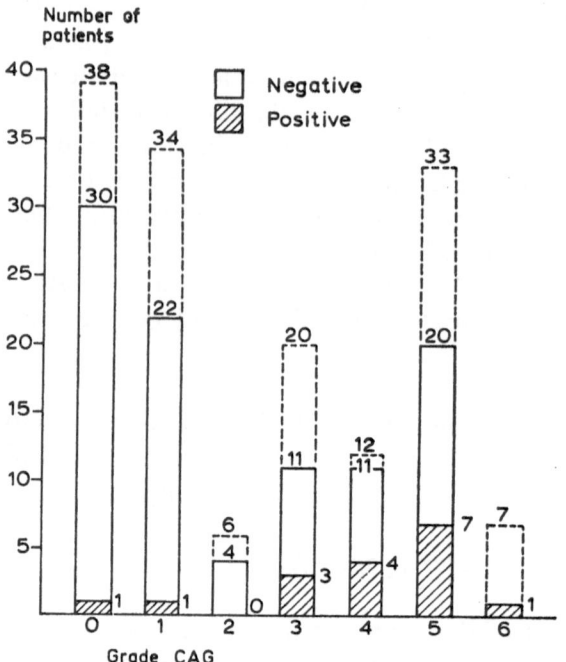

The fraction of correct-negative predictions was 96%; the fraction of correct-positive predictions on the other hand was as low as 35%. The index of merit was 0.31 (± 0.10).

Only ischaemic ST-depressions were found to be discriminative: inclusion of other criteria led to a considerable increase of the number of false-positive diagnoses.

It should be noted that only one precordial lead was recorded by us: it is conceivable recording of multiple leads, that would have yielded a better result.

Werkö: When you use the exercise test you must have some sort of standardization so you will know exactly what kind of load you are putting on the heart, and not only the amount of external work done by the patient. This may be achieved in the future. It is important to emphasize here that patients who are receiving digitalis were excluded from the correlation study of Bruschke. In the clinical situation when you have to evaluate the exercise test and the history, the patient may have been on therapy for a long time and therefore it may be impossible to evaluate the test. Even though there is some correlation of angiographic findings positive results of the exercise ECG it is far from perfect. One of the most important points that has been made here is that a history of anginal pain is very well correlated to the angiograms that you obtain. That is perhaps the very best type of exercise test.

Frick: I think that much depends upon what exercise test that you are doing. If you are doing a maximal exercise test the correlation is better. It also depends upon what leads you are recording during the test. Posterior ischaemia is very difficult to detect. If you are not using the standard leads after excercise but only the bipolar or unipolar leads you will easily miss the signs of posterior ischaemia. I think that the correlation is good in a series but that it is not good for the individual.

Werkö: Is this only your opinion or do you have any facts to support it here?

Frick: I have some facts, but I do not have the slides here. Many other people have shown that the correlation in the series is good but it does not hold for one single individual.

Werkö: This last statement, that the correlation is good for groups but not for individuals, is probably good. Too many people say, as you did now, that if you use this or that lead, or this or that type of exercise you will get a good correlation. This must be tested and correlated in the living patient with coronary angiography before you can be sure of such statements. We have seen too many cases which have had positive exercise tests and who had perfectly normal coronary arteries and who would have been classified as coronary atherosclerosis if we had not performed the angiogram. I noticed in Lichtlen's series that there were three cases where there was unexplainable positive exercise electrocardiogram without any changes in the coronary arteries. It is easy to make sweeping statements but we must try to find more facts before we finally decide on the value of the methods that we are using.

Frick: In Baltimore, the group of Richard Ross has shown that by using multiple leads, the recovery of pathological findings is increased in the excercise test. I think that it is obvious that by using maximal tests you will increase the recovery. It adds to the value of the correlation but when we look at reports of correlation tests we should note what sort of excercise and what leads they are using, etc.

Werkö: I would like to ask the panelists here if they have any experience with the influence of drugs on the coronary angiogram.

Paulin: We, among others, have seen in coronary angiograms the effect of direct intra-arterial application of vasodilators. Nitroglycerine in the normal coronary circulation widens the epicardially located and therefore angiographically demonstrable arteries to a considerable degree. From this finding I would not like to make any specific conclusion concerning the effect upon the coronary circulation because I do not think that angiography is a good method to show an increase in flow, which can and has been shown by other methods. We widened the arteries pharmacologically in order to obtain additional proof that the coronary arteries are normal, i.e. could one observe that the arteries widened, they could not be stiff or sclerotic. In cooperation with Dr. Varnauskas we have also used other stimuli such as hypoxia and we were able to show vasodilation in these circumstances.

Werkö: Didn't you also use blood pressure elevating drugs or were they depressants?

Paulin: We observed in the cases which showed marked vasodilatation, a considerable drop of the aortic pressure.

Werkö: Have you had any experience with drugs, Dr. Bruschke?

Bruschke: We have given a large number of cases nitroglycerine during catheterization and we always saw a dilatation of the coronary arteries after the administration of that drug, but not of the pathological lesions. It, therefore, sometimes makes the diagnosis easier, because it is easier to see the difference between the lesion and normal vessels. We have never seen real lesions dilate with nitroglycerine.

Werkö: In summation, we could say that it is possible to demonstrate that the coronary arteries dilate under the influence of certain substances, but it is impossible with the method to say if the blood flow increases or not. This leads us to the following important question: Could you use coronary angiography to see whether the coronary circulation is improved by surgical means, as in the Vineberg Procedure or other cardiac revascularization procedures?

Lichtlen: We should do as many studies as possible in the patients who underwent surgery. Mainly the group from Cleveland has shown that after the Vineberg Procedure you really can see beautiful filling of the distal vessels in a functioning implant. However, we are still faced with the question whether the coronary flow has really increased or not. It is very helpful to have coronary angiography in these patients but it does not take you any further. It just shows you that the implant is open. On the other hand, in direct coronary surgery, when the surgeon has done a by-pass or a path graft, then, if you see that the vessel is open, it is a very important observation indicating that blood flow is restored. I do not know if it is so important after a Vineberg Procedure.

Werkö: It is quite clear that what you can do with angiography is to demonstrate the anatomy of the coronary arterial circulation and not its physiology.

Finally we should have a few words about the complications seen when this method is used. While discussing this, we should perhaps answer one of the questions that has been submitted to us here. Who should perform coronary angiography, the radiologist, cardiologist or both together?

Bruschke: That is a very difficult question to answer. We have only followed the selective method of Mason Sones in a series of 600 cases. As far as mortality is concerned, we had only one patient who died following the procedure. This was a man with very severe coronary sclerosis and a badly contracting left ventricle. He tolerated the procedure well, but the following day he became decompensated and died five days later because of cardiac decompensation. It is dubious whether there is a direct association here or not. The other complications that we have seen were myocardial infarction, arrhythmias, cerebral complications and thrombosis of the brachial artery. One patient developed myocardial infarction during catheterization. This was probably due to a dissection of the right coronary artery. His clinical picture was remarkable asymptomatic and he made an uneventful recovery and returned to his normal work. Four patients developed ventricular fibrillation and all of these patients could be easily defibrillated. In three cases there was ventricular asystole which necessitated a short period of external cardiac massage. In all of the patients who had the arrhythmias, it was possible to proceed with the catheterization and to complete the procedure. It was never necessary to terminate the procedure after recovery from the arrhythmias. In 200 cases, including the above cases with arrhythmias, we have done enzyme studies and ECG follow-ups. Apart from the one patient who developed myocardial infarction, these studies have always been negative. We feel that this is an indication that the procedure is quite harmless, generally speaking. We have unfortunately had two cases of cerebral vascular accident. In both instances the recovery was quite satisfactory. Early in our series, we saw signs of insufficiency of the brachial artery in about 5% of our cases. We changed our technique of arterial cut-down later in the series and this complication dropped to below 2%.

Practically all of the symptoms of brachial artery insufficiency spontaneously disappeared after a few months. In only two cases was surgical intervention necessary. To sum up our major complications, we had one death, one myocardial infarction, two cerebral vascular accidents and two arterial complications which necessitated surgery. This is a total of six complications in a three years' series of 600 cases or an incidence of 1%.

Paulin: In answer to your question 'Who should perform the coronary arteriography' I would like to state that naturally the person who is most familiar with the technique should do it.

Concerning complications during coronary arteriography one must divide the material into non-selective and selective examinations. We have mainly used what we think is a less complicated technique in almost 700 cases. We have not had any direct and immediate major complication such as fatality, ventricular fibrillation or other long lasting severe impairments of vital functions. We have, of course, followed our patients and it is for natural reasons very difficult to evaluate the results and to draw the correct conclusions. We have had one patient who died in sudden death – probably in cardiac arrhythmia – exactly two days after the uneventful coronary arteriogram. This patient was a very advanced atherosclerotic case and it is impossible to attribute the event to the angiographic procedure with certainty. Again we did not observe any fatality during the same day of the angiographic procedure.

As far as damage to the myocardium is concerned during the more than 700 non-selective angiograms we have had two patients in which we suspected a myocardial infarction after the coronary arteriogram. The patients had some chest pain some hours after the examination and the enzyme reactions were slightly increased. From a clinical point of view these findings had to be considered as questionable myocardial infarctions.

A complication which caused us more trouble, was local damage of the arteries at the site of catheter introduction. This initiated a more precise supervision and registration of post catheter abnormalities in our institution. We found that platelet aggregation at the catheter wall and a strip-off effect when the catheter is removed was the main reason for these arterial thrombotic obstructions. We have tried successfully to prevent these complications by treating our patients with Macrodex infusion prophylactically. Not any complication of this kind was observed in more than 80 pretreated patients.

A direct comparison with our selective examinations is not possible. We perform this technique on specific indications only and our own experience with this technique is therefore limited. We have had one clear myocardial infarction and one suspected infarction among the 25 selective examinations during the last year. No other major complications were noted. In my opinion there is little doubt that the mechanical interference of the catheter with the coronary artery wall and the injection of very high concentrated contrast material must subject the patient to a higher stress and hazard than the non-selective examination.

Lichtlen: In 350 patients, we saw one major incident with ventricular fibrillation. This was a patient with a small right coronary artery which was surely plugged during the injection. He had a small infarction and ventricular fibrillation one hour afterwards but this was easely defibrillated. He left the hospital three weeks later.

We had about a one to two percent incidence of problems with the brachial arteries. There were three patients who required surgery on their brachial arteries. We saw no other major complications.

Werkö: I think that the question of complications could be narrowed down to the statement that this is not an innocuous procedure. Some myocardial damage may be produced, especially with the selective techniques. You must be very alert to the periferal arterial damage which has a much higher incidence than has been earlier suspected. We should take steps to prevent any arterial damage to the peripheral circulation. Dr. Paulin's statement that the one who is familiar with the technique and on whom you can rely should perform coronary angiography is the correct one.

We will now turn this discussion to a consideration of other diagnostic methods. Dr. Hugenholtz will discuss the evaluation of left ventricular function by catheterization methods.

Hugenholtz: see original text, page 176.

Werkö: Thank you very much for a nice demonstration of a very difficult subject. This leads us directly to the question of exercise findings. I now ask Dr. Lichtlen to tell us something about his experience on the hemodynamics of the left ventricle during exercise.

Lichtlen: The techniques shown by Dr. Hugenholtz are very interesting, but not yet adapted to daily routine. We are performing angiograms in every patient undergoing catheterisation, but to get good volume studies you have to achieve left ventriculograms without any extrasystoles, which is not so easy to do in these patients. We therefore still think that exercise is a good way to get a closer look at the hemodynamics. We have learned that when exercising patients with coronary disease you must also look at their left ventricular anatomy, because LV hemodynamics are influenced not only by ischaemia during exercise, but also by left ventricular alterations due to previous myocardial infarctions.

We divided our coronary patients according to their left ventricular anatomy as demonstrated by angiography: patients with a normal LV, those with LV wall dyskinesia resp. incomplete contractions and those with LV aneurysms. A typical example of a 52 years old patient with a normal left ventricle is presented. He suffered from severe angina pectoris for at least six months. In systole, the left ventricle showed normal contractions. There was a complete obstruction of the posterolateral branch of the left circumflex, the distal portion being filled from the right coronary artery. The most important point to be made is that in spite of a normal left ventricle there was an abnormal increase of LV enddiastolic pressure from 13 to 32 mm Hg, whereas stroke work and systolic ejection rate increased in the normal way. At the same time an elevation of the ST-segments were observed and the patient developped angina three minutes after beginning exercise. This is also an important point. In every case studied, enddiastolic pressure rose much earlier than angina pectoris occurred, resp. the increase of enddiastolic pressure – usually beginning 10 to 20 sec. after the onset of exercise – preceeded angina pectoris by 2 to 3 minutes, and had reached its maximal level before angina developped.

An identical behaviour was seen in patients with LV dyskinesia resp. incomplete contractions of the apical area and/or the anterior LV wall. A typical example is given in a patient with a severe lesion of the left anterior descending branch. At LV angiography there was incomplete emptying of the apical area during systole. At exercise, LV enddiastolic pressure increased very markedly, whereas the rise of stroke work and systolic ejection rate was subnormal. The patient experienced also typical angina about four minutes after the begin of exercise with ST-depressions in the precordial leads. In this patient too, the abnormal increase of enddiastolic pressure began about 20 seconds after the onset of the study, much earlier than the manifestation of angina pectoris.

Patients with left ventricular aneurysms show a completely different behaviour. A typical example is given in a 58 years old patient with severe stenosis of his anterior descending branch. A large left ventricular aneurysm, including the apical area and the anterior wall was seen at angiography. LVEDP was elevated already at rest, stroke work, stroke volume systolic ejection rate and dp/dt being markedly reduced. During exercise, LVEDP rose to very high levels (40 mm Hg). Two points should be emphasized: in all patients with coronary disease, even in those with angiographically normal left ventricles, LVEDP increased significantly and abnormally during exercise. However, in coronary patients with a normal left ventricle all other parameters – stroke work, cardiac index, systolic ejection rate and dp/dt – behaved in a normal way. On the other hand, in patients with anterior wall aneurysms stroke work, stroke volume, systolic ejection rate and dp/dt were significantly reduced at rest and their increase during exercise was markedly smaller than in normal patients, patients with normal left ventricles or those with wall dyskinesia. One has to conclude that in these patients ventricular performance has to rely on the Starling Mechanism.

Werkö: We talked earlier about the correlation between or within groups. Is there any overlap between these different groups, or could you use any of these different variables to distinguish between individuals?

Lichtlen: There was some overlap between normals and those with wall dyskinesia, but the means were significantly different. There was no overlap between those with left ventricle aneurysms and those with wall dyskinesia or normal left ventricles.

Werkö: We will continue now with the electrocardiographic changes during and after exercising patients with ischaemic heart disease.

Schweizer: A. M. Master pointed out that in exercise electrocardiography it is not necessary to record during exercise as significant anomalies occurring during exercise are always also present after exercise. Other people have shown that this is not so. We have tried to define our position in this controversy using the information obtained during the Basle Study II.

The electrocardiographic investigation of the 4641 employees was carried out in the following way. *1.* 12 leads at rest, the patient in supine position. *2.* Lead v_5 at rest, the patient standing. *3.* Lead v_5 at 30 second intervals during 3 minutes, the patient performing Master's two-step-test. *4.* Leads I-III and v_4-v_6 at rest, immediately after exercise and at 1 minute intervals during 6 minutes, the patient in supine position. The ECG findings were rated 'positive' if the following changes were observed: 'J'-point and/or ST-segment more than 1 mm below the isoelectric line (q-q) + QX/QT ratio more than 0.5.

The results, shown in the table below, indicate that significant anomalies can occur during exercise only and that we would have missed 10.5% if we had recorded after exercise only. It may well be that the percentage will be even higher if more leads are used during exercise. Our position in the controversy mentioned is clear now. In exercise electrocardiography the number of false negative results can be reduced by recording during exercise. A further reduction might be achieved by increasing the work load. This is illustrated by the fact that in our study the heart rate during the Master two-step-test was below 120/min. in each age group except in young women (aged 15-34) in whom heart rates up to 126/min. were recorded.

Basle Study II. ECG evidence for coronary heart disease* during and after exercise (Master 180 SEC)

During exercise only	10.5%	
During and after exercise	80.8%	
After exercise only	8.7%	

* ST depression more than 1 mm QX/QT ratio more than 50%

Werkö: This leads us directly into the next phase of our discussion, namely, the use of the electrocardiogram during atrial pacing as compared with the results of exercise tests.

Roos: See original text, page 171.

Frick: From the presentation of Dr. Roos, it would appear that this is an ideal procedure. There are, however, some drawbacks, and I will illustrate some of my experiences with this procedure from two years ago. This is a patient with angina pectoris, who was paced three times with increased heart rates until the onset of pain. In these three consecutive pacing runs, this patient had angina pectoris at a very good threshold. We called this type 'Obeyers', because they obey our rules. As a rule, angina occurs when the oxygen consumption of the heart exceeds its supply, as Dr. Roos has said.

This is an example of a 'non-obeyer'. This patient has tension-time indices without pain up here, but with continued pacing he comes down here and has pain. They do not obey our nice rule. They are fortunately in the minority.

The majority of the patients obey the rule that the pain occurs when there is a threshold. Perhaps the explanation for the 'non-obeyers' lies in the heart volume response to this pacing. Heart volumes were taken by triggered x-rays during the various phases of pacing. The normal response is that when you pace, the heart volume goes down with increasing heart rate. With these 'non-obeyers' there is an unpredictable heart volume response. The tension-time index is actually a very rough estimate if you take it from the aortic pressure curve, because the tension is in the ventricular wall with which we are dealing. If there are pathological changes in the heart volume during pacing, then the tension-time index derived from the pressure curve does not tell the truth. The pacing technique can, however, be used to evaluate certain parameters. We know that in the past ten years, since the report of Muller and Rowrick in 1958, it has been generally accepted that during angina pectoris there is left ventricular failure. This view is based on the fact that they observed elevated left ventricular end-diastolic pressures during the angina induced by exercise. If we pace these patients with increasing heart rates and we take the capillary wedge pressure which, in the absence of mitral valve disease, reflects with some accuracy the left ventricular end-diastolic pressure, we see the onset of pain when the pressure is still in the normal range. If we continue the pacing in spite of the pain with increasing heart rates, we see that the end-diastolic pressure goes up. We think that the insufficiency or left ventricular failure is a function of the duration of ischaemia in the ventricle. The same phenomenon has been observed by the group in Bethesda. Using the same pacing procedure, they saw no rise in end-diastolic pressure during angina, but if you apply exercise, as Dr. Lichtlen did, we see an increase in the left ventricle end-diastolic pressure. I think that this is due to the fact that in coronary artery disease there is reduced compliance. The ventricle is fibrotic and during exercise we are increasing the inflow into that fibrotic ventricle. It reacts by raising the pressure. Dr. Lichtlen also said that the Starling system is evident in his experiments. I do not agree. I think that the rise in left ventricle end-diastolic pressure during exercise in these patients is not necessarily due to an increase in volume. It could as well be due to a non compliant left ventricle.

Hugenholtz: You are looking at the entire heart as a pump. As such, as has been made quite clear earlier in this discussion, you are considering several factors at the same time. If you do not know ahead of time what the pressure-volume characteristics are for that ventricle, you cannot derive any conclusions as you are doing here. You can say it is abnormal, but you do not know where the abnormality lies. If you say that there is some indication of failure, I would like to respond with the question: 'What is failure'? It is really a function of what you are attempting to find. If you want only to detect an abnormality that is fine. If you want to draw the conclusion, that this is an indication of bad muscle, I object because I do not think you have the facts.

Lichtlen: What are your thoughts about the changes in volume measurements and what are the implications of the contrast medium on volume, contractility etc? We know that the contrast medium has a very profound effect on left ventricular contractility.

Hugenholtz: They have these effects after about one second, that is after two or three beats, when it really reaches the coronaries.

Lichtlen: That is the time when you measure your volume.

Hugenholtz: No. We measure it right away, before it reaches the coronaries and has its profound effect. You can get in the first two or three beats a very good outline of the ventricle and obtain your data. This is not to say that there are not any side effects of the contrast medium. You do get an increased preloading and all sorts of other things. I do not think that we should go into the technical details of angiographic measurements at this time.

Werkö: This illustrates a very interesting fact. Ever since the time of Starling, as soon as anyone starts to say failure, everyone gets excited and tries to explain the nature of failure. You have supporters on the panel who would also like to know what failure really is.

We have heard a discussion which had the title: 'diagnostic methods in ischaemic heart disease'.

Only one diagnostic method has really been discussed and that was coronary angiography. We have heard about some other methods of evaluation of myocardial function. One very important fact that arose from this discussion is that we cannot diagnose coronary artery disease by indirect means. We can use all kinds of evidence and indices which point to the fact that there is a defect in the myocardium, but we must have much more information about the coronary arteries before we can say that what is wrong with the myocardium is due to coronary artery disease.

Earlier it was usual to diagnose positively aortic stenosis, pulmonary hypertensions, cardiomyopathies, etc. In the absence of such a diagnosis it was assumed that coronary artery disease was present, i.e. diagnosis by exclusion. We will still miss the right diagnosis in some cases. We must have more information about what is occurring in the coronary arteries in the living person before we can rely upon a few bits of indirect evidence to diagnose coronary artery disease. It has been said that the use of atrial pacing is like listening to the drummer instead of listening to the entire orchestra. If we are going to study coronary artery disease, ischaemic heart disease, and myocardial failure, then we do not only want to listen to the drummer or to the orchestra. We wish to know what the other musicians are doing and you may also wish to know about the performance of the conductor too.

THE PLACE OF SURGERY IN THE TREATMENT OF ISCHAEMIC HEART DISEASE

Å. SENNING

The first surgical intervention for angina pectoris was done more than 50 years ago, when Ionescu performed a sympathectomy to interrupt the sensitive and motoric cardia nerves. Since then a large number of surgical methods were tried to reduce the morbidity and mortality from coronary sclerosis, which in spite of improved medical treatment seems still to increase. Because of high mortality or dubious results in most of these earlier surgical methods it is understandable that many internists are still reluctant to refer the coronary patients to the surgeon.

But today there are some definite indications for surgery in coronary sclerosis: Let me illustrate it with an impressive case. A 54 years old man had in december 1968 an anterior wall infarction with a slow electrocardiographic regression. It followed a left heart failure making the patient unable to work. Then a typical angina pectoris occurred increasing to a decubital angina. The ECG in April 1969 still showed the picture of a subacute anterior wall infarction. The x-ray demonstrated an enlargement of the heart with suspected left ventricular aneurysm, that could be definitely demonstrated in the left ventriculogram. The aneurysm comprises the anterior wall, the apex and the distal part of the posterior wall. The affected area showed no contractions, contrasting with the good contractions in the other parts of the left ventricle. The injected contrast medium stayed for a long period of time in the left ventricle.

The left heart insufficiency is well explained by this ventricular aneurysm and the excision of this aneurysm is indicated. To clarify the cause of the anginal pains an additional selective coronary angiography according to Sones was made. It showed a complete stop in the descending branch of the left coronary artery corresponding to the aneurysmatic area. In the right coronary artery a practically complete stop was demonstrated 6 cm from its aortic origin.

It was judged advisable to correct the stenosis in the right coronary artery before excising the left ventricular aneurysm, because of the risk of an additional infarction in the area perfused by the right coronary artery.

The operation – end of April 1969 – consisted in an end-arterectomy of the short occlusion in the right coronary artery and in the closing of the artery by widening it with a saphenous vein patch-graft.

Only then the aneurysm comprising the anterior part of the left ventricular wall and the distal anterior part of the interventicular septum was excised. The opening of the right ventricle was sutured first and then the left ventricle was closed.

As soon as the non contracting left ventricular aneurysm had been excised, the heart took over the circulation. No signs of left ventricular failure remained and the patient is now back at work.

This case comprises the two ideal indications for surgery in ischaemic heart disease, namely occlusion of the right coronary artery and circumscript aneurysm of the anterior wall and apex of the left ventricle. The indication for direct coronary surgery is extremely difficult to make, as we know neither in advance the spontaneous course of the disease nor the long term results of surgical interventions. Of upper most importance for direct coronary surgery is a good coronary angiography and a case history with typical symptoms and signs of coronary insufficiency.

According to the experience of Sones with 10000 ciné-angiographies in 60% the right coronary artery is predominant. Correction of stenosis or occlusion in the right coronary artery within the 6 first centimeters is done relatively easy on the beating heart. Interventions on the left coronary artery on the other hand are technically more difficult and require the use of extracorporeal circulation with hypothermia.

There are four operative procedures of direct approach on coronary arteries:

Endarterectomy per se, endarterectomy with patch-grafting, by-pass-operations and coronary artery resection with grafting.

We don't use endarterectomy as such for two reasons: First of all the orifices of the small branches will be occluded when the intima of the main artery is excised and secondly the endarterectomised part of the vessel seems successively to resclerose. We prefer to do a very restricted endarterectomy, saving orifices of the branches, fixing it to the vessel wall. The artery is closed by widening it with a patch from the vena saphena magna taken above the medial malleolus. (fig. 1).

For bypass operations either the internal mammary artery can be used – as has been done experimentally by Gordon Murray and clinically tried in a few cases. Or one can take according to the method of Effler a piece of the saphenous vein from the malleolar region to perform a bypass with end-to-side anastomosis from the aorta to the coronary artery distal to the occlusion. (fig. 2). This technique seems to have some advantages in long stenosis, specially in the descending left coronary artery. The bypass procedure has a risk specially when used on the right coronary artery, as the vein may be elongated and kinked at the site of insertion. For an operation on the right coronary artery the patient is heparinized and connected to the heart lung machine, but without starting it. The artery is opened over the stenosis and a small plastic cannula is tightly inserted in the proximal and distal part as a temporary internal shunt. Only in one of our cases it was necessary to use the heart lung machine, because of weak cardiac action. Operations on the left coronary artery are always done in extracorporeal circulation, and additional hypothermia is applied to the heart with iced saline solution to interrupt the left coronary circulation for surgery without using an internal shunt, as the septal branches cannot be perfused by this method. The heart is kept in ventricular fibrillation, making exact suturing of the left coronary artery possible.

Since 1962 29 patients underwent direct coronary surgery in Zurich, 13 on the right, 13 on the left coronary vessel and 3 simultaneously on both arteries.

Table 1. Arteria coronaria dextra

	Nr.	Clin. good	Recurr.	Died
Endarterectomy +				
Patch graft	11	10	1*	—**
By pass	2	1	1	—
	13	11	2	—

* 1 Pat. reop.
** 1 Pat. died 7 yrs postop.

Surgery on the right coronary artery (table 1) consisted in 11 patients in end-arterectomy and venous patch-grafting, with ten good results and one recurrence of obstruction, that had to be reoperated. In two patients a venous bypass had been done from the aorta to the post-occlusion coronary artery with one good result and one postoperative thrombosis of the bypass.

13 patients were operated on the left coronary artery (table 2), four of them underwent endarterectomy and path-grafting in the anterior descending vessel.

Table 2. Arteria coronaria sinistra

	Nr.	Clin. good	Recurr.	Died
Endarterectomy +				
Patch graft				
Descend. a.	4	2	1*	1
Circ. a.	3	2		1
By pass				
Ao-Desc. a.	6	3		3
	13	7	1	5

* Reop.

Two of these are clinically good, one suffered a recurrence and was re-operated with good result. One patient died postoperatively. Three operations were done on the left circumflex artery, two with good results, one patient died. From six patients undergoing bypass operations for left coronary artery occlusion three died and three show clinically good results.

In three patients with severe stenosis in the left and right coronary artery, operations were performed simultaneously on both vessels, but all three patients died (Table 3).

Table 3. Two coronary arteries

	Nr.	Died
R. desc. sin. +	2	2
R. circ. sin.		
A. cor. dx. +	1	1
A. cor. sin.		
	3	3

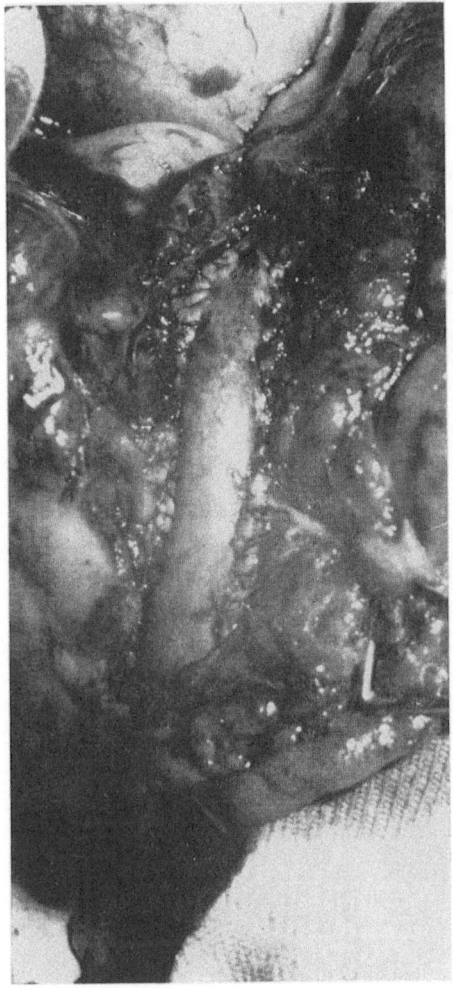

Fig. 1. Venous patch in right coronary artery.

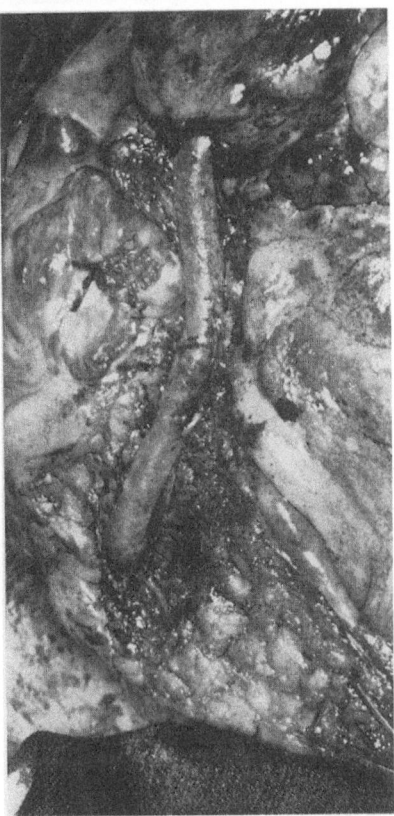

Fig. 2. Aorto-coronary saphenous vein graft bypassing stenosis of right coronary artery.

Summarising the results we note that all 13 patients undergoing direct surgery for right coronary artery occlusion survived, from 13 patients operated on the left coronary artery five died and all three patients operated simultaneously on both arteries did not survive the intervention.

With this experience in mind our indication for direct coronary surgery is as follows:

Interventions in patients with angina pectoris are done on the right coronary artery with severe localized stenosis or occlusion, if this vessel predominates in the blood supply to the heart. Secondly surgery is done on a stenosed right coronary artery, if the left coronary artery is stenosed as well and a filling of the left distal coronary artery occurs through good intercoronary anastomosis.

The more riskful operation on the left coronary artery is done only if direct surgery on the right side is impossible because of diffuse sclerosis and in cases, where the stenosis is located within the first four centimeters of the left coronary artery or its two main branches.

The most popular method for myocardial revascularisation is for the moment the operation according to Vineberg. The whole length of the internal mammary artery is dissected and the distal end is implanted in a tunnel of about 4 cm of length that is made in the left ventricular myocardium.

Sometimes the two mammary arteries are used either for implantation in the right and left ventricular myocardium, or for revascularisation of the left myocardium along the circumflex and the descending branch of the left coronary artery.

The reason, why these implanted arteries do not thrombose, has not yet been fully understood. Very shortly after implantation there cannot be any blood flow through this artery until the first collaterals have been formed between this artery and the small coronary arterioles. In our own experimental investigations we have shown that a perfusion of this artery immediately after insertion with a flow of three to five ml per minute causes a severe myocardial haematoma with ventricular fibrillation. After 3 to 6 months a significant development of collaterals from the implanted vessel to the coronary artery has been demonstrated. It is therefore understandable, that in the very first few months after the operation the incidence of new infarction is as high as in a not operated control group, but according to the results of Dwight Harken – including postoperative mortality and infarction – a Vineberg operated series showed significantly better result after 1½ years postoperatively than a comparable group with conservative medical treatment only. Effler and his coworkers in Cleveland have recatheterized 124 patients one year after a Vineberg operation and the coronary angiographies showed an open mammary artery in all but 8 cases. In 53 of the operated patients the clinical improvement was considered good, and in another 16 patients the improvement was classified as fair. According to Effler the ideal patient for a Vineberg operation has angina pectoris and stenosis of at least 90% either in the descending left coronary artery or in a large diagonal branch with already existing intercoronary anastomosis. The area for arterial implantation has to have normal thickness of the myocardial wall with good contractility. It is useless to make an implantation in a non contracting myocardial area. The maximal blood flow through an implanted artery has been measured with 50-60 ml/min. This flow seems not to change under physiological stimuli as exercises or under medicaments. In Zurich we have been reluctant to the Vineberg operation and have done only 21 (table 4) cases.

Table 4. Revascularisation after Vineberg

	Nr.	Op. results	Clin. +	±	?	Died
Implantation of one mamm. art.	6	6	3	2	1	0
Implantation of two mamm. art.	12	12	4	8		0
Vineberg L +Patchgraft R	2	1			1	1
Vineberg L + Patch A. cor. dext. + sin.	1				1	
Total	21	19	7	2	10	2

+ = good
± = not improved
? = Observation time not sufficient

Two of these patients died during surgery, apparently of myocardial ischaemia. Direct coronary surgery was attempted in these cases without success. Another patient died within a week after the operation. Only four of the Vineberg patients have been controlled postoperatively with angiograms, all 4 implants are open. Seven patients showed four months postoperatively a clinical improvement, in two the conditions remained unchanged. In one of the unimproved patients the post-operative angiography showed an open internal mammary artery, but there was no formation of anastomosis to the coronary vessels. Our own experience with this operation is yet too small to allow any definite conclusion, but because of the good results reported by several Ameri-can authors we are decided to proceed at the Vineberg operation in some selected cases and to evaluate this method further with a very precise follow up. This operation is definitely contra-indicated in cases with severe cardiac insufficiency, in patients with a recent infarction and in those with another non treatable systemic disease.

VENTRICULAR ANEURYSM

Ventricular myocardial aneurysm developing after an ischaemic heart disease has a relatively poor prognosis. Surgery is indicated in aneurysms that cause left heart failure and in cases with multiple embolization. Relatively often an aneurysmatic myocardial wall ruptures during the first week after the infarction, very seldom at a later date. A rapid growth as a sign of imminent rupture is a clear indication for surgery. Recurring episodes of tachy-arrhythmia may force us as well to resect the aneurysm. The Cleveland group has done around 200 ventricular aneurysmectomies with a mortality of less than 13%. Heimbecker in Toronto resected a great number of ventricular myo-cardial aneurysm in the apical area with only one death. The resection of an aneurysm located in the base of the left ventricle, that is the area of the most important myocardial contraction has a much higher risk. In Zurich only four cases have been referred to surgery. They have all been operated upon with good results. The ordinary chronic aneurysm is really easy to resect and as we do leave a margin of fibrotic area a safe suture can be accomplished. Immediately after resection of the non contracting aneurysmatic area the heart shows again a very strong action with improvement of the circulation.

The exact place of surgery in acute myocardial infarction has not yet been established. Surgery may seem useful as the Beck's trigger zone would be abolished and the relatively stiff gangrenous myocardial wall would after resection no longer impeed the contraction. In some few cases of acute infarction resection has been done for instance by Heimbecker, but the mortality rate has been relatively high. In acute infarction it is very difficult to detect the borderline in between definitely dead myocardium and parts where a recovery of the muscle might be possible.

ACUTE SEPTUM RUPTURES

A patient survives relatively seldom a rupture of an infarcted interventricular septum. In some few cases surgical closure of the rupture has been successful, when performed immediately. Several patients that survived the rupture were successfully corrected at a later date. Our only attempt of surgery in a severely ill patient with acute rupture of the interventricular septum ended with a failure, as the patient died with signs of a new infarction.

Most cardiologists and even cardiac surgeons are still reluctant to surgery for ischaemic heart disease. Quite a different attitude is seen in some places in the United States, as for exemple in the Cleveland Clinic. This slide shows their statistics of 2000 operations for ischaemic heart disease performed till May 1968. 1600 consisted in Vineberg operations, the other 400 were direct interventions on coronary arteries and resection of ventricular myocardial aneurysms.

We know that surgery will not cure the coronary disease, but it can in some selected cases dramatically improve a patient's situation. A much more frequent use of coronary angiography is mandatory, specially in young patients with angina pectoris or after infarction. A careful selection of patients for these newer and improved surgical interventions will give better clinical results.

To summarize we think that surgery seems to have its given place in the following situations of ischaemic heart disease:
1. Direct interventions on coronary artery in isolated stenosis in the proximal 6-8 cm in a predominant right coronary artery;
2. in occlusion of a right coronary artery in combination with stenosis of the left coronary artery;
3. in stenosis in the proximal 4 cm of the left coronary artery branches, when inoperable lesions of the right coronary artery exist.

4. A Vineberg operation is indicated in diffuse coronary artery sclerosis, specially of the left descending branch, if the myocardial contraction is good and intercoronary anastomosis are present.
5. Aneurysmectomy is indicated in left ventricular myocardial aneurysm in the apical area, when causing left heart failure, and if there is adequate blood supply to the contracting myocardium through the right coronary artery.

DISCUSSION

Dubost: Concerning the Vineberg procedure, I agree with Dr. Senning's position completely. We do not trust it despite the fact that several fine teams have shown very interesting improvements and angiograms after the operation. For a long time, we have tried to do something for anginal pain included resection of nerves, ligation of arteries and putting talcumpowder into the pericardium, and we have observed very dramatic improvements. I saw a patient about 12 years ago on whom I was able to make only a small cutaneous incision because he was in such a poor condition that it was impossible to do anything else. He has remained cured since that time and all doctors familiar with this disease have seen many such cases. Since we cannot scientifically determine the degree of improvement after surgery, it will always be a subjective decision.

There is another treatment for coronary disease that has not been mentioned, namely, heart transplantation. This is not a simple procedure nor a simple decision, but it can be chosen if all other surgical procedures are of no use. In our three cases of heart transplantation, all of the patients were bedridden with intractable heart failure and intractable anginal pain. The best cardiologists in France were unable to improve their condition. That was the reason why those patients were referred to us. Two of them have survived the operation; the first one is now 13 months and the second one is now six months after surgery. These are acceptable figures.

Concerning ventricular aneurysms I'd like to present a few cases. When you open this aneurysm the wall is very thin and many clots are sometimes present. After resection of the fibrosis it is sufficient to close the ventricle with two pledgets of teflon. After this procedure. as Dr. Senning did mention, the contraction of the left ventricle is very much improved.

Turning our attention to that very interesting disease, interventricular defect after myocardial infarction, I think that the failures of the previous surgical procedures are due to the approaches which have been used. The majority of surgeons have used the right ventricular approach. This is a very difficult one. Since the defect lies at the apex of the heart, it is very difficult to expose it from the right side because of the many muscles which are hiding the defect. On the contrary, if you approach it from the left ventricle, the ventricular defect is easily seen and it is not hidden by the chordae. You see the defect very close to the apex of the heart. It is very easy to suture your prosthesis in this way with separate stitches which perfectly occlude the defect. This is a very simple operation, since at the end you can resect a part of the left ventricle to reduce fibrosis. We have used this procedure on six patients and have lost only one. The problem is to know when to operate; immediately after the infarction, during the first days, or later on when the edges of the defect become fibrosed. It is better for the surgeon to operate when the edges are fibrosed, but in a recent case we operated four days after infarction because the patient was in intractable heart failure. This was a surgical success. We are enthusiastic about this approach and we think it could increase the patient's chances of survival.

Direct coronary artery surgery can be done in a peculiar disease due to the blocking of the coronary artery ostium by syphilis. This disease is not very common, but it gives to the surgeon his best successes. The disease involves one or both of the coronary ostia and very often leads to modification of the aortic leaflets with slight degree of aortic insufficiency. This is, in fact, not a true disease of the coronary arteries, but only of the aorta. The ostia are blocked but the trunk and branches are perfectly normal. This explains why the surgical successes are quite good. It is a very simple procedure to by-pass the circulation, open the aorta, to resect the thickened portions of the aortic intima that blocks the ostia. Occasionally, the coronary ostium is so obstructed that you must dissect the trunk free and trace its lock to the aorta in order to find the true area of the ostium. The first patient on whom I did this procedure in 1959 is still alive and has had no attacks of angina since the surgery. He is perfectly normal. We have operated on five other patients. Two of them received a Starr valve because of a high degree of aortic insufficiency. One of these has died after surgery because of emboli to his brain.

In February, I have had the opportunity of operating a case of atherosclerotic aneurysm of the right coronary artery in a woman, 37 years old.

She was complaining of angina and the coronarography showed a huge aneurysm involving the two-thirds of the length of the right coronary artery.

The operation consisted in the resection of the aneurysm, the restauration of the continuity of the artery being assured by an autogenous saphenous vein graft bridging the two ends of the artery.

The post-operative coronarography showed a perfect patency of the graft and a normal visualization of the distal end of the coronary artery.

Finally, I would like to show you one example of the aorto-coronary by-pass technique, using a venous saphenous autologous graft between the aorta and one of the coronary arteries.

There is a case of a complete block in the descending interventricular artery. You can see the saphenous graft between the aorta and the distal part of the descending interventricular artery.

We believed, from the x-ray that showed only a limited narrowing of the artery, that we would have a very simple operation. In fact, the descending interventricular artery was quite bad. We dissected it free almost to the apex of the heart and it was quite bad, almost all along the way. We did however perform and end-to-side anastomosis under these poor conditions. This patient is doing well and has had no pain to date. This by-pass procedure, as Senning, has mentioned, is probably the best one that we can do and which we can offer to our patients. It will probably replace the Vineberg procedure in the future.

But we feel we must be very careful about the estimation of the results obtained by this technique. For the moment, we estimate that the aorto coronary venous shunt should remain an experimental procedure, reserved to few cases, well investigated and whose results should be judged only by the medical team.

Duchosal: Our surgeon in Geneva, Professor Hahn, has operated on 17 cases of coronary occlusion. He believes that the best procedure is to put a graft from the aorta to the distal part of the coronary. He does not consider too much about the length of the graft and has done by-passes in to 14 centimeters in length. He has lost two of these patients; one, three weeks after surgery due to splanchnic bleeding and the second a few days after surgery due to insufficiently evaluated aortic incompetence. It is his opinion that these anastomatic by-passes from the aorta to the distal coronary, whatever the distance involved, are very rewarding. Fourteen patients were operated on their right coronary arteries and one on the left decending anterior artery. These procedures were not particularly difficult and have given very few post-operative complications.

Hellerstein: The institution that I am associated with is about three-quarters of a mile geographically and about ten miles philosophically from the Cleveland Clinic. It is, however, true that in Cleveland, whether at the University Hospital or Western Reserve University or the Cleveland Clinic, implantation of internal mammary arteries will produce a significant improvement of regional blood flow in 60 to 70 percent of the cases. When you challenge such patients with exercise or pacing, to produce angina pectoris, as shown by Gorlin, there is decreased lactic acid production.

On many occassions, I have approached Dr. Effler about the development of a good control series which is obviously needed today. He replied that we must answer the basic question: 'can we improve regional blood flow in a deficient area?' There is reasonable evidence that we can do this. However, I would second the suggestion that since you are on this side of the Atlantic Ocean, before you get involved and do as many cases as the Cleveland Clinic, you must set up a control series with rigid criteria. You should not have the surgeons involved in the post-operative evaluation of the patients because their enthusiasm may be reflected in the results that they report.

I would like to ask Dr. Dubost and Dr. Senning whether they are willing to do something even more exciting? We are seeing patients with acute myocardial infarction within a few minutes of its onset when they have monophasic s-TT elevations. Are you willing to go in to relieve the obstruction, and if not, why not?

Senning: It all depends on how early you refer the patient to me. We have done studies in dogs and have shown that if you clamp the coronary artery for more than one hour, it is difficult to get this myocardium back. If you clamp the coronary artery for more than two hours, more than 50% never work well again in that area. After three hours, none of the animals survived but they all died of myocardial infarction. We therefore, should have the patient within one hour of infarction.

Dubost: It would be possible to put a tube into the coronary artery and to suck out the clot. That would be better than resection.

Dubost: What is the action of Propanolol in angina, and what is your opinion on the electric stimulation of the carotid sinus in decreasing anginal pain?

Hellerstein: Propanolol is a very fine drug which has a negative inotropic effect, it slows the heart rate. There have been various reports on its effect in reducing angina pectoris and it may objectively improve cardiovascular function. It surely does relieve angina in about 60 to 70 percent of cases. It does increase the end-diastolic pressure and is therefore dangerous to use in certain patients with posterior wall infarction with bradycardia. Nevertheless, it is a major advance in the treatment of symptomatic angina. Dr. Gorlin claims that the mortality rate of a series of patients treated over several years is lower than those receiving Propanolol. This is related to the comment that I made yesterday. The consequence of coronary disease may be rhythmic and have nothing to do with the coronary disease itself. Apparently, the β-adrenergic blockers does do something to the epinephrine related arhythmias. In reference to the carotid sinus stimulation that Braunwald is doing, for some reason we have not seen a patient in which we thought it necessary to put in an electrical pacemaker to stimulate the carotid sinus area. Therefore, we have not used that equipment.

CHAPTER IV

ISCHAEMIC HEART DISEASE AND PHYSICAL ACTIVITY

CENTRAL HEMODYNAMIC EFFECTS OF PHYSICAL TRAINING IN HEALTH AND IN ISCHAEMIC HEART DISEASE

M. H. FRICK

After almost 50 years of study on the haemodynamic effects of physical training in normal subjects it would seem clear that this problem is largely solved. However, when interest arose in the circulatory effects of physical activity in coronary artery disease (CAD) it appeared that the data on responses in normal subjects were insufficient in many respects. One of the drawbacks is that the normal series are strongly biased by young subjects in the age considerably lower than the patients with CAD. While it can be anticipated that the training responses are largely the same over a rather wide age range, this is not necessarily true, and, in fact, may be quite different in many respects. Furthermore, many of the 'normal series' are composed of comparisons between athletes and sedentary subjects, a design not necessarily revealing the effect of training.

Knowledge on the haemodynamic determinants of myocardial oxygen consumption is relatively recent, and many studies on normal subjects, especially many of the early ones, have not been designed to give this sort of information and the data are not amenable to a retrospective scrutiny in this respect. The data on normal responses to physical training, collected into table I, are subject to all the above stated handicaps.

As is evident from the table, many aspects crucial for the understanding of responses at functional level are unknown in normal subjects. This is apparently due to reluctancy to place catheters in ventricles especially when physical exercise is applied simultaneously. As a result the question of 'contractility' of the normal trained heart is unanswered. This item combined with the behavior of the size of left ventricle during exercise is in key position when the economy of the trained heart is evaluated.

Table 1. Effects of physical training on central circulation in healthy subjects and in patients with coronary artery disease

	At rest Normals	At rest Coronary	Upon exertion Normals	Upon exertion Coronary
Heart rate	— or + —	+ —	—	—
Stroke volume	+ or + —	+ —	+	+
Cardiac output	+ —	+ —	+ — or —	+ — or —
Aortic pressure	+ —	+ —	+ —	+ —
Pulmonary art. pressure	+ —	+ —	+ —	+ —
Heart volume	+ or + —	+ —	?	?
Rate-pressure products	— + —	— + —	—	—
Right ventricular end-diastolic pressure	+ —	+	+	+
Left ventricular end-diastolic pressure	+ —	+	+	+ —
Right ventricular function	?	+	?	+
Left ventricular function	?	?	?	+

Abbreviations: — = decrease, + = increase, + — = no change, ? = not known.

The data on patients with CAD come from few small series and must be considered preliminary. In addition many aspects still remain to be explored to complete the picture. Especially the crucial question of enhanced coronary collateral development as a result of training must be solved.

REFERENCES

1. Bevegård, S., A. Holmgren & B. Jonsson, *Acta physiol. scand.* 57, 26 (1963).
2. Freedman, M. E., G. L. Snider, P. Brostoff, S. Kimelblot & L. N. Katz, *J. Appl. Physiol.* 8, 37 (1955).
3. Frick, M. H., A. Konttinen & H. S. S. Sarajas, *Amer. J. Cardiol.* 12, 142 (1963).
4. Frick, M. H., *Amer. J. Cardiol.* 22, 417 (1968).
5. Frick, M. H. & M. Katila, *Circulation* 37, 192 (1968).
6. Hanson, J. S., B. S. Tabakin, A. M. Levy & W. Nedde, *Circulation* 38, 783 (1968).
7. Hellerstein, H. K., T. R. Hornsten, A. Goldbarg, A. G. Burlando, E. H. Friedman, E. Z. Hirsch & S. Marik, *Canad. Med. Ass. J.* 96, 758 (1967).
8. Mitchell, J. H., 18th Annual Scientific Session, *Amer. Coll. Cardiol.* (1969).
9. Varnauskas, E., H. Bergman, P. Houk & P. Björntorp, *Lancet* 2, 8 (1966).

PERIPHERAL HAEMODYNAMIC EFFECTS OF PHYSICAL TRAINING IN HEALTH AND IN ISCHAEMIC HEART DISEASE

E. VARNAUSKAS

Discussing at length the cardiac performance in health and in ischaemic heart disease and how this performance is modified by physical training it is appropriate for a moment to consider other sections of the cardiovascular system than the heart pump itself.

The primary function of the circulation is to furnish an adequate blood flow through the tissue capillaries. In essence all other parts of the cardiovascular system including the heart subserve the regulation of capillary flow. Many complex changes in the functionally different cardiovascular sections must occur and must be integrated for example in heavy muscular exercise in order that oxygenated blood is delivered at a suitable perfusion pressure to the muscle capillaries. If this integrated control fails in any of its links, this may derange the performance completely. A strenuous physical training may modify some mechanisms of this control as suggested by earlier studies in this field.

Unfortunately the information is very limited concerning the effect of physical training on the integrated control of the capillary blood flow in the tissues. Measurements of regional flows are fewer than the few studies on total haemodynamics. Much of the knowledge about the regulatory mechanisms of the peripheral circulation while exposed to physical training must be therefore to a large extent deduced from the indirect measurements in man or from the animal experiments.

In the first part of my presentation I will discuss some aspects of peripheral circulation based on indirect evidences. In the second part I will present to you pre- and post-training results from a study in progress. This study comprises measurements of femoral muscle blood flow during a standard exercise on bicycle ergometer and measurements of enzymatic activity in the biopsies of the femoral muscle obtained from the other leg.

Table 1. The effect of physical training in four studies

+ = *increase*   — = *decrease*   NS = *no significant change*   IHD = ischaemic heart disease

	Normal			IHD	
	Max. work	Submax. work		Submax. work	
	(4) sitting	(4) sitting	(6) supine	(5) sitting	(7) supine
Oxygen uptake	+	—		NS	NS
Cardiac output	+	—	NS	—	NS
Arterio-venous oxygen difference	+	+		+	NS
Mixed venous oxygen saturation	—	—		—	NS
Arterial blood pressure	+	+	NS	—	NS

In table 1 a summary of the four studies (2 from Helsinki, 1 from Stockholm and 1 from Gothenburg) on the effect of physical training in health and in ischaemic heart disease is presented. The methodological similarities and differences between the investigations may play a significant role in comparing the results. These studies have been chosen because of the following reasons.

They all are longitudinal investigations. Each man serves as his own control. The length of the training period was similar in all studies. Bicycle ergometer has been used by all groups to perform the tests.

These studies split into two groups with respect to the body position in which the measurements were performed. The two Helsinki studies 3 and 4 were done in *supine* position while the Stockholm and Gothenburg studies, 1 and 2 respectively, were performed with the subjects in *sitting* position. This allows the assessment of the body position effect on the results of physical training.

Furthermore it must be remembered that the number of subjects studied in each investigation is comparatively small, which actually reflects the general situation in the literature up to day. This may have some influence on the statistical interpretation. Our conclusions from these studies probably must be more hesitant than we may wish.

It is by now well documented that the physical training results in an increased maximal aerobic power or maximal aerobic capacity in healthy subjects. This is represented in table 1 by the oxygen uptake during maximal work. It is quite understandable that such information is lacking concerning patients with ischaemic heart disease.

On the submaximal exercise levels the post-training oxygen uptake tends to decrease, probably as a result of improved mechanical efficiency. The decrease is not a consistant finding.

The post-training maximal cardiac output is augmented in normal subjects.

During a given constant submaximal exercise level the cardiac output is reduced both in normal subjects and in coronary patients in the two studies performed in sitting position while it is unchanged in studies performed in supine position.

Whether or not the body position alone explains these differences, is difficult to assess. In study 4 two loads of exercise were used and during the first load which was less heavy than the second a significant decrease of cardiac output was recorded. During the second work load there was a substantial but not significant increase of cardiac output. The general changes during exercise have been interpreted as not significant. No such discrepancies in the post-training cardiac output values can be found in study 1 in which also several steps of exercise were performed in sitting position.

The arterio-venous oxygen difference in sitting position increases after the training consistantly while it remains unchanged if measured in the supine position in the coronary patients. The data from the study 3 are not available.

These changes and lack of changes in arterio-venous oxygen differences respectively are entirely dependent on the behaviour of the oxygen saturation in the mixed venous blood. No changes in arterial blood are found at submaximal exercise level. The mixed venous blood is more desaturated with oxygen after the physical training than before according to the measurements made in sitting position but it is unchanged in measurements obtained in supine position.

The intra-arterial recordings of the blood pressure exhibit most interesting changes following physical training. There is a slight but significant blood pressure increase in normal subjects during maximal and submaximal work levels, while the blood pressure in patients with ischaemic heart disease shows a significant decrease when recordings are made in sitting position. The two supine studies disclose no significant changes in blood pressure following physical training. These differences in blood pressure behaviour are difficult to explain at the present time.

Thus, from the data of this table can be concluded that the effect of physical training on the total blood flow to the tissues and on the oxygen exchange between blood and tissues as visualized by the mixed venous oxygen content is principally the same in health and in ischaemic heart disease, provided the comparisons are made between methodologically comparable investigations. A probable exception to this rule consists of the blood pressure response.

Let us now examine possible control mechanisms of the blood flow changes and those of the mixed venous saturation changes obtained in sitting position (studies 1 and 2). Study 3 is in this respect lacking some very necessary information. This makes the comparisons incomplete between the studies 3 and 4.

First of all the possibility of a placebo effect must be considered. Anxiety and nervous tension which may be present in connection with the first investigation can disappear during the subsequent period of training and repeated measurements. This might be particularly apparent in patients with ischaemic heart disease. Establishing close and confident patient-doctor-relationship may change the pattern of haemodynamic response to exercise by changing the sympathomimetic tone.

A separate study was performed in our laboratory (1) in which 10 coronary patients suffering severe and frequent attacks of angina pectoris were investigated before and after one month of placebo medication and frequent visits to the doctor. A small general tendency towards a more hypokinetic circulation was noticable in the post-training results. However, the only significant change was found in the heart and in the product of heart rate and systolic blood pressure. Both these variables decreased by 8 and 12 per cent respectively while all the others including cardiac output and arterio-venous oxygen difference showed no significant changes. The placebo effect is thus comparatively small and essentially limited to the lowering of the heart rate. This implies in turn that an estimation of the physical training effect from changes in heart rate alone can sometimes be affected by considerable pitfalls. This effect may then be overestimated.

From the view point of the peripheral circulation there are at least two alternatives to explain the post-training reduction of cardiac output and the reduction of oxygen saturation in the mixed venous blood.

ALTERNATIVE 1

The physical training may alter arterial blood flow distribution to the regional circulations or to the different capillary sections within the same regional circulation, for example working muscle.

The mixed venous blood is a mixture of many end-capillary bloods which may vary widely in composition depending on the oxygen uptake/blood perfusion ratios in the individual capillary sections. This situation is analogous to that in the lung, in which the composition of pulmonary venous blood may be dependent on the distribution of various ratios.

It can be assumed that the physical training improves the blood distribution so that the previously overperfused capillary sections may afterwards receive less blood flow allowing the oxygen uptake/blood perfusion ratios to approach unity. In other words, the perfusion of the capillaries would become more adequately adjusted to the oxygen needs in various vascular sections. All unnecessary and luxurious perfusion would be then eliminated. This type of changes takes place in the lungs during exercise. The validity of the assumption that the physical training is accompanied by such changes in the peripheral circulation is not as yet established.

ALTERNATIVE 2

Enhanced oxygen extraction from the capillary blood by the tissue cells, preferably mitochondria of muscle cells may take place following physical training. Increased oxygen extraction capacity may then have consequences on the amount of the capillary blood flow needed to supply tissues with the same oxygen amount; same amount of oxygen can be extracted from less volume of arterial blood per unit time.

To investigate the validity of this hypothesis a following pilot study was carried out.

Five male and two female medical students in the age of 20 to 25 years were submitted to strenuous physical training on bicycle ergometer on the average three times a week during a time period of six weeks.

Before the training was started and at the end of the training period a needle biopsy from vastus lateralis of the quadriceps muscle was taken and the measurement of succinic dehydrogenase activity was performed.

Muscle blood flow was also measured in the same muscle as the biopsy but on the other leg using Xenon clearance technique. These flow measurements were performed during a submaximal exercise level corresponding to 60% of the maximal oxygen uptake. The muscle blood flow study was made in duplicate one day prior to the biopsies and once more in the middle of the training period.

Heart rate was recorded more or less continuously during the special exercise-test runs and during the Xenon studies by means of ECG.

This investigation was carried out in co-operation with doctors Björntorp, Fahlén, Přerovský and Stenberg.

Figure 1 comprises the results of the maximal aerobic power calculated from the heart rate increase on two submaximal work loads during the separate test runs. It also includes the results of the heart rate recorded during a given submaximal exercise load when the muscle blood flow was measured. The results are expressed as mean values ± standard deviation.

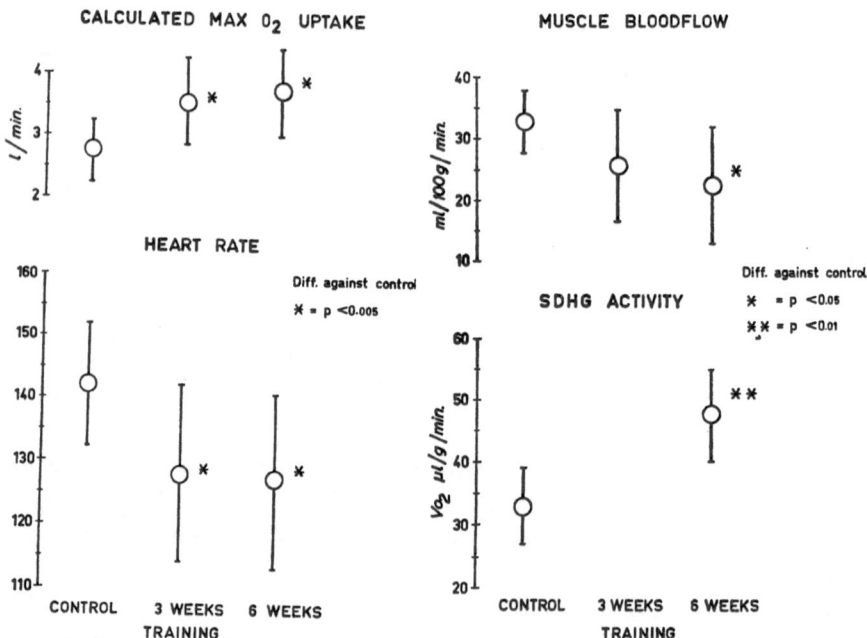

Fig. 1. Calculated maximal oxygen uptake and heart rate during submaximal exercise before, during and after physical training.

Fig. 2. Muscle bloodflow and succinic dehydrogenase activity before and after physical training.

There was an increase of maximal aerobic power parallelly with a decrease of heart rate. In other words the heart rate decreased whether the heart rate values were recorded during testing procedures or during the muscle blood flow measurements. The present absolute values of maximal aerobic power should be taken with a great reservation (remember the placebo results!) but it is undisputable that the directional and qualitative changes of maximal aerobic power are realistic. The suggestion is strong that a significant effect of physical training was achieved by the above mentioned training program.

The results of muscle blood flow measurements and those of succinic dehydrogenase activity are presented in figure 2.

The capillary blood flow in the working muscle is significantly lower after the six weeks' training than before. The decrease takes place already after 3 weeks' training similarly to what is happening with the heart rate and maximal aerobic power.

The reduction of muscle blood flow during a given exercise level has been reported to occur also in 2 patients with coronary artery disease after a 6-8 weeks training program (2). The method for blood flow measurement was the same as in the present study. The conclusion

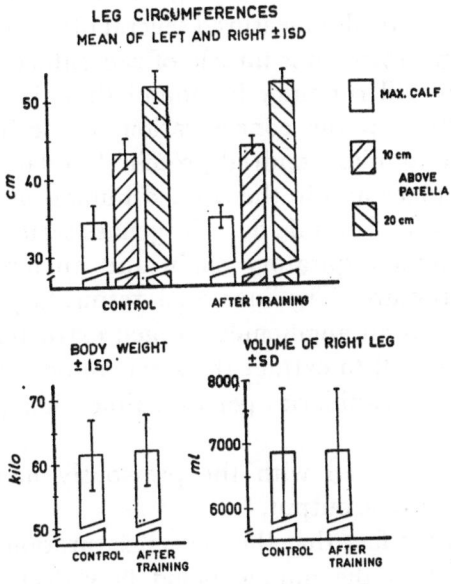

Fig. 3. Leg circumferences, body weight and leg volume before and after physical training.

is that the adjustment of muscle capillary blood flow in submaximal exercise after the physical training is qualitatively the same in health and in ischaemic heart disease.

In this connection it is important to consider the possibility of an increase in muscle mass as a consequence of training. Such an increase would result in a decreased blood flow per 100 grams of muscle tissue because the pre-training level of work would be lower if calculated per 100 grams of muscle tissue. The assessment of muscle mass was made by the measurements of volume and circumference of the leg.

The results are presented in figure 3 together with the values for body weight. No changes of any of the variables were recorded. These results do not support the assumption that muscle mass increased in the present experimental set up. On the other hand these measurements are too unspecific to allow any definite statement in one or other direction.

The succinic dehydrogenase activity rose markedly at the end of the training period just as the muscle blood flow was reduced. No muscle biopsies and no measurements of the succinic dehydrogenase activity were performed after 3 weeks' training.

The present finding of increased enzymatic activity is in agreement with the results reported by Holloszy (3) who in addition to the succinic dehydrogenase activity also measured several other respiratory enzyme activities in the gastrocnemius muscle of rats subjected to a strenuous program of tread-mill running. He found that the physical training induced an increase in the concentration of specific mitochondrial enzymes and in total mitochondrial protein. Similar changes might be expected to take place also in the trained human muscle as suggested by the present results. Succinic dehydrogenase seems to be an integral part of the proximal respiratory chain and an integral part of the mitochondrial structure. The increased respiratory enzyme activity most likely results in an augmented oxygen extraction capacity. This enables the muscle cell to extract the same amount of oxygen from a less blood volume in capillaries per unit time after the training than before.

This reasoning fits well with the previously mentioned physical training effect on cardiac output.

It also fits with the fact that the oxygen saturation of mixed venous blood drops and that the muscle blood flow decreases during submaximal exercise levels.

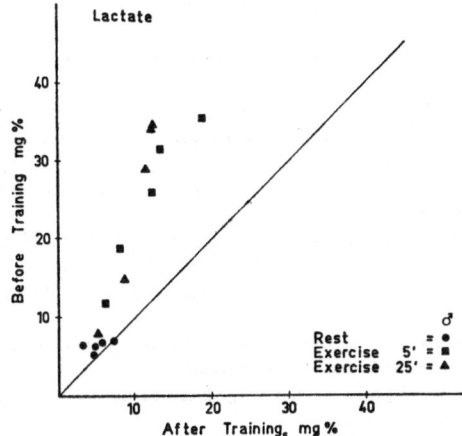

Fig. 4. The effect of 6 months physical training on lactate concentration in the arterial blood (1).

Furthermore the post-training decrease of lactate levels during sub-maximal exercise as illustrated in figure 4 (from study 2) can partly be explained on the basis of increased enzymatic activity. According to Holloszy's suggestion 'Most likely during moderate exercise the rate of aerobic metabolism of pyruvate in the muscles of sedentary individuals is limited not by the supply of oxygen but by the capacity of the mitochondria for pyruvate oxidation'.

In summary the improvement of circulatory adjustment in exercise as a result of physical training is apparently brought about by a number of physiological and biochemical mechanisms. The net effect is a more effective peripheral circulation contributing to cause a more efficient and economic work of the heart. This in turn results in an ability to perform heavy work with less feeling of discomfort in health and with less cardiovascular symptoms of insufficiency in ischaemic heart disease. To what extent the physical training also has a primary effect on the regional circulation supplying the constantly working heart muscle is difficult to assess. No direct evidence has as yet been presented in support of improved coronary blood flow or increased enzymatic activity in the myocardium.

Finally it must be kept in mind that the physiological and biochemical responses to training may be significantly altered by age of the subjects, by long term training, by training intensity and probably by the frequency of training-sessions.

REFERENCES

1. Bergman, H. and E. Varnauskas, *Hemodynamic effects of training in coronary patients.* Tel-Aviv, (okt. 1966).
2. Clausen, J. P. and J. Trap-Jensen, Effect of training on muscular blood flow during exercise. *Acta Physiol. Scand.* Vol. 74, 23A (1968).
3. Holloszy, J. O., Biochemical adaptation in muscle. *J. Biol. Chem.* 242, 2278 (1967).
4. Ekblom, B., Effect of physical training in oxygen transport system in man. *Acta Physiol. Scand.* Suppl. 328 (1969).
5. Varnauskas, E., H. Bergman, P. Houk and P. Björntorp, Hemodynamic effects of physical training in coronary patients. *Lancet*, July 2, 8-12 (1966).
6. Frick, M. H., A. Konttinen and S. Sarajas, Effects of physical training on circulation at rest and during exercise.
7. Frick, M. H. and M. Katila, Hemodynamic consequences of physical training after myocardial infarction. *Circulation* 37, 192 (1968).
8. Björntorp, P., M. Fahlén and V. Szostak, *Studies on succinic dehydrogenase activity in human skeletal muscle.* (To be published).
9. Ekblom, B., P.O. Åstrand, B. Saltin, J. Stenberg and B. Wallström, Effect of training on circulatory response to exercise. *J.A.P.* 24, 518 (1968).
10. Folkow, B., C. Heymans and E. Neil, Integrated aspects of cardiovascular regulation. In: *Handbook of Physiology*, section 2: Circulation, Vol. III. Ed. W. F. Hamilton and P. Dow. Am. Physiological Society. Washington, DC, pp 1787-1823 (1965).
11. Hanson, J. S., B. S. Tabakin, A. M. Levy and W. Nedde, Long-term physical training and cardiovascular dynamics in middle-aged men. *Circulation* 38, 783 (1968).
12. Otis, A. B., The control of respiratory gas exchange between blood and tissues. In: *The Regulation of Human Respiration.* Ed. D. J. C. Cunningham, and Lloyd, pp. 111-119, Blackwell, Oxford (1963).

EVALUATION OF EXERCISE TOLERANCE AND WORKLOAD. I

F. H. BONJER

INTRODUCTION

The relationship between physical activity and ischaemic heart disease can be discussed in many ways.

Epidemiologists have studied the hypothesis that habitual physical activity is a protective factor against ischaemic heart disease.

Physical training becomes more and more an important feature in treating myocardial infarctions. The progress made in such a training program can be assessed by means of repeated exercise tolerance tests.

It is the aim of this paper to explain how results of an exercise tolerance test at the end of the training period can be used for the decision what kind of a job or profession can be resumed or assumed, if physical activity is taken as a criterion. For that reason this paper belongs to the field of rehabilitation.

EXERCISE TOLERANCE TEST

The essence of such a test is to provide the subject with appropriate means for physical exercise. Nevertheless he should be kept stationary in order to allow the investigators to make physiological measurements. Treadmills and bicycle ergometers do serve the purpose. The bicycle has the advantage that external work can be measured more readily and that the pattern of movements is so well defined that the mechanical efficiency has a constant and known value. The emerging questions: how heavy should the test be and for how long should it be continued, can be answered by the introduction of a steadily increasing load. An increase of 10 watts after each minute has proved to be the optimal slope (fig. 1).

The ECG, heart rate, blood pressure, ventilatory minute volume and oxygen uptake should be observed throughout the test. In principle, it is possible to record all these phenomena automatically in the near

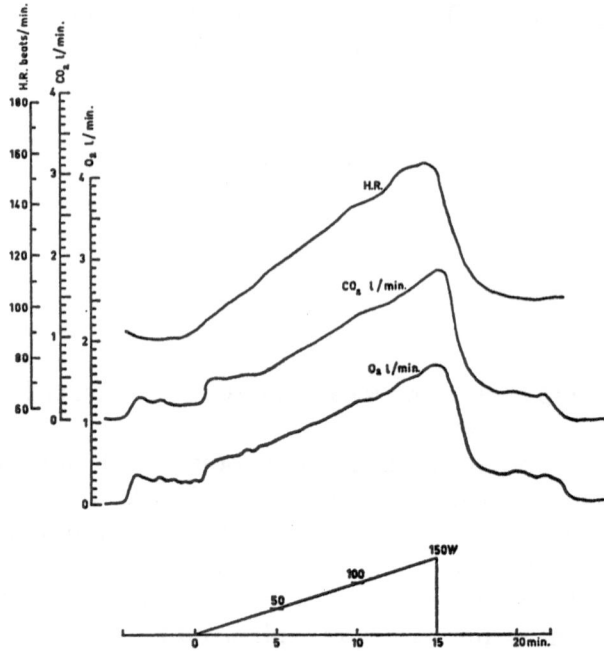

Fig. 1. Record of physiological responses of oxygen uptake, carbondioxide excretion and heart rate to a steadily increasing load.

future. The test should be discontinued if maximal heart rate (according to sex and age) is reached, blood pressure decreases, ST-segment shifts exceed 2 millivolt, cardiac rhythm changes, or the subject complains about chest pain. The oxygen uptake measured in the final stage of the test is considered as the maximum oxygen uptake, which is not necessarily equal to the aerobic power.

ALLOWABLE ENERGY EXPENDITURE

A short lasting heavy exercise test may yield to the maximum oxygen uptake. This gives information about the physical working capacity, but not the answer to the question what energy expenditure over any longer period of time would be allowable. Studies of the relationship between working time and the level of energy expenditure which is still acceptable for such a working time, have revealed that there exists a linear relation between the acceptable level of oxygen uptake and the logarithm of the working time in minutes:

$$\text{Å}_t = \frac{\log 5700 - \log t}{3.1} \times \text{Å}_4$$

in which Å_t represents the allowable mean level of oxygen uptake during time t and Å_4 stands for the maximum oxygen intake, both expressed in l/min. It may be mentioned that log 5700 − log 480 is almost equal to one. Therefore the mean oxygen uptake for 480 minutes is about ⅓ of the maximum (fig. 2).

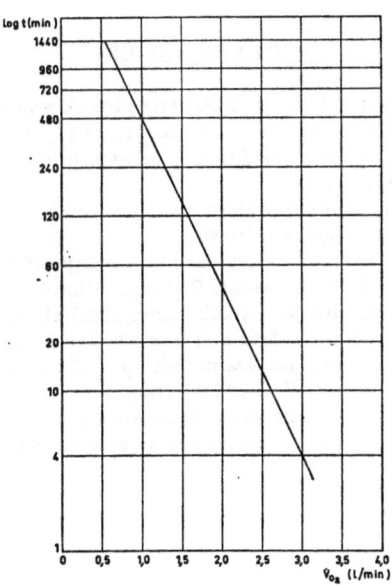

Fig. 2. Allowable mean level of oxygen uptake as a function of working time in case of a maximum oxygen uptake of 3.0 l/min.

COMPARISON OF ACCEPTABLE AND REQUIRED ENERGY EXPENDITURE

Maximum oxygen uptake can be measured during an exercise tolerance test. From this and from the proposed or usual working time a value can be calculated for the acceptable level of energy expenditure.

Field studies can result into data about the mean energy expenditure during the working day. The ratio between the latter (= $/\text{Ṁ}$ for metabolism expressed in kcal/min) and Å_t (for acceptable mean level of activity for a working time of t minutes here to be expressed in kcal/min):

$$\frac{\dot{M}}{\dot{A}_t} \text{ is called the } \textit{degree of loading}$$

and provides an opportunity to match the required and the acceptable energy expenditure. The value of this ratio should never exceed unity. How the energy expenditure of different activities throughout a working day can be assessed, will be explained in the next paper. (H. van der Sluys, Evaluation of exercise tolerance and workload. II).

REFERENCES

1. Bink, B., F. H. Bonjer and H. v. d. Sluys, Het physiek arbeidsvermogen van de mens (Human physical working capacity) *T. Eff. Doc.* 31, 526 (1961).
2. Bonjer, F. H., Actual energy expenditure in relation to the physical working capicity. *Ergonomics*, 5, 29 (1962).
3. Bonjer, F. H., Measurement of working capacity by assessment of the aerobic capacity in a single session. *Fed. Proc.* 25, 1363 (1966).
4. Bonjer, F. H., Physical working capacity and energy expenditure. In: Ergometry in cardiology. Denolin, H. et al. eds. *Studienreihe Boehringer*, Mannheim (1968).
5. Bonjer, F. H., Relationship between working time, physical working capacity and allowable caloric expenditure. In: Muskelarbeit und Muskeltraining, hrsg. W. Rohmert. p. 86-98. Proc. Internat. Kolloquium Darmstadt 1968. *Schriftenreihe Arbeitsmed. Sozialmed. Arbeitshyg.* Bd. 22. Stuttgart, A. W. Gentner Verlag.
6. Bonjer, F. H., Uitvoering en interpretatie van de inspanningsproef bij hartpatiënten. (Procedure and interpretation of exercise test in cardiac patients). *Arts en Soc. Verz.* 7, 14 (1969).

EVALUATION OF EXERCISE TOLERANCE AND WORKLOAD. II

H. VAN DER SLUYS

Generally speaking one may state that suitable work is good for everybody. This applies even more when the worker is stricken by a myocardial infarction. Our work classification unit started its activities three years ago.

Why do we want to know the workload? There are five reasons:

1. To know if patients with IHD can resume their former job for a normal working day.
2. To find out if they can do their former job only part time.
3. To decide if it would be better to have another job or
4. if they are unemployable.
5. Finally it is important to know what kind of sparetime activities are allowed to maintain a good condition.

How can we get an insight in the allowability of the workload? Here we can mention four procedures:

1. First there is the clinical judgement based on sound logic. I believe this method will be applied in most cases. This method of trial and error is very easy, but there is the disadvantage that in the case of doubt one takes the safe side. That means that in all cases when the cardiologist does not know the nature of a patient's job, he will say that the man is unemployable.
2. The second method is to assess the workload by means of energy expenditure tables.
   I should like to remind you of the tables of Passmore and Durnin, Consolazio, Rose, Edholm and Spitzer and Huttinger (see fig. 4).
3. The third method, which is actually the best one is to measure the oxygen consumption during the actual work. The disadvantage of this method is that it takes a lot of time and it is impossible to continue measuring for an entire day. And last but not least you want to know the workload at a time when the patient is not yet working.

4. Therefore we developed a method by using a structured interview
   based on an indirect time and motion study. (For description see
   appendix). In general, the energy expenditure for each activity can
   be calculated by multiplying the time spent in minutes by the oxygen
   consumption per minute.

   In our approach not only the time spent on each activity is determined but also the kind of activity.
   In order to obtain the oxygen consumption each activity is analysed
   in terms of posture and movements.

   Combination of these factors with body weight, the weight of
   loads to be carried and the speed provides the nett oxygen consumption for each activity.

   Basal metabolism is derived from standard tables.

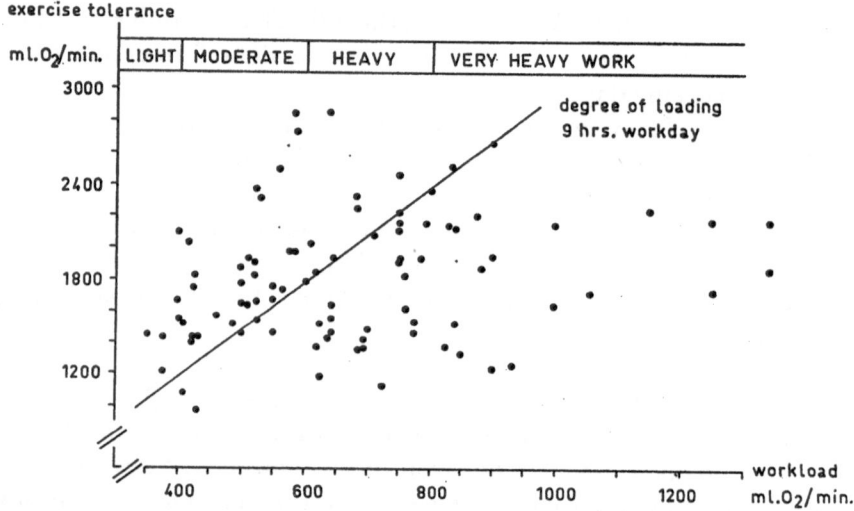

Fig. 1. Workload former job vs. exercise tolerance in IHD, n = 97 males.

Figure 1 shows what we found regarding the workload with our
method in 97 male patients with IHD. On the abscissa the assessment
of the workload in ml.o$_2$/min is plotted against the maximum oxygen
uptake.

   The line shows the degree of loading for a normal workday of 9
hours. From this graph the conclusion can be drawn that there is a
wide variation in the exercise tolerance after the infarction as well as
in the workload of the former job.

There are men with a high maximum oxygen uptake and a low workload and conversely those with a high workload and a low maximum oxygen uptake.

In the heading a classification is given of light, moderate, heavy and very heavy work.

This categorization is drawn up on our experience of the last three years and it is based on the workload in terms of oxygen consumption. At this moment the question arises whether it is sufficient to know just the name of the occupation with a view to estimating the workload.

For instance is teaching to be considered light work?

Generally speaking yes, but in a special case the workload was calculated at 500 ml O_2/min.

So in that case teaching had to be regarded as moderate work. Another example, the workload of a printer was rated at less than 400 ml O_2/min. In that particular case printing corresponded with light work.

So the name of an occupation can be misleading and one has to individualize. At present you have to make allowances for the changing character of work as a result of increased specialization, mechanization and the advent of new jobs.

For example a painter. In the good old days this occupation covered the whole scale of work. Nowadays one sees more and more specialization, for example men who only prime and men who only paint.

An example of mechanization is a level crossing keeper. In former days the gates were opened and closed by hand. Nowadays they are worked mechanically and the keeper only has to press the button.

Finally, more and more new jobs are created that did not exist before. For example, the job of operator in the process industry. So our conclusion is that a classification of jobs in the categories light, moderate and heavy work only gives a rough idea of the workload and sometimes may be misleading. As I mentioned we started three years ago with the method of structured interview and made some control measurements of the oxygen consumption during the actual work and we found the measurement and the calculation corresponded satisfactorily. But perhaps the best proof lies in the fact that for all patients we advised to resume working, nearly all were able to do the work we had calculated.

What can be done if both values are available? (fig. 2).

On the abscissa the workload in ml O_2/min. and on the ordinate the

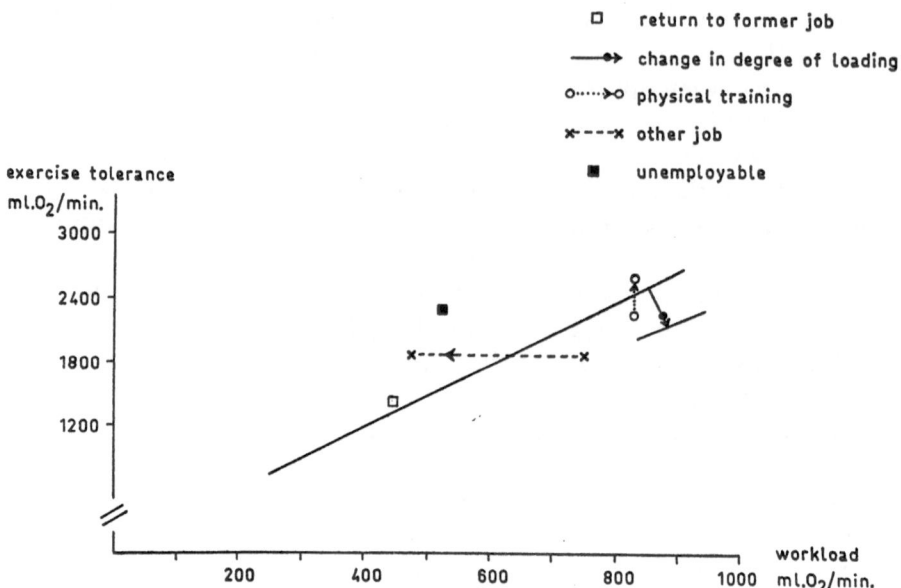

Fig. 2. Interplay between exercise tolerance and workload.

exercise tolerance also in ml o_2/min. The line shows the limit of the degree of loading for a normal workday of 9 hours. The points, which are lying above this line, denote patients who are physically able to resume work.

Five alternatives are given:

1. Firstly the case of a 43 years old teacher. His maximum oxygen uptake was 1400 ml o_2/min. and his workload 420 ml o_2/min. So we advised him to go back to his former job where he has now been working for more than a year.

2. The second alternative you can apply is to give physical training with the intention of increasing the maximum working capacity. An example of this is a bricklayer, who had a maximum oxygen uptake of 2245 ml o_2/min. His workload was calculated as 830 ml o_2/min. So he could not do his former job for a full working day. We gave this man, 53 years of age, a physical training of two months and after the training his maximum oxygen uptake was measured again and found to be 2615 ml o_2/min. So we advised him to resume his former job. We started cautiously and let him work half days, gradually extending his working day. Now he has been working

half a year on full days. This is a good example which can be achieved by training, but not all patients who received physical training had an increase in their maximum oxygen uptake.

3. Then you can follow the third alternative namely to change the degree of loading by decreasing the number of working hours. In the case of a 48 years old plasterer who had a maximum oxygen uptake of 2200 ml O_2/min. and a workload of 870 ml O_2/min. and could not do his former job. It was possible to resettle him as a part time worker in consultation with his employer. We calculated that for him part time should be 5 hours a day. Now he has been working for a year to the full satisfaction of his boss and himself.

4. Fourthly the case of a baker, 52 years of age, whose working time could not be shortened. Nevertheless, we could resettle him in other work with a lower workload. Now he has been working in industry full days for more than a year.

5. The last case is that of a man, 47 years of age. He was a film operator in cinema. His maximum oxygen uptake was 2400 ml O_2/min. and his workload 520 ml O_2/min. So physically he was able to do his work easily, but he did not return to his former job, because of psycho-social factors. This illustrates that there is not only the physical aspect, but also a psycho-social aspect; this last point is of great importance for the workresumption.

A general view is given on the figure 3.

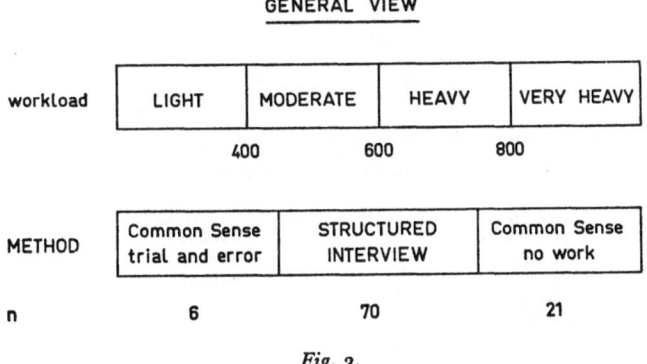

Fig. 3.

70 out of 97 patients belonged to the middle categories, so this is a rather important part.

The conclusion can be drawn that light work on the one side and very heavy work on the other side, can be sufficiently handled by common sense. But the method of structured interview – or any other more precise evaluation of the workload and the exercise tolerance – is particularly of great help to the cardiologist in dealing with all kinds of moderate and heavy work.

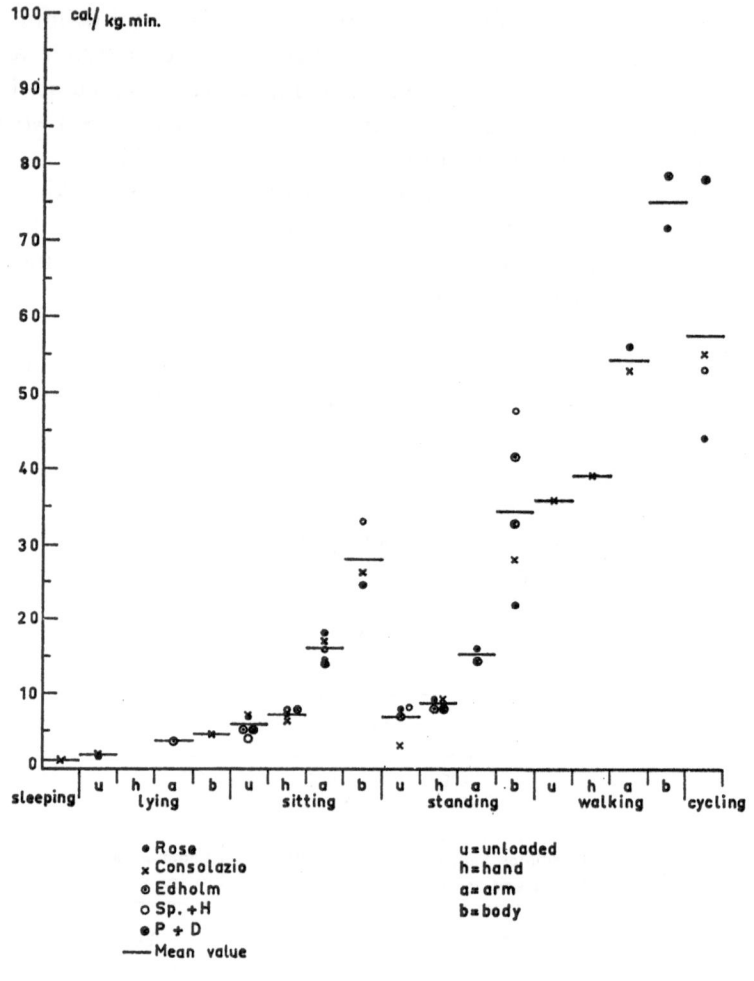

Fig. 4

REFERENCES

1. Bink, B., F. H. Bonjer and H. van der Sluys, Het physiek arbeidsvermogen van de mens (Human physical working capacity) *T. Eff. Doc.*, 31, 526 (1961).

2. Bink, B., F. H. Bonjer and H. van der Sluys, Assessment of the energy expenditure by indirect time and motion study. In: *Physical activity in health and disease*, Proc. Beitostölen symposium 1966, ed. by K. Evang, and K. Lange Andersen, Oslo, Universitetsforlaget, 207-14 (1966).

3. Sluys, H. van der, Het menselijk activiteitspatroon tegen de achtergrond van de leeftijd. In: *Functionele leeftijd van industrie-arbeider. De ontwikkeling van een meetmethode*. Nederlands Instituut voor Preventieve Geneeskunde. TNO, Wolters-Noordhoff, 44-52. (1968).

4. Sluys, H. van der, Assessment of energy expenditure. In: *Progress Report 1966-1967 Cardiac rehabilitation Research Leyden*. Academisch Ziekenhuis (NIPG-TNO), Leiden, 14-19 (1967).

ASSESSMENT OF THE ENERGY EXPENDITURE BY INDIRECT TIME AND MOTION STUDY

Introduction

Human physical activities are different from minute to minute and from hour to hour. Moreover, the pattern of physical activities on workdays differs from the one on saturdays and sundays.

Energy expenditure may be assessed by direct measurement of the oxygen intake and the time spent to each activity. Such measurements during all activities, however, require a large number of experiments. The following essay provides a substitute to avoid this time consuming procedure: assessment of the energy expenditure from time and motion study. In general the energy expenditure for each activity in kilocalories (M) can be calculated by multiplication of the time spent in minutes (t) and the number of kilocalories expended per minute ($\dot{M}$):

$$M = t \cdot \dot{M}$$

It is the aim of this paper to demonstrate how both elements can be determined in a satisfactory way without direct measurements on the spot.

ASSESSMENT OF TIME EXPENDITURE

To assess the time induced by the daily physical activities an anamnestic method has been developed employing a questionnaire (protocol I). The 24 hours of the day can be divided into different periods which can be determined by asking for generally well-known marking points in clocktime, such as:
– at what time do you get up,
– at what time are you leaving home for work,
– at what time are you starting work,
– at what time do you take rest pauses,
– at what time do you go home,
– at what time do you have dinner,
– at what time are you going to bed?

By fixing these clocktimes it is possible to determine the durance in minutes of the intermitting periods of the different parts of the day. Such periods have been indicated in protocol I.

In the practical application of this assessment of time it should be born in mind that the real time of any specific activity uses to be much shorter than the total time spent on such an activity. Two examples may illustrate this. The work of a navvy consists of digging grooves and refilling these after placing cables, tubes, etc. He works without official pauses for 525 minutes per day. When allowing 6 kcal/min. ($\dot{M}$) for this kind of work, the total load (M) for this man equals 525 . 6 = 3150 kcal. But from the length, the depth and the width of the groove digged it appears that only 5 m³ have been displaced. The required time for displacing 5 m³ is known to be 300 minutes. So the rest of the time must be spent by the navvy to small rest pauses. The calculation of the work now becomes:

300 . 6   = 1800 kcal
225 . 1.7 =   383 kcal (for standing during rest pauses)
_____
    total = 2183 kcal

This example illustrates that there may be a large variety in the individual 24-hours caloric expenditure even within a group of people with the same profession, simply because they will work according to different *time schedules*.

The next example is taken from playing tennis. Tennis was played from 9 till 12 o'clock, or during 180 minutes. When allowing for tennis a caloric expenditure of 7 kcal/min. ($\dot{M}$), the total metabolism (M) would be 180 . 7 = 1260 kcal. The number of sets played, however was three, while the time expenditure of one set is about 20 minutes; apparently the rest of the time was spent by looking to the play on the next tennis court, sitting on a chair, or other minor activities. The calculation should be modified:

60 . 7   = 420 kcal
120 . 1.6 = 192 kcal (for sitting)
_____
    total = 612 kcal

This second example proves that what has been demonstrated for professional activities is also applicable to leisure time activities.

THE ENERGY EXPENDITURE PER ACTIVITY

Many data have been published about the energy cost of different act-

ivities. For the sources of literature used for this study: see references
2, 3, 4, 5, 6, 7 and 8. Most of the authors include basal metabolism in
their data on energy expenditure for different activities and indicate
the body weight of their subjects. In many cases, however, no reference
is made to the body height or age. Nevertheless these data have been
adapted for our purpose in such a way that basal metabolism was
subtracted and nett energy expenditure was expressed in kcal/kg min.
The resulting list of caloric expenditures related to different activities
according to the authors mentioned was considered as a less appropriate
tool for the assessment of energy expenditure for all forthcoming
activities. For this reason all activities, as they are referred to in
literature, have been classified according to work posture and movements.

Hand-writing for instance is classified as:

sitting posture – hand movement.

It is obvious that many different data were at hand for some postures
and movements and only few for others. In the case more data were
available for the same activity the mean value has been chosen.
Original data of different authors and mean values have been plotted
in a diagram. The classification used in this diagram and the mean
values in kilocalories per kg min. are listed in the next table. To improve legibility of the diagram all values are expressed in small calories.

posture	movement	kcal/kg min.	
sleeping		0.0011	
lying	unloaded	0.0019	
	hand	—	
	arm	0.0037	
	body	0.0045	
sitting	unloaded	0.0058	
	hand	0.0076	
	arm	0.0160	
	body	0.0279	
standing	unloaded	0.0069	
	hand	0.0089	
	arm	0.0154	
	body	0.0345	
walking	unloaded	0.0361	100 steps/minute (3.96 km/hour)
	hand	0.0390	
	arm	0.0543	
	body	0.0750	
cycling		0.0575	15 km/hour

ASSESSMENT OF THE TOTAL ENERGY EXPENDITURE

The total energy expenditure for 24 hours or any shorter period consists of the nett energy expenditure of all activities included and the basal metabolism of the subject. The latter may be derived from sex, age, and body size. For any shorter period of 24 hours the daily amount of kilocalories should be corrected by the term $\frac{t}{1440}$. As all data about the energy expenditure for different activities have been expressed in kcal/kg.min. ($\dot{M}$), the mentioned formula for the energy expenditure:

$M = t \cdot \dot{M}$ should be written as:

$$M = \frac{t}{1440} \cdot BM + \dot{m} \cdot W \cdot t,$$

in wich M stands for total metabolism for a given period in kilocalories,

BM   for basal metabolism in kcal/day,
t   for duration of the period in minutes,
$\dot{m}$ for nett metabolism resulting from the activity per kg body weight and per minute,
W   for body weight in kg.

Sometimes additional data have to be taken into account such as the weight to be carried or the external force to be exerted and the working rate. If the additional weight or external force (w) is indicated in kg and the influence of the speed of work (s) is introduced in such a way that a normal speed is represented by unity and abnormal speeds are indicated by a fraction of unity, the final formula for the total energy expenditure for a given period covering one specific activity reads:

$$M = \frac{t}{1440} \cdot BM + t \cdot \dot{m} \cdot (W + w) \cdot s.$$

EXAMPLE OF APPLICATION

How time and motion study can be used for the assessment of the energy expenditure during actual work and other activities is demonstrated by the analysis of the daily activities of a cooper (protocol II). Apart from the basal metabolism, which is derived from Carpenter's tables (2), and sleeping for which the additional metabolism has been indicated in the list, activities like dressing, washing and transportation are evaluated in terms of caloric expenditure according to the posture and movements concerned. The same applies to the professional work, which is done for a period of 525 minutes with a series of rest pauses amounting to 45 minutes. During the remaining 480 minutes 40 tubs are constructed. The mean time spent to one tub amounts to 12 minutes and contains the following components:

1.	to place staves	0.5 min.
2.	to ram down these staves	0.5 min.
3.	to fasten by turning the toggle	1.0 min.
4.	to fix tapes	2.0 min.
5.	to put in the bottom	1.0 min.
6.	to fix 2 tapes and ram on	2.0 min.
7.	to fix 3 tapes and ram on	2.0 min.
8.	to fix 1 tape and put in the top	1.0 min.
9.	to fix finally the tapes	2.0 min.
		12.0 min.

These activities can be converted into terms of posture, movement, weight and speed:

	posture	movement	weight	speed
1.	standing	arm	1	1.00
2.	,,	body	5	1.00
3.	,,	body	4	1.00
4.	,,	arm	3	1.00
5.	,,	arm	3	1.00
6.	,,	body	5	1.00
7.	,,	body	5	1.00
8.	,,	arm	5	1.00
9.	,,	body	7	1.00

In behalf of the calculation code numbers 2, 6 and 7 are combined as numbers 4 and 5. The result is introduced into protocol II under the heading of work. Spare time activities are dealt with in the same way as the professional ones. The protocol contains additional space for recording week-end activities. The last section of this protocol summarises the energy expenditure on normal workdays, saturdays and sundays. The mean value per day is calculated by taking five times the workday expenditure, adding the expenditure on saturdays and sundays, and by dividing the sum by seven. In this case the mean daily caloric expenditure amounts to 2764 kcal.

The absolute value is an information of limited significance as there is a wide variety in body size. If we want to evaluate the physical activity of men, more relevant information can be obtained from the quotient mean caloric expenditure divided by basal metabolism than from the mean caloric expenditure itself. We propose to call this

quotient, which can be calculated for in our example as $\dfrac{2674}{1530} = 1,75$,

the coefficient of activity.

This coefficient is thought to be important for many studies in the field of epidemiology of cardiovascular and other diseases, social and preventive medicine and for the study of the relationship between physical activity and working capacity.

REFERENCES

1. Bink, B., F. H. Bonjer and H. van der Sluys, Assessment of the energy expenditure by indirect time and motion study. *Physical activity in health and disease, Proc. Beitostölen Symposium 1966,* ed. by K. Evang and K. Lange Andersen. Oslo, Universitetsforlaget, 207-14 (1966).
2. Carpenter, T. M., *Tables, factors and formulas for computing respiratory exchange and biological transformations of energy;* 3rd ed. Washington, Carnegy Institute (1939).
3. Consolazio, C. F., R. E. Johnson and L. J. Pecora, *Physiological measurements of metabolic functions in man.* New York, McGraw-Hill (1963).
4. Edholm, O. G., J. G. Fletcher, E. M. Widdowson and R. A. McCance, Energy expenditure and food intake of individual men. *Brit. J. Nutr.* 9, 286-300 (1955).
5. McDonald, I., Statistical studies of recorded energy expenditure of man. Part II. Expenditure of walking related to weight, sex, age, height, speed and gradient. *Nutr. Abstr. Rev.* 31, 739-62 (1961).
6. Passmore, R. and J. V. G. A. Durnin, Human energy expenditure. *Physiol. Rev.* 35, 801-40 (1955).
7. Rose, M. E., *Foundation of nutrition,* 4th ed. rev. by G. McLeod and C. M. Taylor. New York, McMillan, (1946).
8. Spitzer, H. and T. Hettinger, *Tafeln für den Kalorienumsatz bei körperlicher Arbeit,* 4e Aufl. Sonderheft der Refa Nachrichten. Darmstadt, Beuth Vertrieb (1964).

PROTOCOL I

Name:	P. A. Coolen	Age:	1903	Code number: 158
Address:	Buitensingel 63	Weight:	75 kg	
Profession:	Cooper	Height:	170 cm	

	Normal workday		
	speed	clock time	time in minutes
1. At what time do you get up?		6.20	
2. How much time takes your dressing?			15
3. How much time takes your breakfast?			15
4. Do you walk in the morning (with your dog)?	—		
Do you do some home work?			
Do you sit down a while before leaving home (morning paper)?			
5. At what time do you leave home for work?		6.50	
Walking? Distance?	—		
Cycling?	—		
Is use made of autocycle, scooter, motor, car, bus, streetcar, train?			5
Time for changing?			
6. At what time do you arrive at your work?		6.55	
Do you have any activities before you start? sitting			5
7. At what time do you start your work?		7.00	
8. Lunch time: 12.00-13.15			75
Spare time: coffee 9.45-10.00, tea 15.45-16.00			30
Do you go home for lunch?			
Are you doing this in the same way as going to work?			
If you do not go home, do you have a walk in lunch time?	—		
Or are you doing something else?			
9. At what time do you go home?		17.30	
Walking? Distance?	—		
Cycling?	—		
Is use made of autocycle, scooter, motor, car, bus, streetcar, train?			5
Time for changing?			
10. At what time do you arrive home?		17.35	
11. What are your activities until dinner?			
Washing and dressing?			
Sitting, reading the newspaper?			25
Have a walk?	—		
12. How much time takes your dinner?			30
13. At what time do you finish dinner?		18.30	
14. Do you assist in dish-washing?			
15. How do you spend the evening?			
Reading the newspaper?			
SUBTOTAL			205

| | Normal workday | | |
	speed	clock time	time in minutes
TRANSPORT			205
Television?			
Sitting?			
Hobbies?			270
Social Activities?			
Do you work overtime?			
Extra work?			
Sport?			
16. At what time do you go to bed?		23.00	
17. At what time are you in bed?		23.15	15
18. How many staircases do you perform a day?			
4×	—		
19. Other peak loads?			
20. Are you doing sport?			
Sleeping time			425

WORK DESCRIPTION

How long are you in this job?　　30 years

Mechanisation?
Season?
Piece work?
Time you start?　　　　　　　　　7.00
Dressing before work?

| Posture | movement | | | weight | distance | | |
	hand	arm	body				
sitting	hand			0 kg	m		45
standing				kg	m		
walking				kg	m		

| Posture | movement | | | weight | distance | | |
	hand	arm	body				
sitting				kg	m		
standing		arm		1 kg	m		20
				3 kg	m		120
				5 kg	m		40
walking				kg	m		

| Posture | movement | | | weight | distance | | |
	hand	arm	body				
sitting				kg	m		
standing			body	4 kg	m		40
				5 kg	m		180
				7 kg	m		80
walking				kg	m		

| | TOTAL | 1440 |

		Saturday	
	speed	clock time	time in minutes
1. At what time do you get up?		8.30	
2. How much time takes your dressing?			15
3. How much time takes your breakfast?			15
4. What are you doing between breakfast and lunch?	sitting	9.00	240
5. At what time do you have lunch?		13.00	
6. At what time do you finish lunch?		13.30	30
7. What are you doing between lunch and dinner?	sitting		270
8. At what time do you have dinner?		18.00	
9. At what time do you finish dinner?		18.30	30
10. How do you spend the evening? sitting TV			330
11. At what time do you go to bed?		24.00	
12. At what time are you in bed?		24.15	15
13. Are you doing sport?			
Sleeping time			495
		TOTAL	1440

		Sunday	
	speed	clock time	time in minutes
1. At what time do you get up?		8.30	
2. How much time takes your dressing?			15
3. How much time takes your breakfast?		9.00	15
4. What are you doing between breakfast and lunch?	sitting		240
5. At what time do you have lunch?		13.00	
6. At what time do you finish lunch?		13.30	30
7. What are you doing between lunch and dinner?	sitting		270
8. At what time do you have dinner?		18.00	
9. At what time do you finish dinner?		18.30	30
10. How do you spend the evening? sitting TV			270
11. At what time do you go to bed?		23.00	
12. At what time are you in bed?		23.15	15
13. Are you doing sport?			
Sleeping time			555
		TOTAL	1440

PROTOCOL II

Name:	P. A. Coolen			Code number: 158	
Address:	Buitensingel 63				
Profession:	Cooper				
Age:	1903				
Weight:	75 kg				
Height:	170 cm				

Normal workday

Activities				kcal/ kg min.	kcal/ min.	time in minutes	kcal
1. Basal metabolism (BM)				—	—	—	1530
2. Sleep				0.0011	0.0825	425	35
3. Personal activities							
• getting up, dressing, washing				0.0154	1.1550	30	35
• meals, coffee, tea				0.0076	0.5700	150	86
4. Going to and from work							
	speed						
• walking				0.0361			
• cycling				0.0575			
• autocycle, scooter, car				0.0170	1.2750	10	13
• bus, tram, train				0.0133			
• time for change				0.0069			
5. Work							

posture	movement	weight	speed				
sitting	hand	0		0.0076	0.5700	45	26
	arm			0.0160			
	body			0.0279			
standing	hand			0.0089			
	arm	1		0.0154	1.1704	20	23
		3			1.2012	120	144
		5			1.2320	40	49
	body	4		0.0345	2.7255	40	109
		5			2.7600	180	497
		7			2.8290	80	226
walking	hand	—		0.0390			
	arm	—		0.0543			
	body	—		0.0750			
stairs				0.2716			

6. Spare time							
— sitting, TV etc.				0.0058	0.4350	300	131
— hobby and home work				0.0255			
— gardening				0.0345			
— walking				0.0361			
— standing				0.0069			
— car driving				0.0170			
— stairs $4 \times (4/3 \times 0.2716 \times 75)$				0.2716			27

					TOTAL	1440	2931

Saturday

Activities		kcal/ kg. min.	kcal/ min.	time in minutes	kcal
1.	Basal metabolism (BM)	—	—	—	1530
2.	Sleep	0.0011	0.0825	495	41
3.	Personal activities				
	• getting up etc.	0.0154	1.1550	30	35
	• meals etc.	0.0076	0.5700	75	43
4.	Spare time				
	• sitting, TV etc.	0.0058	0.4350	840	365
	• hobby and home work	0.0255			
	• gardening	0.0345			
	• walking —	0.0361			
	• standing	0.0069			
	• car driving	0.0170			
	• stairs 4	0.2716			27
			TOTAL	1440	2041

Sunday

		kcal/ kg. min.	kcal/ min.	time in minutes	kcal
1.	Basal metabolism (BM)	—	—	—	1530
2.	Sleep	0.0011	0.0825	555	46
3.	Personal activities				
	• getting up etc.	0.0154	1.1550	30	35
	• meals etc.	0.0076	0.5700	75	43
4.	Spare time				
	• sitting, TV etc.	0.0058	0.4350	780	339
	• hobby and home work	0.0255			
	• gardening	0.0345			
	• walking —	0.0361			
	• standing	0.0069			
	• car driving	0.0170			
	• stairs 4	0.2716			27
			TOTAL	1440	2020

metabolism in kilocalories							
	BM	sleep	personal activities	going to work	work	spare time	total
Normal workday	1530	35	121	13	1074	158	2931
Saturday	1530	41	78	—	—	392	2041
Sunday	1530	46	78	—	—	366	2020
Mean per day							2674

PANEL DISCUSSION ON ISCHAEMIC HEART DISEASE AND PHYSICAL ACTIVITY

MODERATOR: H. K. HELLERSTEIN

Hellerstein: From a historical point of view we have gone almost full circle in our consideration of exercise. In the age of the ancient philosophers, of Maimonides and Plato, it was well-known that one should exercise daily and should keep one's body and self in the best possible condition. In the modern era physical fitness was relegated solely to athletes and champions and rarely prescribed in the treatment of patients.

In the period of 1925 to 1950, exercise was used to test cardiovascular function. The original test of Oppenheim and Master measured the heart rate and blood pressure responses to 1.5 minutes of step climbing. With the availability of the electrocardiogram, Master changed the emphasis of his test from cardiovascular function to coronary arterial structure. His exercise test has proved valuable in the detection of coronary insufficiency, which in most instances is due to coronary arteriosclerosis. In the past decade, interest in exercise has broadened from that of testing for diagnosis to that of testing of function in order to have a scientific basis for the prescription of training and work classification of cardiac subjects.

Physical training and fitness are now in vogue. It is a marvelous thing that we have again recognized the wisdom of the ancients. Maimonides advised the son of the Sultan of Egypt to exercise daily to the point of breathlessness and follow other good health practices. Centuries later Heberden reported that he had nearly cured a patient with angina pectoris by having him saw wood for 30 minutes daily.

Our studies and those of other members of this panel have confirmed the value of supervised physical activity for subjects with ischaemic heart disease.

The first question for the panel's consideration is: How can a clinician measure maximum oxygen uptake in his office?

Varnauskas: Maximum oxygen uptake is the maximal level of oxygen uptake that the organism can attain. I know of no clinician who is determining this in his office and I don't think that the clinician has to do so. Maximum oxygen uptake is a physiological definition. It should not be confused with the maximum amount of work that a patient can perform. The patient may show signs of circulatory insufficiency which would cause the doctor to stop the exercise before reaching the physiological maximal oxygen uptake. That would be the maximal work load determined by clinical symptoms and signs. This particular level of exercise certainly gives sufficient amount of information from clinical point of view.

Frick: I fully agree that the maximum oxygen uptake is the highest amount of oxygen that the subject can consume in a unit of time. In ischaemic heart disease it is my understanding that it means the maximal level of oxygen that he can consume up to the point of pain or distress. He is unable to tolerate anymore. This is quite different from the physiological definition of maximum oxygen uptake.

Pool: I think it is impossible to measure maximum oxygen uptake without the proper equipment. Clinicians can use other tests with which they can make estimates within certain limits.

Bonjer: We might think in terms of aerobic power. It is an index of to what extent the circulatory and respiratory system can transport oxygen to the muscular system. It is not necessary to measure the oxygen uptake if a calibrated bicycle ergometer is used, as the mechanical efficiency of bicycling is known.

Hellerstein: Maximal aerobic power is that condition which is reached when a person does increasing amounts of work and yet fails to increase his oxygen uptake. Many patients have a limiting feature which prevents them from achieving their maximum oxygen uptake. In such instances, the maximal performance would not be equivalent to maximal power. In dealing with patients with coronary disease we must understand that we do not generally push them to true maximal oxygen uptake. Unfortunately the linear relationship between heart rate and work performance cannot be applied unreservedly in cardiac patients as in normals.

Åstrand extrapolated heart rates at submaximal work levels to estimate the maximum oxygen uptake. For normal subjects, the Åstrand's method is accurate within plus or minus 5-10 per cent, for ischaemic patients within plus or minus 10-15 per cent. Some measure of aerobic power can be gotten from the performance of a simple office step test according to the method of Bruno Balke. The patient makes, for example, 15 ascents and descents on a 30 cm step per minute for three minutes, while a single bipolar EKG lead and arm blood pressure are recorded. After two minutes rest, the number of ascents is increased to 20, 25, 30, or 35 etc. The oxygen cost can be calculated from Balke's formula and the relation of heart rate response to oxygen cost can be plotted. As I recall, the oxygen cost is approximately 3.5 ml O_2/min./kg body weight for each meter the body is elevated. Thus the cost of 15, 20, 25, 30, 35 and 40 ascents/minute on a 30 cm step is 16, 21, 26, 32, 37 and 42 ml O_2/min./kg B.W. The oxygen cost of resistance bicycling is also remarkably constant per kilopond meter or watt. Thus, the practicing physician can evaluate in his office the heart rate, blood pressure and ECG responses to work of known magnitude for given period, facts necessary to determine a rational load for training.

Varnauskas: In our studies we have been interested to evaluate the haemodynamic effects of a relatively moderate exercise load which is usually well – tolerated by the patient during a time period of 30 minutes. Our aim was thus not to push the patient to work as hard as possible but rather to expose him to a more frequent and more regular physical activity than he has been used to before the training period. The results of our investigation disclosed that the moderate exercise of 30 minutes' duration performed three times per week produces measurable haemodynamic changes after one month of training. These changes are more pronounced after six months of training.

In general we suggest that the patients should be more active, for example do more walking, than they have been practicing before.

Hellerstein: I don't think that the audience is satisfied with our answers. Let us assume that you have exercised a patient and find that he is able to do work up to an equivalent of two liters oxygen intake per minute with a heart rate of 160. What do you tell him if he asks you how much work he is permitted to do?

Frick: There are two main problems here. The first is anginal pain. We hope to stop anginal pain completely with this procedure. Our second aim is to prolong life. Hypoxia is the main stimulans for collateral formation. Therefore our training should be hard enough to induce hypoxia and the formation of new collaterals. This should help us to prolong the life of these patients. I do not think that a reduction in heart rate as improved function of the ventricles prolongs life, although they might be important factors in the reduction of pain. We train the patient for two months under hospital supervision and then discharge him.

Pool: Our intentions have been to increase the work tolerance of the patient and not more than that. We see an average improvement of about 25 percent of the maximum oxygen uptake after a training period of two months.

Hellerstein: In view of the fact that most physicians cannot give their patients the same training that is available in large hospitals what advise can we give them?

Van der Sluys: One practical method you can use is to advise walking. You can calculate from the patient's weight the oxygen consumption required for a walk with a certain speed. If you know the maximum oxygen uptake you can calculate how many minutes he is allowed to walk using the formula by Dr. Bonjer.

Hellerstein: If you evaluate the patient, measure his heart rate, ECG and blood pressure you will find a level at which he shows signs of strain i.e., significant ST displacement, arrhythmias, or disproportionate changes in blood pressure. You will know that this is close to his maximum tolerable level.

How can we equate this level to his performance when walking? The easiest thing to do is to count his heart rate. If the patient develops coronary insufficiency or other evidence of strain, at a heart rate of 120 per minute, his walking pace should be adjusted to produce a heart rate below this level. For the many patients who don't develop angina or premature beats, you can prescribe a target level which is approximately 70 per cent of their age determined maximal rate. For middle-aged people the latter is about 165 to 170 beats per minute.

70 per cent is therefore approximately 120 beats per minute. We know that 70 per cent of the maximal heart rate is equivalent to 50 per cent of the maximal oxygen uptake. The work physiologists have arrived at the same figure as the physical trainers in terms of what is necessary to produce a training effect.

Returning to Dr. Frick's statement the aim of training is to relieve angina, to improve cardiovascular function and to improve the peripheral circulation. In 1957 Dr. M. Karvonen predicted that a large part of the benefit of training will be found in the periphery rather than centrally. The exercise induced increase in mitochondrial density is very important in the periphery because the oxidative enzymes have increased in the skeletal musculature. The methods of training are rather empirical. The frequency of training varies from two to five times per week. We should know the minimum training time required to achieve the maximum effect. We do not know it at this time.

Frick: I think that it depends upon the intensivity of the training. This brings me back to the question of prescribing training for an average person outside the hospital. He should measure his heart rate and work so that he remains mostly below his pain threshold. If we are going to promote collateral circulation it is important that he takes one spurt of activity up to pain. We have about 60 patients now following this advise and we have seen no ill effects at all. The question of how often one must train is related to the nature and intensity of the training. I think that one half hour three times a week is quite sufficient if the patient goes nearly up to pain.

Hellerstein: We have now identified the strain level. A person should exercise below it for the biggest part of his exercise period but he can approach it.

Pool: Not all patients, who have had a myocardial infarction have anginal pain. Only about 30 percent of our patients has angina pectoris. The others are trained in the normal way up to a heart rate that is much higher than in patients with anginal pain.

Hellerstein: Patients who do not have coronary insufficiency can be trained as if they were almost normal individuals using the fundamental principle of pushing them to 70 to 80 percent of their maximal heart rate. We must remember that the maximal heart rate decreases with age. A teenage child can exercise up to 220 beats per minute, a 60 years old man can go up to 160. Therefore, when we relate heart rates, we should not relate fixed heart rates but the rate for the particular age.

Varnauskas: If we assume that the high work intensity which frequently may cause anginal pain promotes the development of collateral coronary circulation then the question may arise whether or not the same effects are achieved by mental stress which produces blood pressure rise, heart rate increase and eventually anginal pain?

Hellerstein: Dr. E. Braunwald has asked that same question: What is the difference between the acceleration in heart rate and blood pressure and electrocardiographic changes induced by emotion versus those due to physical effort? In psychiatric terms a person who has angina feels and reacts as though he were running, but his body is at a standstill. It is like a racing disengaged motor, using a lot of fuel but not getting any mileage from it. There is a fundamental difference in adaptive phenomena that are called upon by emotion compared to that effort.

Varnauskas: Robinson has nicely shown what happens with work of the heart when the patient is exposed to mental stress. The work of the heart as it is defined by the arterial blood pressure and heart rate product at the time for angina pectoris reaches the same level during the stress situation as during the bicycle work. The circulatory mechanisms which are assumed to be of major importance for the development of collateral coronary circulation seem thus to be in operation in both situations.

Pool: The difficulty here is in deciding on what you are aiming to train. Do you only want to promote collateral circulation, do you wish to prolong life or do you want to give your patients a better work capacity. It may be that different types of training are required.

Frick: It is nice to have a pain-free patient but that is only part of our goal. We should aim to prolong his life. The question is whether we can promote collateral circulation by training. The few studies with coronary angiography have been disappointing. The same principle applies here as in making coronary angios after the Vineberg procedure. They have been done in rest and not in an ischaemic situation. The angios should be performed in hypoxia or during atrial pacing. In rest the collaterals may be closed because they are not needed.

Hellerstein: Dr. Frick has stated that coronary arteriography does not measure blood flow; it measures structure. Until we use methods which measure flow we will not know whether training modifies coronary flow. Such studies are urgently needed.

Frick: The findings of improved function might be due to anatomical changes or functional changes. We know that in almost every heart with a myocardial infarction there is some degree of asynergy in the contraction. If we are producing a more organised contraction by training programs we could have improved function without much hypertrophy.

Hellerstein: We are agreed that training changes some easily measured parameters like heart rate and stroke volume in a majority of people. We also know that the morbidity is decreased, that these patients have less angina and they also feel better. We do not have definite data on the effects on mortality. We know that it does not change coronary structure in many cases. It does change myocardial structure because there is good evidence that the heart volume may decrease and the heart mass probably increases.

We must now consider the criterion of benefit. Who should exercise? What are the criteria for training? Whom would you exclude?

Pool: We exclude all patients who are in heart failure. We have chosen an age limit of about 65, mainly because of practical reasons.

Hellerstein: I don't think that practising physicians agree with that. They can train these people outdoors, by prescribing them walking and cycling.

Pool: We do give them such advise, but that is not really training. It is difficult to advise patients to exercise to a heart rate of 165 per minute when you have no opportunity for supervision.

Bonjer: We should keep in mind that, even in those cases, where a training program is not absolutely necessary, we should still train them if they are to resume work.

Frick: It has been our experience that if a patient has pain with a heart rate below 100 per minute it is very hard to train him. We use that heart rate as a threshold for accepting patients. We also do not train patients with a clear bulging of the left ventricle.

Hellerstein: It is my feeling that only 25-35 per cent of coronary patients are eligible for a formal, high level physical reconditioning program. My contra-indications are: rapidly progressing angina pectoris, impending infarction, massive ventricular aneurysm, congestive heart failure not responding to treatment, arrhythmias, patients with paroxysmal ventricular tachycardia, patients with a 2nd or 3rd degree A-V block, patients with fixed ventricular rate pacemakers, untreated atrial fibrillation with a rapid ventricular rate, frequent ventricular premature beats at rest which increase with activity, moderate to severe valvular disease, outflow left ventricular obstructive disease, certain neuro-muscular and mental diseases.

There are certain precautions that should be taken if you are training patients who are receiving drugs, (reserpine, beta-blocking agents, quinidine etc.), because these agents modify many of the patients responses.

As far as indications are concerned, I think we can agree that normal persons who are highly coronary prone would be eligible for training programs. I would also include reconditioning, neuro-circulatory asthenia, coronary disease without contra-indications, and intermittent claudication. Reconditioning is certainly useful in preparing patients for surgery and in rehabilitating them after surgery.

Varnauskas: I have seen no accidents which could be attributed more to the training than to the disease itself. The question is how far going limitations with respect to physical training should be imposed on the patients exhibiting some of the previously mentioned contra-indications. How much de-training do you advocate? I feel that even a low physical activity implies physical training in contrast to bed rest and this is also beneficial for the patient unless the medical treatment as such requires complete bed rest.

Frick: In the last 1000 tests that we have done up to pain on the ergometer, we had one short burst of ventricular tachycardia, which stopped when we stopped the test. We also had one case of a pathological Q-wave wich disappeared the next day.

Pool: All of the patients whom we trained had previously performed a maximum exercisetest. Nevertheless in five cases out of a total of 50 cases we found during the training ventricular ectopic beats and in two a burst of ventricular tachycardia. These were unexpected because they did not occur during the previous maximum exercise test.

Hellerstein: In our 10 years experience we have tape-recorded ECGs for 48 consecutive hours in several hundred subjects. We found that many had arrhythmias in non-exercise periods. We are not quite sure that the events would not have occurred without training. We advise patients who develop ST changes at the target heart rate to take nitroglycerin prior to the effort. We can show that one nitroglycerin tablet is equal to improvement in performance of 150 kgm/min. The patients with ventricular ectopic beats are given anti-arrhythmia therapy. In our own experience we have not had a single patient die in many thousands of exercise tests over a period of 10 years. It is probably more dangerous to wait to get into the program than to participate in the training program.

A member of the audience has asked: How long a time interval do you want to elapse between an acute myocardial infarction and the beginning of the training program.

Pool: We start the heavy training three months after the infarction. Before that time one can prescribe some slight exercises.

Frick: I think that the scare is complete in six weeks and therefore two months after infarction is an appropriate time to begin training. We also give the patients some light exercise before that time.

Varnauskas: The expert group of WHO has worked out a program for rehabilitation. It consists of several stages depending on the course of the disease. Some physical activity can be started from the very beginning, i.e. already in the coronary care unit. The amount of the activity is increased with progression of the recovery. In our studies we do not start regular controlled physical training on bicycle ergometer before three months have elapsed from the onset of the disease. This is because we want to assess the biochemical and physiological effects of physical training and thus we want to start from the point where the influence of the disease itself on these variables has disappeared. No unmotivated limitations of physical activity are imposed on the patients at any time of the disease.

Hellerstein: We must individualise our decision based on whether the patient has had a massive coronary or a very minor one a 'coronette'. If the patient has had no congestion or arrhythmias we do not allow him to become deconditioned. In six or seven weeks we can enter him into a fairly high level program. When patients develop ventricular tachycardia during training, (we have seen only two or three out of about 250 patients), we detrain them slightly and put them on anti-arrhythmic drugs.

Hellerstein: This afternoon, the panel has tried to define some basic concepts about the training of patients with ischaemic heart disease. We wish to encourage you and to convince you that it is possible to measure aerobic power without elaborate equipment. There is a basis for prescribing exercise training and work prescription as a certain percentage of the patient's maximum capacity. We think that training is good in selected cases who do not have contra indications. Physical conditioning enhances performance, certain psychological parameters and reduces morbidity in these patients who have angina. We do not know about its effects on mortality yet. We also do not know about changes in coronary flow although we are quite certain that coronary structure does not change grossly. We think that there is some change in the myocardium in terms of its size and volume. There are many things that we still do not know and there is obviously the need for much research. We do not know how long a person should exercise and what the intensity of training should be. There are other points of disagreement. We all do agree on one point, that physical training is a positive approach to the treatment of a terrible disease (ischaemic heart disease) and there is need for substantial research on every level to learn more about the adaptation that takes place in the person, in his heart, in his circulation and in the periphery with all grades of physical training.

CHAPTER V

EPIDEMIOLOGY AND PRIMARY PREVENTION

Chapter V and VI contain the proceedings of the symposium organized by the Netherlands Heart Foundation,
which has been held in connection with the Boerhaave Course on Ischaemic Heart Disease.

INTRODUCTION*

R. J. H. KRUISINGA

MR. CHAIRMAN, DEAR COLLEAGUES

It is a pleasure to welcome you on behalf of my Government. A special welcome to our foreign guests, coming from USA and most European countries. We highly appreciate that Dr. Pisa, as representative of WHO, is attending this meeting. And is taking an active part in it. It is a well-known fact that my Government seized all possible opportunities to stimulate WHO's activities in the field of cardiovascular diseases.

In the two previous days your approach to the problem was more or less theoretical. This day – sponsored by the Netherlands Heart Foundation – is devoted to public health problems in relation to coronary heart disease. I therefore gladly accepted the invitation to open this session.

You will be interested in the situation in the Netherlands. This country is densely populated. In the different provinces the density is between 170 and 1000 people per km². Originally a rural country the Netherlands have been industrialising rather rapidly after World War II.

Hand in hand with urbanisation, and hand in hand with the change of mode of life from the rural to the modern urban pattern, mortality from coronary heart disease is increasing year by year. Only since the early sixties we are aware of this situation. In the past few years a survey brought to light the raising prevalence of coronary heart disease in male and female civil servants.

This survey was part of a prevalence study held in several European countries by the WHO. My Ministry has given a threefold support to this survey by providing the subjects, a grant-in-aid and advices in organization of the project.

Our knowledge about the morbidity pattern of coronary heart disease in the Netherlands is far from complete. We must try to fill the

* Address given at the opening of the symposium of the Netherlands Heart Foundation.

gaps. We must become aware of the fact that in our country coronary heart disease is the most important single cause of death. Most probably it is also the most important cause of serious illness in middle aged men. From our analysis of changing mortality patterns it is now known that cardiovascular diseases, neoplasms, and respiratory diseases contribute 45%, 35% and 10% respectively to the increase of total mortality in adult men. The increase of mortality from cardiovascular diseases in men manifests itself already at the age of 35. The present rates for men under 55 are now as high as for more than ten years older women. In the Netherlands the annual death toll of ischaemic heart disease is at present 15000 men and 9000 women. Of those 9000 men and 3500 women are under 75. Passing the decades from 45-54 and from 55-64 the Dutch man has a risk of 2% and 5% respectively of dying from ischaemic heart disease.

Ischaemic heart disease and cerebrovascular and hypertensive diseases show a quite different mortality pattern.

The conclusion may be drawn that the high risk factors underlying these diseases must be quite different. On the other hand mortality and morbidity rates from coronary heart disease are in Holland still lower than in other Western countries. Our rates, however, are rather rapidly increasing.

One remark concerning one of the causes why. Physical inactivity differs from other Western countries. Pedal cycles are in daily use here but are being replaced by mopeds.

In 1950 Holland had one car in 75 and one moped in 100 inhabitants. At present one car and, or one moped in every two families. The post war generation is physically far less active than their parents were. Will for this reason alone the incidence of ischaemic heart disease continue to increase?

We should not close our eyes for the following two facts:

1. the average food consumption has increased substantially to 3000 calories daily;
2. cigarette consumption per capita per year increased from 913 in 1952 to 1321 in 1967.

However, as I stated the situation in some other countries like Finland, u.s.a., Scotland is still worse. The increase during the sixties in our country is, however, very substantial. Furthermore the low rate in France deserves our attention.

Primary prevention is not intensively practised in our country.

Little is still known about the Dutch pattern of high risk factors. We are therefore very interested in your conclusions on primary prevention.

In the first place to adapt our programme of health education on coronary heart disease to modern views. Within the next few years, we hope to become better informed about the pattern of high risk factors in the Netherlands. We hope to do this by stimulating epidemiological field work and standardization of methods of investigation.

Physical inactivity, inadequate diet and cigarette smoking are undoubtedly important risk factors also in our country.

We don't know the weight of each factor in relation to ECG-abnormalities, blood pressure, obesity, cholesterol-, lipid- and glucose-levels. Still less we know about the Dutch pattern by sex and age.

The curative approach of doctors generally explains, why until now more attention has been given to the treatment of coronary patients and to secondary prevention than to primary prevention.

Rehabilitation meets much interest of our cardiologists. Coronary care units are now under construction in some of our large hospitals.

Prevention of reinfarction by anti-coagulant treatment has become common knowledge in the Netherlands, both among doctors and patients.

The first out-patient service in this field started already in 1949.

We lack sufficient data on sudden death from coronary heart disease in the Netherlands. But we cannot do without it. Therefore we gladly accepted WHO's invitation to participate in an international study on coronary heart disease registers, partly focused on sudden death.

In one of our university centres a medical team will register all cases of coronary heart disease in a region of 200.000 inhabitants. Cases of sudden death and of patients treated at home or in hospital will be registered. This study will be possible through financial and material aid by the Ministry of Social Affairs and Public Health. The organisation will set us a heavy task.

Before we were informed about WHO's plan on coronary heart disease registers, the Netherlands Government Health authorities planned to organise the registration of cases of coronary heart disease in a two-fold way. Firstly registration of hospitalized patients all over the country and secondly registration of patients of anti-coagulant services was planned.

The analysis of mortality data will be continued.

We need this combination of data for planning the policy in relation to coronary care units and to secundary prevention. We should, however, keep in mind that primary prevention is our ultimate aim.

Cardiological departments in this country have a long tradition in research, directed to clinical and laboratory problems. We are aware of the fact that this kind of research is also of value from an epidemiological point of view. Therefore my Ministry will from time to time give grants to cardiological departments.

In this connection it is relevant to remind you of the fact that in a laboratory in this city, not far from the place where this meeting takes place, the *electrocardiograph* has been discovered. The names of Einthoven and Wenckebach are for ever connected with clinical research in the field of cardiovascular diseases.

Among the different projects in the field of cardiovascular diseases which will be supported by my Ministry, I mentioned some, among which, the large scale epidemiological research in an area of 200.000 inhabitants.

cal point of view. Therefore my Ministry will from time to time give

I would also like to mention the experiment with the mobile coronary care unit, for today I would stress not only preventive measures, but also curative activities because of the Dutch medical tradition in this field, which should not be entirely forgotten.

For this reason I like to mention the research on effectivity of 'anticoagulant therapy, in which we just decided to support a new project by Professor Snellen.

Mr. Chairman, it was a pleasure to make these few introductory remarks. I wish you every success on behalf of my Government. The Netherlands Heart Foundation is sponsoring this day. It is offering you a booklet with basic facts on coronary heart disease in the Netherlands. From the graphs and tables it will be clear that from a public health point of view coronary heart disease is one of the most important public health problems.

Certainly this is the case in the older Dutch male population. The problem is of increasing importance. Especially it is increasing at that age on which men reach the height of their achievements.

Based on a rational policy it will be our duty to reverse this frightening development. Without well planned preventive measures mortality and morbidity from ischaemic heart disease will show a further fast and substantial rise.

Mr. Chairman appropriate measures will have to be taken.

ISCHAEMIC HEART DISEASE PROGRAM OF THE WHO REGIONAL OFFICE FOR EUROPE

Z. PISA

The present programme of the WHO Regional Office for Europe started in 1968 and will continue in its present form for five years. Its purpose is to develop and test methods and forms of organization that will enable the introduction of efficient cardiovascular control programmes on a national basis. For technical as well as financial reasons it has been necessary to concentrate, in this first phase, on ischaemic heart disease, the most common of the cardiovascular diseases in Europe (fig. 1).

The programme includes projects dealing with the prevention of the disease, the improvement of mortality statistics, the collection of more and better information on the incidence of ischaemic heart disease in the community, the assessment of the contributions of coronary care and different rehabilitation programmes for patients who have suffered myocardial infarction. These projects are complemented by intensive training programmes in epidemiology and statistics, in coronary care and in rehabilitation.

Under a project for epidemiological studies on ischaemic heart disease several centres in different European countries, including the Department of Epidemiology at the London School of Hygiene and Tropical Medicine, are now concentrating on a cardio-respiratory preventive trial in connection with cigarette smoking. In December 1969 a workshop is to be held in London, at which those participating will be made acquainted with the methods to be used. The trial is expected to be in full operation by 1970.

Another project for health education of the public on the prevention of cardiovascular diseases aims at studying the possibility of conducting really effective health education. At present a consultant is collecting information on the work done in different European countries in this field and on the facilities available there.

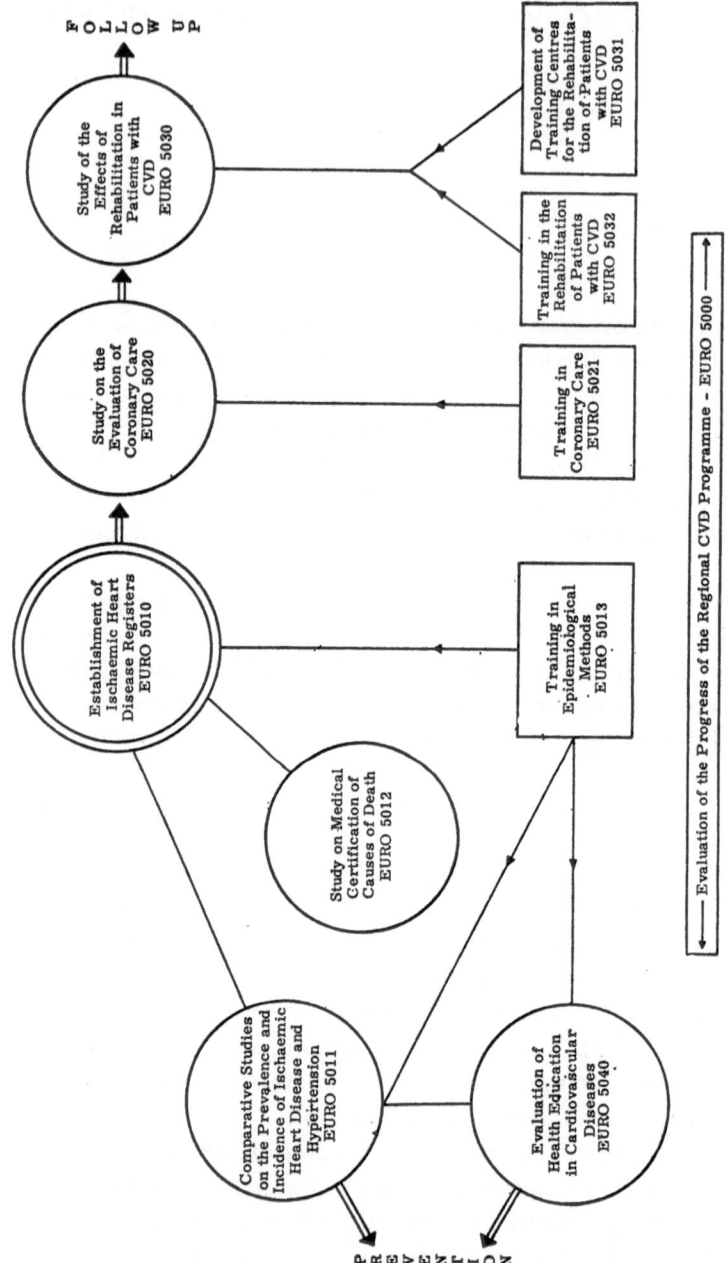

Fig. 1.

A project on Medical Certification of Causes of Death is also being conducted with a view to improving information from death certificates for purposes of mortality statistics. It is being developed in two phases. In the first phase, an assessment is being made in five selected areas, of the information available to the doctor certifying death and the use made of it. In the second stage of the project a set of standard medical histories will be circulated to the collaborating centres in different countries, to test how the information they contain is used by doctors for completing death certificates in various countries influenced by different medical schools. The key project for the development of future cardiovascular control programmes is that on the Establishment of Ischaemic Heart Disease Registers. Well-defined areas have been selected and in them every case of myocardial infarction, whether fatal or not, attended or unattended by a doctor, is to be registered to enable long-term follow-up in all cases of survival.

The data provided and kept up-to-date in this register will make it possible:

1. to determine the exact clinical presence of the disease in the community, from the standpoint of both mortality and morbidity;
2. to study the natural history of the disease;
3. to establish the effect of the disease on work capacity, absentecism and social costs generally:
4. to establish the efficiency of different forms of treatment and methods of prevention, their economic costs and benefits;
5. to establish local treatment requirements from emergency and intensive care to rehabilitation and long-term follow-up;
6. to make available an extensive series of well-defined cases for any future investigation.

This project is closely linked with others and can provide valuable methods and information for them, especially as regards coronary care and rehabilitation. It is, in fact, intended to introduce it into the pilot areas where facilities in those fields are also available. A working group, held in May 1968, has designed a study and adopted an operating protocol as well as record forms for the registration of patients for this purpose. This design is based on experience gained in the Edinburgh Community Study. Two feasibility studies, each of three months' duration, were conducted in Gothenburg and Prague at the end of 1968 and at the beginning of this year. At working groups held in mid-April and mid-May this year a final version of the operating protocol and record forms were prepared, based on experience gained in the pre-pilot areas as well as Edinburgh. In several areas in Europe and overseas great interest has been shown in starting these registers. This project, like the others, is being organized in close co-operation with the relevant units at WHO headquarters in Geneva. Provision is made for the pooling of data in Geneva and for the use of headquarters' computers for analysis.

Another project on the Evaluation of Coronary Care will, to a great extent, benefit from the information collected in the registration areas. A working group, meeting in February 1969, prepared recommendations for the organization of coronary care units. Its report sets out requirements for and standards of design, equipment, staffing, documentation and staff training for coronary care units. At present the project is concentrating on study of the pre-admission period and on the contribution and effectiveness of mobile coronary care units to the community.

A project on the evaluation of rehabilitation programmes will also benefit from the information collected by the ischaemic heart disease registers. In co-operation with the Council on Rehabilitation of the International Society of Cardiology it has been possible to collect, at least in part, information on the situation regarding rehabilitation of cardiac patients in different European countries, especially of those with myocardial infarction. The present situation does not correspond to our present scientific knowledge in this field. As a first step, therefore, a working group composed of experts in the rehabilitation of cardiovascular patients and representing different European schools, has proposed a programme of physical rehabilitation for patients with myocardial infarction. This programme provides for rehabilitation of these patients as an integral part of their treatment. It covers the period from the very first day of the disease up to post-convalescence. Recently, a Working Group discussed the psychological aspects of rehabilitation of these patients. It dealt with the role of psychologists in different phases of rehabilitation and related their action to the previously defined phases of the programme of physical rehabilitation. It also suggested several research projects which might enable assessment of the influence of psychological and social factors on the rehabilitation of patients with myocardial infarction.

In October 1969 a meeting is to be held to review the findings of several studies at present in progress in different European laboratories and to make an objective evaluation of the rehabilitation on patients with myocardial infarction. It is expected that this group will agree on a set of methods which will help in assessing the progress of the patients with myocardial infarction who undergo different rehabilitation programmes.

An extensive teaching programme has also begun. Using existing facilities in leading European centres, courses have been organized in epidemiology and medical statistics, specially covering cardiovascular disease problems. A manual for teaching the epidemiology of cardio-vascular diseases has been prepared and, since autum of 1967, six courses on coronary care have been organized in English, French and Russian for fellows from different European countries. In the field of rehabilitation special courses on the use of work capacity tests have been held in French and English and next year a similar course is to be held in Russian. Further, provision is made for individual fellowships in each of the fields concerned.

In addition to the above measures a project is being run for the evaluation of the cardiovascular disease programme, covering the collection of information on existing services for cardiovascular patients in different European countries. Its purpose is also to establish a net-work of contacts in those countries to inform this office about develop-ments in this field and also disseminate the results of different studies quickly to their own countries.

The programme of the WHO Regional Office for Europe in the field of cardiovascular diseases is being conducted in close collaboration with WHO Headquarters in Geneva, with the International Society of Cardiology and the European Society of Cardiology. Public health authorities in European countries have evinced considerable interest in the programme and several countries have already given financial and administrative support to the centres collaborating with the WHO Regional Office in Europe.

RESULTS OF THE EPIDEMOLOGIC INVESTIGATION OF ISCHAEMIC HEART DISEASE: ILLUSTRATED BY THE FRAMINGHAM STUDY

W. B. KANNEL

INTRODUCTION

The utility of an epidemiologic approach to the study of chronic disease is that it provides the most comprehensive appraisal of the manner in which the disease arises, evolves and terminates fatally in its natural environment. Prospective epidemiologic studies of coronary heart disease (CHD) in a variety of population samples have focused attention on a broader spectrum of coronary disease than that which is clinically manifest. This has resulted from intensive medical surveillance which has yielded not only those cases coming under medical care, but those not hospitalized as well, including those dying too suddenly to reach the hospital. This has revealed the true nature of the disease as an extremely lethal process characteristically striking down the victim unheralded by prior symptoms.

Epidemiologic studies have pointed to a need for a preventive approach and possible means for delaying its onset and premature death by interrupting the chain of events associated with its occurrence.

The efficacy of epidemiologic information for the practice of medicine is often less immediately apparent to most than is information concerned with the diagnosis and management of already symptomatic disease. From a study of the premorbid personal characteristics and living habits of those who have gone on to develop CHD in comparison with those who have remained free of the disease for long periods, it has been possible to identify factors which appear to predispose and to characterize highly susceptible persons. As a result of prospective epidemiologic studies, both at Framingham and elsewhere, a portrait of the prime candidate for coronary disease has emerged. This has enabled the construction of a 'coronary profile' which allows an estimate of the probability of developing the disease as well as identifying the risk factors which need correction. They have yielded information concerning the incidence of the disease, death rates attributed to it, the probability of an attack and an undistorted picture of its natural history, i.e. the chain of events leading to its occurrence. Clues to the pathogenesis of CHD have been provided by these studies and many of the major hypotheses concerning the etiology of this disease have been tested prospectively. On occasion, new hypotheses have been suggested.

The purpose of this report is to review the findings of epidemiologic studies of coronary heart disease, using Framingham data as an illustration. The preventive and therapeutic implications of this epidemiologic information will be emphasized.

METHODS

Since the findings of epidemiologic investigations of coronary heart disease will be illustrated with data from the Framingham Study, a brief description of the methods employed is relevant. The Framingham Study is a straightforward prospective longitudinal study and it can serve as a model since the methods employed are reasonably characteristic of those used in such epidemiologic investigations. An extensive description of methods employed in prospective epidemiologic studies in general, and at Framingham in particular, has been published elsewhere for consideration in extenso (1-13). Briefly, the methods followed at Framingham were as follows:

1. Study design

A sample of 5.127 men and women examined and found free of CHD at time of initial examination were classified at that examination and biennially thereafter according to a variety of living habits and biochemical and physiologic personal attributes believed possibly important in atherosclerosis. At biennial intervals thereafter they were examined for development of evidence of CHD.

Medical surveillance was quite complete and included, in addition to examination in the clinic, daily surveillance of hospital admissions in the only general hospital in town, evaluation of death certificates, medical examiner's reports, and information from spouses and physicians concerning the health of participants. It is unlikely that any sizeable number of myocardial infarctions or deaths due to CHD escaped detection.

2. Follow-up

After 14 years of biennial cardiovascular surveillance follow-up has been gratifyingly complete. Over 97% of subjects took more than one examination in the clinic. Of those who took the initial examination and survived the 14 years of follow-up, about 80% took all seven biennial examinations. Less than 2% of the original population sample examined are unaccounted for having been completely lost to follow-up.

3. Criteria for CHD

The diagnostic criteria employed have been described in detail elsewhere (11,14-17). A diagnosis of ANGINA PECTORIS was based entirely on subjective complaints. Minimal criteria consisted of brief duration of substernal discomfort clearly related to exertion or excitement and relieved by rest or nitroglycerine. The symptoms must not have occurred regularly during rest and must not last more than 15 minutes. Symptoms had to be sufficiently clear so that two independent medical examiners could elicit from the patient the same information. MYO-CARDIAL INFARCTION was accepted as a diagnosis when documented by serial ECG changes of an evolving infarction or, on occasion, when transient elevations of serum enzymes (SGOT and LDH) in an appropriate clinical setting occurred in the absence of unequivocal ECG findings. All ECG's were examined by the study personnel comparing the pre-morbid ECG's with those obtained during and subsequent to hospitalization. A syndrome of CORONARY INSUFFICIENCY was included when clinical findings suggesting a myocardial infarction occurred in the absence of evidence of myocardial necrosis but accompanied instead by transient ECG evidence of myocardial ischemia or injury. SUDDEN UN-EXPECTED DEATH was attributed to CHD when it occurred in persons not suffering from some potentially lethal disease under circumstances suggesting death in a matter of minutes from onset and documented to have occurred in less than one hour.

4. Examination procedures

Biennial cardiovascular examination was performed which included a 13-lead ECG, physical examination, detailed cardiovascular history, a chest x-ray, body weight and skinfold thickness, a lipid profile, blood sugar and hematocrit, among other observations. Three blood pressures were obtained on each participant with the subject seated, arm resting on a desk. Physical activity assessments were obtained on the fourth biennial examination based on a 24 hour history of usual activity. A 'physical activity index' was computed for each subject representing the sum of the products of weighted hours spent at various levels of physical activity, ranging from basal (assigned a weighting factor of 1.0) to 'heavy activity' (assigned an energy expenditure weighting factor of 5.0). Biochemical laboratory methods employed have been detailed elsewhere (16,18). Long-term dietary assessment was obtained by a nutritionist in a subsample of the population at the time of the fifth biennial examination using the method of Burke (6, 7).

5. Statistical methods

A variety of statistical methods have been employed over the years including multivariate analysis, quantal response curves, discriminant function analysis, multiple logistic function, linear multiple regression and simple age-adjusted incidence rates (19-22). When the effects of variables on the incidence of CHD for large age subgroups were compared, age-adjustment for differences in age composition of the subclasses was made using 'morbidity ratios'. The population free of CHD was subdivided according to the various personal attributes or living habits being considered in relation to subsequent incidence of CHD. The number of cases of CHD observed during the ensuing 14 years was then determined for each subgroup. This number was then compared to a calculated expected number of cases obtained by applying the age-specific incidence rate for the whole population to the various subgroups under scrutiny. For convenience, the 'morbidity ratios' were multiplied by 100, so that a morbidity ratio of 100 (cases observed equal to cases expected) represents the standard risk of the population.

IMPLICATIONS OF THE NATURAL HISTORY OF CHD

Epidemiologic studies have revealed in stark reality the way CHD occurs in the general population. As a result it has become clear that patients who reach the hospital alive represent the survivors of a lethal process that has already exacted the bulk of its deadly toll. Hospital statistics alone provide a much too benign assessment of this death-dealing illness. An examination of the pattern of medical care afforded all 'heart attack' victims (i.e., initial attacks of CHD excluding angina pectoris) reveals that fully 40% are not hospitalized even in a

community such as Framingham where even mere suspicion of a myocardial infarction is cause for hospitalization. The major reasons for
failure to receive hospital care is the occurrence of *sudden unexpected
death* or the fact that the myocardial infarction went *unrecognized*. The
case fatality rate in those hospitalized was about 17% in the precoronary care unit era. That in those who did not reach the hospital
was 50% (fig. 1). In fact, one in every five attacks presented with
sudden death as the first and last symptom of CHD.

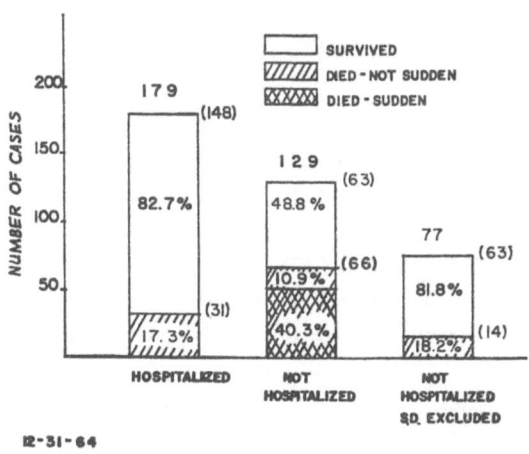

Fig. 1. Immediate mortality following initial episode of CHD (exclusive of a.p.), men and
women 30-62 and free of CHD at entry: Framingham heart study.

Of potentially greater importance than modern innovations in
medical technology (including cardiac transplantation) to the future
reduction in mortality from CHD is the growing appreciation that the
bulk of deaths from CHD are occurring before it is possible for the
patient to receive intensive coronary care in the hospital. An examination of all CHD deaths during initial attacks reveals that fully 65%
were sudden and unexpected, the entire course of the illness terminating
in a matter of minutes (fig. 2). Consequently, efforts confined entirely
to improving the management of already symptomatic disease surviving long enough to reach a hospital facility, no matter how successful
or ingenious, cannot be expected to have a major impact on mortality
in this leading cause of death.

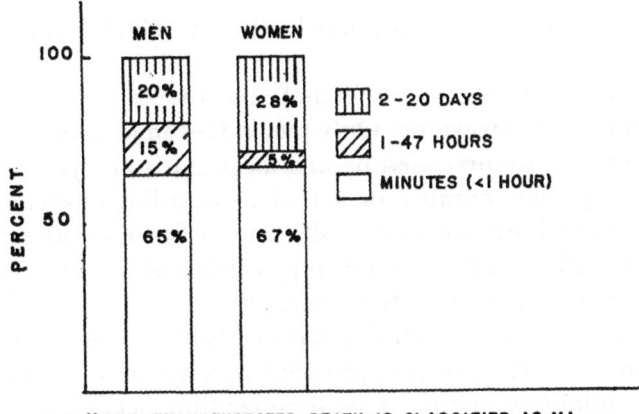

Fig. 2. Immediate mortality of initial myocardial infarction*, men and women 30-62 at entry: Framingham heart study 14-year follow-up.

As a result, efforts are being made to determine the events that are likely to precipitate the lethal episode and to reduce the time interval between the onset of symptoms and the availability of comprehensive, sophisticated emergency facilities. Mobile coronary care units are being developed to rapidly bring life-saving equipment to the victim at the onset of the attack. However, even this may be too little and late.

Coronary heart disease is an extremely common disease and myo-

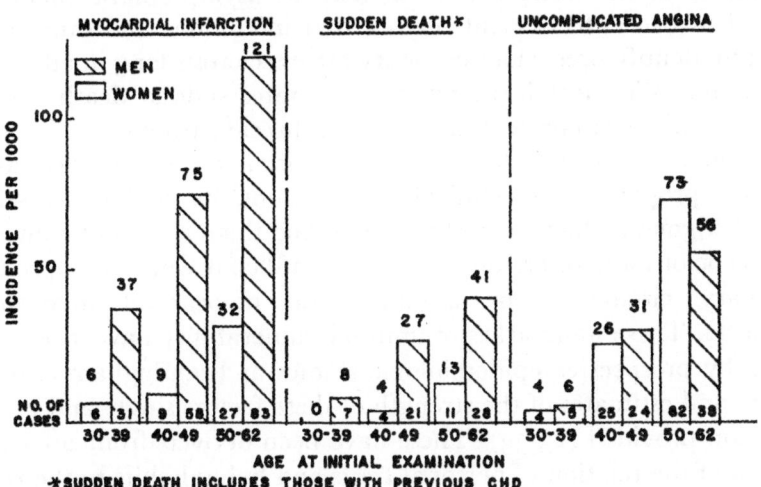

Fig. 3. 14-year incidence of clinical manifestations of CHD by age and sex, men and women 30-62 at entry: Framingham heart study.

cardial infarctions are its principal clinical manifestation in men (fig. 3).

In addition to being highly lethal, the disease characteristically strikes without much warning. Only one in four myocardial infarctions or sudden deaths are preceded by angina pectoris one year before the attack. A surprising number of actual myocardial infarctions never even reach the clinical horizon. Fully one in five such attacks go *un-recognized*, half silent and the rest so atypical that neither the victim nor his physician even considered the possibility.

In a disease with this natural history early diagnosis of still asymptomatic coronary artery disease provides a possibility for salvage of the bulk of potential CHD victims. Highly susceptible persons with accelerated coronary atherosclerosis, persons with a compromised coronary circulation, and those with occult, asymptomatic CHD should be detected in the general population and effort made to correct the biochemical and physiologic predisposing factors and to modify contributory faulty living habits. We must learn to anticipate the disease on its way to happening and intervene effectively long in advance of the first symptoms which, all too often, may also be the very last. Such primary prevention is facilitated by a thorough knowledge of the epidemiology, or chain of events leading to the occurrence of the disease. At the very least, the clinical concept of the spectrum of the disease must be broadened to include its asymptomatic phase. We must learn to detect 'silent' myocardial infarctions and other occult CHD; to identify precocious coronary atherosclerosis long in advance of symptoms. We must learn what precipitates sudden deaths in such persons and how to protect them against this catastrophe.

While most myocardial infarctions occurred unheralded and a sizeable proportion are clinically inapparent, its victims are seldom free of stigmata which could have identified them as highly vulnerable to precocious atherosclerosis, or already afflicted with a compromised coronary circulation or asymptomatic myocardial involvement (table 1). These hallmarkes of unusual vulnerability have been identified by prospective epidemiologic studies at Framingham and elsewhere and estimates of the strength of these factors singly and in combination provided (23-33). These have been derived from an examination of the relation of personal traits and living habits to the rate of subsequent development of CHD under observation in a variety of population samples. The findings of these studies can be exemplified by

Table 1. Proportion of coronary heart disease with abnormalities* on initial examination

No. of abnormalities	Men		Women	
	No.	%	No.	%
None	81	25.5	34	20.8
One	113	35.5	59	36.2
Two	87	27.4	43	26.4
Three or more	37	11.6	27	16.6
Total	318	100.0	163	100.0

Note: Eleven persons did not have all measurements done, so are not included in above table.
* Abnormalities – hypertension, cholesterol $\geq$ 250, ECG abnormal, smoking $>$ 1 pkg. cigarettes, diabetes, obese (20% above median).

data from the Framingham Study which follows. Asymptomatic persons with these high risk traits can be readily identified by the practicing physician using ordinary office procedures and simple laboratory tests. From these observations a profile of susceptibility can be constructed and the probability or risk of an attack estimated, simply or using computers, to define as much as a thirtyfold range of risks.

Host factors: Stigmata associated with accelerated atherogenesis
The concept of chronic disease arising from a single cause is becoming obsolete. Evidence to date in CHD strongly suggests that it derives from the contribution of a variety of interrelated host and environmental factors which operate over many years. Epidemiologic investigation into the causes of CHD has provided information concerning the biochemical and physiologic precursors of accelerated atherosclerosis. In persons so predisposed it has also been possible to identify factors which appear to precipitate attacks, those which affect survival once an attack occurs and which predispose to recurrences and shorten life.

While it is now possible, using coronary cine angiography, to directly assess the extent of involvement of the coronary arteries with athero-thrombotic disease, this procedure is costly, unpleasant and not without hazard. It cannot in its present form be justified for evaluation of the coronary circulation in asymptomatic persons not being considered as possible candidates for surgical revascularization of the myocardium. Significant coronary atherosclerosis can be assumed from autopsy studies carried out in war casualties to be ubiquitous in persons beyond age 25 (34-37). Since a rather pronounced narrowing or actual occlusion is required to compromise the coronary circulation to an extent that ischaemia and infarction occurs, symptomatic CHD is uncommon before the age of 40. It is in this interval that preventive measures have greater potential than after the disease has progressed to the point where symptoms appear.

The rate at which coronary atherosclerosis is likely to be accumulating and the probability of having advanced coronary atherosclerosis can be estimated from measurements of certain atherogenic biochemical and physiologic precursors. This provides an indirect but useful approach to the detection of asymptomatic coronary artery disease. A multiplicity of host factors have been identified which are associated with an increased incidence of clinically overt CHD. To what extent these are genetic or environmentally determined has not been clearly established.

Age and sex

Age and the male sex constitute the most powerful atherogenic host factors which have yet been identified. Age could very well be atherogenic with susceptibility determined at the moment of conception. Susceptibility to overt CHD and the extent of coronary atherosclerosis clearly increases with age in both sexes. It is possible that age also affects myocardial irritability, myocardial reserve or blood coagulability. While age may well be atherogenic per se, it very likely also reflects the length of exposure to acquired biochemical abnormalities or physiologic disturbances and exposure to adverse living habits. The immunity of women to coronary disease is only relative since even in the female CHD is quite common. Sex may well play a biologic role since the relative immunity of the premenopausal woman apparently becomes attenuated after the menopause. Hormonal factors would seem the most likely explanation. The sex ratio comes closer to unity with advancing age, the gap in incidence closing with advancing age. Only 20 years later in life do women develop myocardial infarctions at a rate comparable to that seen in men (fig. 3).

It is clear that coronary atherosclerosis is not simply a consequence of age and sex since, at any age in either sex, some persons have proved more vulnerable, based on a number of personal attributes, than others (23-33). The chief hallmarks of vulnerability which have been linked to precocious coronary atherosclerosis are the serum lipids and the blood pressure. Together these interact to determine the rate of atherogenesis and they constitute key factors in assessing the magnitude of the risk of developing CHD. At any level of one the risk of CHD was noted to increase in proportion to the level of the other (fig. 4).

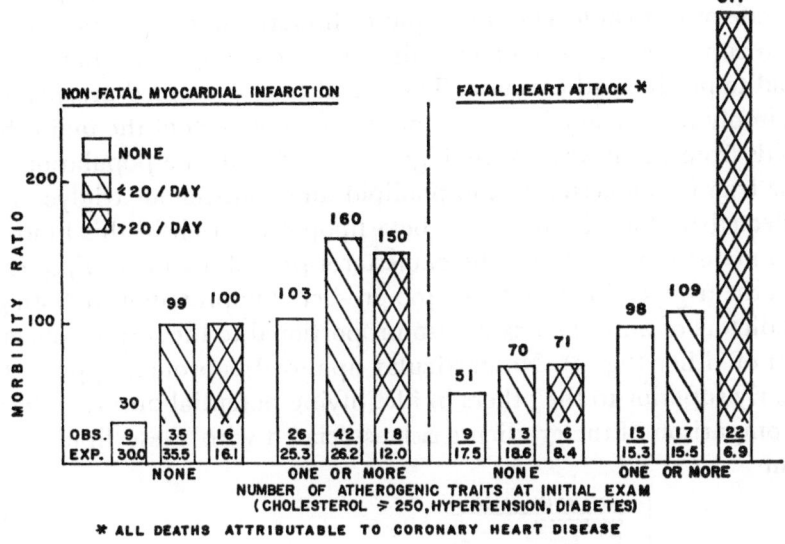

Fig. 4. Risk of coronary heart disease (14 years) according to lipoprotein concentration and blood pressure status, men 30-49 at entry: Framingham tudy.

Serum lipids

The preponderance of evidence seems to emphasize a multifactorial causation of atherosclerosis, but if a single common denominator does exist, then some aberration of the metabolism or transport of lipid must be regarded as the chief contender. An appraisal of the evidence accumulated from animal experiments, laboratory research, clinical observation, autopsy studies and epidemiologic research leaves little doubt of a major role of lipids in atherogenesis (15, 16, 18, 33, 38-47). However, despite the considerable volume of research, the single lipid among those implicated which is most basic in atherogenesis is still not established, if such a lipid indeed exists. Virtually every lipid encountered in the blood has been incriminated in atherosclerotic disease (16,40-50).

Prospective epidemiologic data comparing the strength of the relationship of the major lipids and lipoproteins to the incidence of CHD is scarce. Prospective data from Framingham concerning the incidence of CHD over 14 years in relation to antecendent premorbid serum lipids and their lipoprotein vehicles appears to shed some light on the role of the various lipids in the development of CHD.

Within the range of lipid values encountered in affluent populations, no safe or critical level of any lipid or lipoprotein can be identified. In such populations, given enough time, everyone appears to have enough lipid to produce atheromata. The risk of CHD, examined prospectively, is simply proportional to the concentration of each of the major blood lipids from the lowest to the highest recorded in the population. This was true for cholesterol, phospholipid and endogenous triglyceride as reflected by the Sf 20-400 pre-beta lipoprotein rich in this lipid. The two major lipid vehicles, the cholesterol-rich Sf 0-20 beta lipoprotein, and the triglyceride-rich Sf 20-400 pre-beta lipoprotein were both good predictors of CHD, the risk of CHD proportional to the serum concentration of either (fig. 4). No particular lipid or lipoprotein appears to be clearly superior to the others in identifying potential CHD as judged by a comparison of the gradients risk associated with these lipid components.

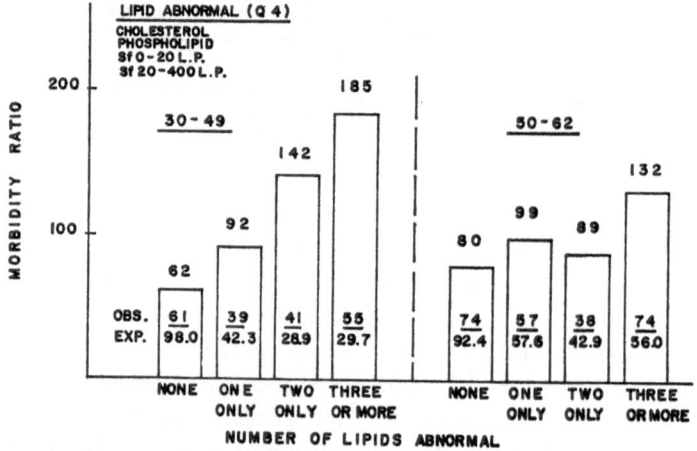

Fig. 5. Risk of coronary heart disease (14 years) according to number of abnormal lipids, men and women 30-62 at entry: Framingham heart study.

If the upper quartile of the distribution of each lipid and lipoprotein vehicle is designated arbitrarily as 'abnormal' and the risk of CHD is determined according to the number of such abnormalities present in each subject's blood, then it appears that risk increases in proportion to the number of lipid 'abnormalities' present (fig. 5). However, it is not clear from this that each lipid separately contributes to risk since the mean level of each particular lipid also rose with the number of lipid abnormalities present (table 2).

Table 2. Mean lipid and lipoprotein content according to number of lipid 'abnormalities'

Men 30-62 at entry – Framingham Heart Study

Men 30-49 No. of lipid Abnormalities	No.	Mean serum lipid content			
		S_f20-400 Lipoprotein	S_f0-20 Lipoprotein	Serum cholesterol	Serum phospholipid
None	746	126.7	363.6	197.2	143.8
One	309	189.8	434.9	222.5	178.7
Two	211	259.5	479.1	248.0	200.0
Three	136	339.7	501.2	285.4	236.5
Four	65	345.9	567.2	293.0	249.9
Men 50-62					
None	277	121.8	363.8	197.2	149.6
One	151	188.5	447.0	223.4	178.5
Two	94	221.7	480.4	253.5	205.7
Three	80	274.6	523.4	280.9	225.4
Four	25	357.8	586.6	291.8	258.2

While risk of CHD was distinctly and impressively related to the lipoprotein content of the blood, the risk of CHD could largely be accounted for by the degree of accompanying hypercholesterolaemia. Detailed analysis of the net contribution of each lipid and its lipoprotein vehicles to risk of CHD suggests that elevated serum cholesterol content, regardless of how transported or partitioned among the lipoprotein vehicles, is associated with an increased risk of CHD, the risk determined essentially by the total cholesterol concentration. After accounting for the level of Sf 20-400 pre-beta lipoprotein and other factors related both to blood lipids and to CHD, there was still an appreciable gradient of risk proportional to the serum cholesterol concentration. On the other hand, when risk of CHD was examined according to Sf 20-400 pre-beta lipoprotein level, adjusting for the concomitant *serum cholesterol* level, no residual risk gradient could be discerned in men (fig. 6). Knowledge of both the lipoprotein pattern and the serum cholesterol level proved no better in discriminating potential coronary victims than a knowledge of the cholesterol level alone.

Those persons with the usual degree of 'hypercholesterolaemia' encountered in the general population (i.e. 250-350 mg%) had a two to

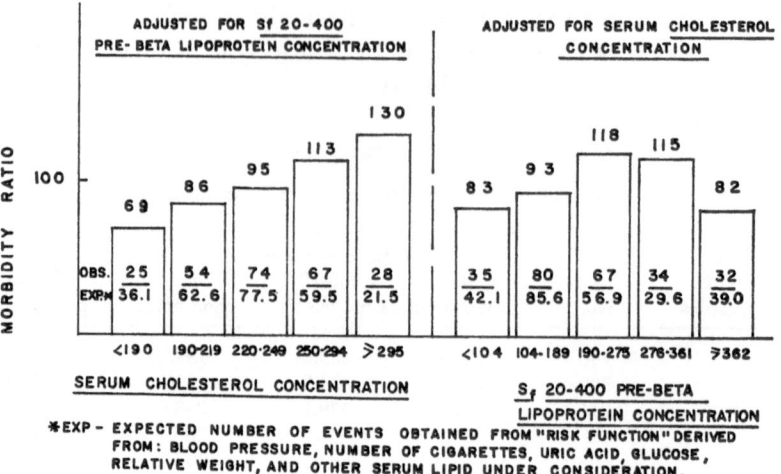

Fig. 6. Risk of coronary heart disease (14 years) according to serum lipid adjusted for associated variables, men 38-69 years: Framingham study.

five-fold increased risk of CHD, depending on age and sex, and this was true regardless of whether the 'hypercholesterolaemia' was of the carbohydrate sensitive variety (associated with Sf 20-400 *pre-beta* lipoprotein elevation), or of the saturated fat and dietary cholesterol sensitive type (associated with Sf 0-20 *beta* lipoprotein increase). The usual variety of 'hypercholesterolaemia' found in the general population, a common and potent contributor to the abundance of CHD which occurs in the general population, was equally often associated with elevation of both types lipoprotein.

It has been held in the past that a high concentration of cholesterol is more serious when not accompanied by a commensurate elevation of phospholipid. This has never been demonstrated prospectively, nor has it been consistently found in clinical studies (55-57). Continued advocacy of the cholesterol/phospholipid ratio as an index of atherogenesis cannot be defended since no trend in risk of CHD according to C/P ratio can be demonstrated among hypercholesterolaemic persons (15).

Lipoprotein patterns are now easily determined using paper or agarose electrophoresis. Determination of the lipoprotein pattern in persons with 'hypercholesterolaemia' is of more importance for diagnosing the nature of the lipid disorder and in selecting the most efficacious therapy to correct it than for estimating the risk of CHD. Any particular lipid can be used for assessing vulnerability to CHD, but none would appear superior to the simple total cholesterol for this purpose. Only in older women is it possible that the Sf 20-400 pre-beta lipoprotein (or endogenous triglyceride) is superior for predicting CHD (fig. 7).

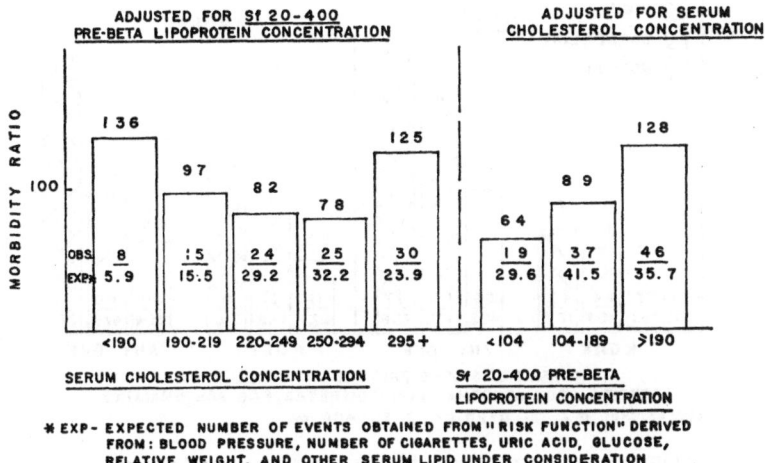

Fig. 7. Risk of coronary heart disease (14 years) according to serum lipid adjusted for associated variables, women 54-69 years: Framingham study.

It remains to be clarified whether the moderate hypercholesterolemia encountered in the general population is principally a heterozygous state for one or more inborn errors of lipid metabolism, or simply an acquired state. It may well be both. While it is likely that the blood lipids are intimately related to the general rate of atheromatous deposition in the arterial intima, local factors appear to play an important role in determining sites of predilection. These factors include the anatomy and caliber of the vessel, the integrity of the vascular intima, the metabolism of the vessel wall, factors which promote fibrin deposition, turbulence and dynamics of blood flow and the pressure in the vascular circuit (58-66).

Blood pressure
More than the associated lipoprotein pattern, concomitant blood pressure status had a marked influence on the risk of CHD associated with either high cholesterol or high triglyceride (Sf 20-400 lipoprotein) (fig. 4). Blood pressure elevation appears to accelerate lipid-induced

atherosclerosis whether elevated casually or basally. Risk of CHD increased in proportion to the antecedent blood pressure level even excluding atherogenic conditions related both to blood pressure and to development of CHD (fig. 8). There was no indication that elevated

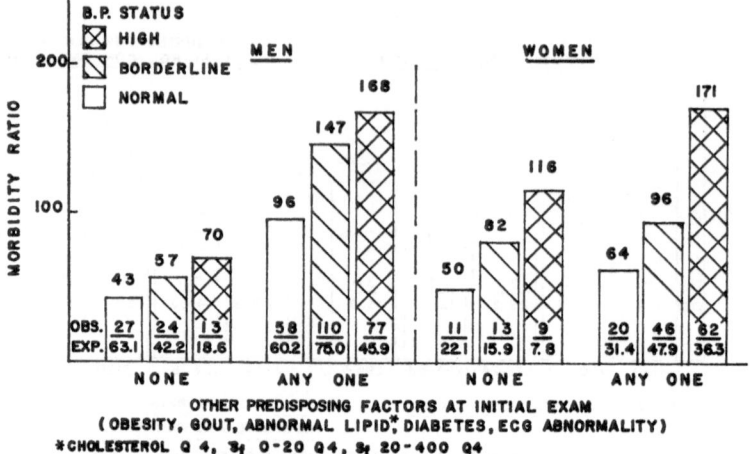

Fig. 8. Risk of CHD (14 years) according to blood pressure status and conditions predisposing to CHD, men and women 30-62 at entry: Framingham heart study.

blood pressure in general, and systolic pressure in particular, was innocuous in older persons. As indicated by discriminant analysis, overall, the *systolic pressure* appears to discriminate better than the diastolic those destined to develop each manifestation of CHD. The standardized mean deviations** were actually higher for systolic than for diastolic pressure (table 3). Only in younger persons is the diastolic pressure

Table 3. Average standardized mean deviation of systolic and dasitolic blood pressure for various manifestations of CHD.

| | | Men 38-69 | | | |
| | CHD-total | Myocardial infarction | Uncomplic- ated angina | CHD-Deaths | |
				Sudden	Non-sudden
No. of cases	252	124	65	22	21
Age range	38-69	38-69	42-65	50-61	50-65
Deviation					
Systolic	0.41	0.34	0.19	0.83	0.74
Diastolic	0.28	0.20	0.13	0.56	0.53

Note: The number of cases includes only age groups with at least four cases. Hence the age range differs from one CHD manifestation to another.

** Standardized mean deviation = mean of cases – mean of those free – standard deviation.

superior to systolic in discriminating potential CHD cases. There appears to be a declining influence of diastolic pressure and a corresponding increase in the contribution of the systolic component of the blood pressure with advancing age. Both components of the blood pressure together and the mean arterial pressure discriminated potential cases of CHD no better than did the systolic pressure alone. Evidently the commonly accepted notion that the cardiovascular consequences of hypertension derive principally from the diastolic component of the blood pressure requires re-evaluation.

The casual blood pressure level, systolic or diastolic, is a major contributor to risk and a good predictor of CHD. Since in older persons the net contribution of systolic pressure is, if anything, greater than diastolic, the commonly held view concerning the innocuous nature of systolic blood pressure elevation in the elderly requires re-evaluation. The common practice of discounting isolated systolic pressure elevation as inconsequential would seem premature. Whether it is a cause or consequence of arteriosclerosis, or both, remains to be determined.

Hypertension is both a potent and common contributor to CHD and the one factor which is effectively controllable. Also, there is already evidence that its control is associated with a substantial reduction in morbidity and mortality from its cardiovascular sequelae (67). There is every reason to believe that its early vigorous control, particularly in those with lipid abnormalities, will result in a substantial reduction in the risk of CHD.

Impaired carbohydrate tolerance

It has long been recognized that diabetics have an unusual propensity to precocious atherosclerosis. While only a small minority of patients with CHD have clinical diabetes, a large proportion have been demonstrated to have impaired carbohydrate metabolism as revealed by various tests of glucose tolerance and serum insulin levels (68-71). There is evidence to suggest that latent ketoresistant hyperinsulinaemic adult onset diabetes is a common precursor of coronary atherosclerosis. The mechanism is obscure. A number of pathogenetic mechanisms may be hypothesized. Diabetes is known to be associated with primary arteriolar changes, with obesity, hypertension and with lipid abnormalities. The latter could explain a propensity to accelerated atherogenesis. An examination of serum lipids in persons developing clinical diabetes in Framingham reveals that lipid abnormalities were present not only at the time of development of diabetes but as much as *10 years before* the onset of overt diabetes. Both cholesterol and more strikingly, Sf 20-400 pre-beta lipoprotein values were higher in potential diabetics than in matched controls (fig. 9).

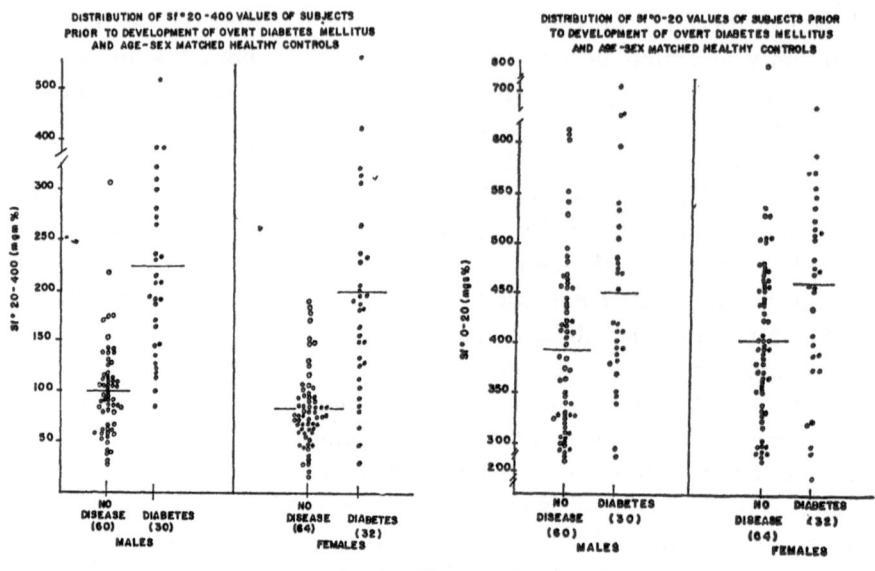

Fig. 9.

This suggests that diabetes may be as much, or more, a lipid than a carbohydrate metabolic problem. This may in part explain the association of diabetes with the excess development of CHD. Diabetes, however defined, was associated with an increased rate of development of CHD, particularly with a fatal outcome. There was some evidence to suggest that a hyperinsulin phase characterized by low casual blood sugars was also associated with an excess risk. This requires confirmation by prospective studies employing serum insulin response to a carbohydrate challenge.

Gouty individuals have been found to have a modest increase in propensity to development of CHD (72). Those with a gouty diathesis have been shown to have higher blood pressures, abnormal blood lipids and obesity to a greater extent than the general population and these appear to account for the increased propensity to CHD.

The more of these atherogenic traits present, the greater the vulnerability to CHD. Risk increased with the degree of abnormality of each of these and with the number of 'atherogenic' abnormalities present; fatal outcome in attacks was also more likely (fig. 10).

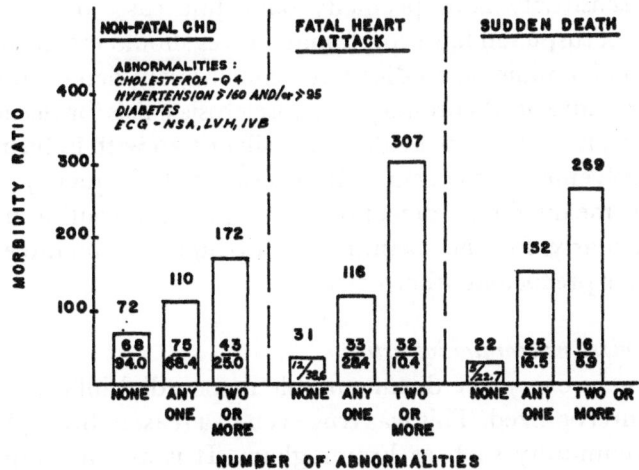

Fig. 10. Risk of immediate mortality in initial heart attack (12 years) according to factors predisposing to CHD, men and women 30-62 at entry: Framingham heart study.

DETECTION OF OCCULT CORONARY DISEASE
In persons with such atherogenic traits the appearance of ECG abnormalities either at rest or provoked by exercise heralds the onset of a functionally important impairment of the coronary circulation. Aside from the ECG, no safe, inexpensive, atraumatic diagnostic method currently exists which can justifiably be used for the detection of advanced coronary atherosclerosis in asymptomatic persons.

Detection of a functionally compromised circulation
The earliest evidence that coronary atherosclerosis has progressed to the point where the coronary circulation is functionally compromised in persons with stigmata associated with accelerated atherogenesis is provided by the post-exercise ECG. Robust asymptomatic persons manifesting ischaemic S-T segment depression provoked by a standard exercise load have been convincingly demonstrated in prospective studies of military and insurance affiliated populations to have a substantially increased risk of coronary morbidity and mortality compared to cohorts not exhibiting ECG abnormality (73-75).

Detection of occult established CHD

The methods available for the diagnosis of clinically overt CHD are quite adequate and if systematically applied, will detect with a high degree of sensitivity and specificity bona fide cases of CHD. With a high index of suspicion few symptomatic cases should escape detection. However, epidemiologic studies have conclusively demonstrated that just as silent advanced coronary atherosclerosis exists for decades prior to symptoms, it has become evident that silent CHD with ischaemic myocardial involvement also occurs with considerable frequency. The only practicable means for its detection is the periodic routine use of the ECG, particularly for the examination of highly vulnerable persons likely to have precocious atherosclerosis.

The unrecognized myocardial infarction

At least one in every five documentable myocardial infarctions which occur go unrecognized. This was true even in a reasonably sophisticated medical community such as Framingham. It is also a sample of the community which is under continuous periodic medical surveillance. Consequently, this is apt to be an underestimate of the frequency with which these occur. The rate of occurrence of such painless or atypical infarctions can be ascertained with validity only from an investigation of a general population sample under routine periodic ECG surveillance. Such infarctions are likely to be especially prevalent in non-hospitalized living patients whose atypical, mild or painless complaints may not come to medical attention. This information was available in the Framingham Study. An examination of the nature and clinical course of these unrecognized myocardial infarctions has identified factors particularly associated with its occurrence as compared to recognized, symptomatic attacks. An unrecognized or silent myocardial infarction was said to be present when on the regular return visit to the clinic the subject's ECG revealed unequivocal evidence of a myocardial infarction in comparison to his previous ECG, but no history was obtained to suggest that either the patient or his physician had even entertained the possibility.

Comparisons made between those who have sustained unrecognized myocardial infarctions and matched non-coronary controls have revealed the same excess of 'risk factors' as observed in persons with overt symptomatic CHD. More relevant, however, is a comparison of the characteristics of those sustaining clinically unrecognized versus overt symptomatic attacks. Such a comparison has revealed a number of features unique to the development of atypical or silent attacks. Persons with angina only rarely had unrecognized myocardial infarctions. Since angina was not significantly less frequent *after* a silent myocardial infarction, an excess of unrecognized myocardial infarctions in those without prior angina cannot be attributed entirely to an unusual propensity of such persons to myocardial ischaemia unaccompanied by pain. Those with prior ECG abnormalities, with hypertension or diabetes, although they might be expected to alert the physician and patient to the possibility of a coronary attack, appeared more prone, if anything, to silent or unrecognized attacks. Age, between 30 and 79 and sex was not related to the rate of occurrence of unrecognized myocardial infarctions. Diaphragmatic or inferior ECG location was not associated with a higher rate of unrecognized attacks.

Such unrecognized, atypical myocardial infarctions cannot be dismissed as innocuous. Survival was no better in persons sustaining these apparently mild attacks than that of their cohorts who had sustained symptomatic attacks and left the hospital alive. Within five years one in three attacks recurred and half the recurrences were fatal whether the attack was symptomatic or unrecognized (fig. 11).

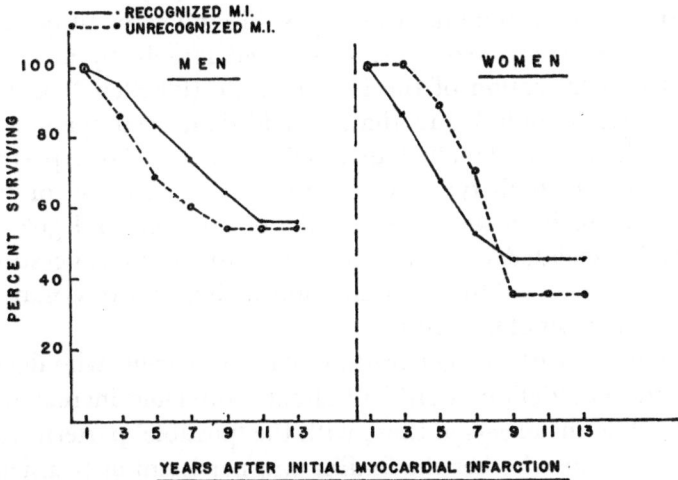

Fig. 11. Subsequent survival in persons surviving one year following initial myocardial infarction, men and women 30-79: Framingham heart study.

Essential for the early detection of asymptomatic myocardial infarctions is the frequent periodic use of the ECG and a high index of suspicion. Routine periodic ECG's are especially indicated in persons particularly vulnerable to CHD because of atherogenic traits such as diabetes, hypertension or prior ECG abnormalities. Even vaguely suggestive complaints in such persons should be an indication for prompt serial ECG examination aimed at demonstrating the evolution on an acute myocardial infarction.

Other ECG abnormalities at rest

The appearance of ECG evidence of infarction, even in completely asymptomatic persons, provides unequivocal evidence of CHD. It has been demonstrated that this is neither a rare nor an innocuous occurrence. Other ECG abnormalities not currently considered diagnostic of CHD also occur without symptoms with considerable frequency in the general population. Such ECG abnormalities including left ventricular hypertrophy, intraventricular block and non-specific abnormality, when they occur without other explanation in asymptomatic persons vulnerable to precocious coronary atherosclerosis have been shown to be associated with a distinct increase in propensity to symptomatic CHD and premature death.

Electrocardiographic left ventricular hypertrophy has been studied in some detail at Framingham as a possible indicator of occult CHD. Two types were compared: that manifested largely by an increased voltage of depolarization of the left ventricle (labelled 'possible' left ventricular hypertrophy) and that, in addition, accompanied by S-T and T wave depression (labelled 'definite' left ventricular hypertrophy). The prevalence of both types rose in proportion to blood pressure in all age groups in both sexes. Only 35% of the men and 50% of the women had associated cardiac enlargement on x-ray suggesting that some mechanism in addition to anatomical hypertrophy may be involved in the genesis of ECG-LVH.

In comparison with the general population, persons who developed an ECG pattern of 'definite LVH' had about a threefold increased risk of overt CHD while the excess in those with the 'possible' pattern was twofold. This was true whether the finding was persistent or transient. Not only did they develop more attacks, but the outcome was more likely to be fatal. The excess risk in those with the 'possible LVH' pattern (voltage alone) but not the 'definite' (with S-T and T wave) can be attributed entirely to the severity and duration of the associated hypertension. Adjustment for the contribution of blood pressure to risk of CHD failed to attenuate the observed effect of 'definite' LVH while it virtually obliterated the effect of the 'possible' (voltage) pattern (fig. 12).

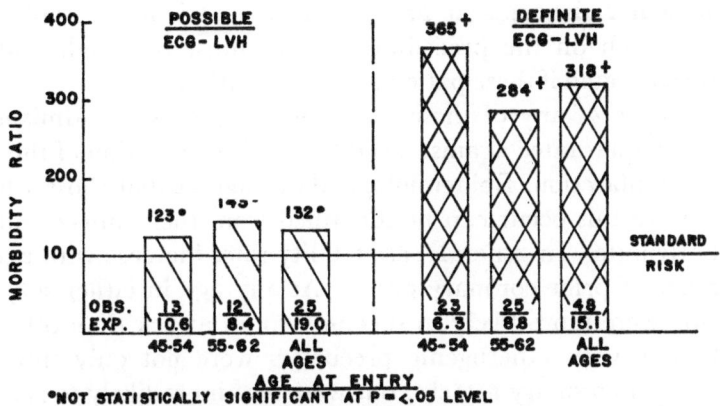

Fig. 12. Factor of increased risk of CHD (14 years) according to ecg-lvh status adjusted* for blood pressure, age and sex, men and women 45-62 at entry: Framingham heart study.

A comparison of the risk of a new CHD episode in those having sustained an actual myocardial infarction versus those acquiring 'definite' ECG-LVH revealed the latter to be almost as serious a finding. Also, mortality from all causes subsequent to development of ECG-LVH was every bit as great as that observed following a myocardial infarction considering only those surviving to appear for one reexamination after their infarction.

It is tempting to hypothesize from the foregoing that only the 'possible' (voltage) ECG-LVH is an expression of hypertension and cardiac hypertrophy while definite ECG-LVH (with S-T and T wave abnormality) reflects in addition, ischaemic myocardial involvement.

FACTORS AFFECTING SURVIVAL IN MYOCARDIAL INFARCTION

It is well appreciated that in patients with an acute myocardial infarction certain clinical findings on admission have an alarming connotation as regards survival. Thus, those with recurrent myocardial infarctions are more likely to succumb than those are with their initial attack. Findings such as shock, pulmonary edema, tamponade, loud systolic murmurs and persistent ischaemic pain auger ill for the patient. In

addition, the development of cardiac arrhythmias from those as
serious as ventricular tachycardia to those as mild as ventricular premature beats can lead to ventricular fibrillation and sudden fatal termination of the illness. Harbingers of sudden fatal termination such as
atrioventricular dissociation and frequent ventricular ectopic beats
which encroach on the preceding T-wave must be sought out and
promptly corrected if these patients are to be salvaged.

The absence of any of these alarming symptoms on admission is,
however, no quarantee against a sudden fatal termination of the acute
myocardial infarction. Epidemiologic data suggest that those who are
likely to have this occur can be identified from their antecedent pre-
morbid attributes. In general, case fatality rates increase with age and
the number of prior coronary events. At any age in either sex, however, some were more likely to succumb to an attack than others. In
general those with atherogenic precursors were not only subject to
more frequent coronary attacks, but were also more likely to succumb
during the attack. Hence, persons who are hypertensive, hypercholesterolaemic or diabetic are more likely to have a fatal outcome in an acute
myocardial infarction. Even occult manifestations of CHD such as a
prior unrecognized myocardial infarction, or only electrocardiographic
left ventricular hypertrophy or intraventricular block were prone to a
lethal termination of the illness. Furthermore, the more of these host

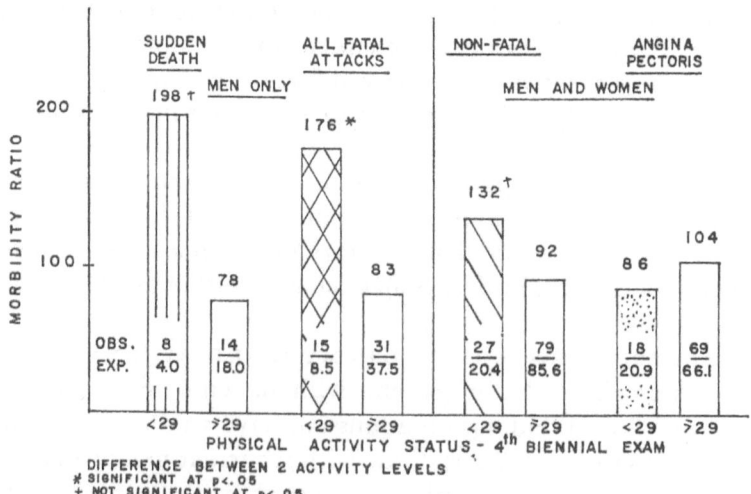

Fig. 13. Risk of manifestations of coronary heart disease (8 years) according to physical
activity status, men and women 35-69 on exam 4: Framingham heart study.

factors present, the more likely was the outcome to be fatal. Such persons warrant careful monitoring in a coronary care unit and require careful attention regardless of how benign their condition on admission. Certain living habits also predisposed to a lethal outcome and appeared to trigger a fatal episode. Thus, persons who smoked cigarettes heavily were prone to sudden death at five times the rate of their nonsmoking cohorts. In addition, those who were sedentary were less likely to survive an attack than their more active cohorts. They were especially prone to fatal attacks in general, and to sudden death in particular (fig. 13).

Persons who are sedentary, are more likely to be overweight, breathless and to have a rapid pulse rate at rest. Whatever the reason, such persons have been found to have a disproportionately high risk of fatal attacks while exhibiting only a modest propensity to non-lethal attacks. The more such traits present, the more likely a fatal outcome (fig. 14).

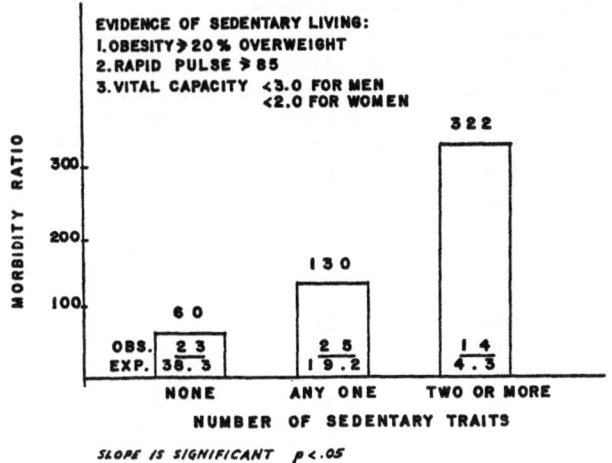

Fig. 14. Risk of coronary heart disease death (12 years) according to evidence of physical activity status, men and women 30-62 at entry: Framingham heart study.

Such persons would also appear to be good candidates for careful monitoring in a coronary care unit. It is likely that persons who have a compromised coronary circulation and who have failed to stimulate the opening of collateral channels are more likely to succumb when an occlusion occurs.

Even should the victim of a myocardial infarction manage to survive and leave the hospital his troubles are far from over. Disability as a result of angina or congestive failure is surprisingly light afflicting only one in three sustaining their initial infarctions. The principal hazard lies in the marked propensity to recurrences with an even greater likelihood of a fatal attack. This propensity to recurrences appeared to be unrelated to the severity of the initial attack, and those with unrecognized or silent attacks faired no better beginning one year after the attack than did those whose attacks were symptomatic and necessitated hospitalization (fig. 11). About one-half of all attacks recurred within six years; a risk from five to ten times that of the general population. Also the likelihood of a fatal óutcome was greater, increasing from about 30% to about 50%. Mortality after development of manifestations of CHD was three times that of the general population, the mortality rate, but not the relative risk, increasing with age (table 4).

Table 4. Incidence of death according to presence of definite coronary heart disease at exam, by sex and age: Framingham study, 14-year follow-up.

Sex and age at exam.	Population at risk at exam. with CHD	No. of deaths in exam. interval with CHD	Average annual rate per 10000 with CHD	Relative risk with CHD
Men	838	80	477	3.0*
30-44	66	1	76	(3.4)
45-54	202	17	421	6.4
55-64	387	40	517	3.4
65-74	183	22	601	2.1
Women	495	27	273	3.0*
30-44	9	0	0	
45-54	88	1	57	(1.2)
55-64	265	12	226	3.5
65-74	133	14	526	3.7

* Age-adjusted by indirect method using as standard rates the sex-age-specific incidence rates (in 5-year age groups) for the entire study.
( ) Based on only one death.

LIVING HABITS

A number of living habits appear to contribute to the development of coronary heart disease and some appear detrimental to survival once an attack occurs. Sedentary living and over-nutrition undoubtedly promote obesity, high blood lipid values, hypertension and impairment of carbohydrate tolerance. These, in turn, predispose to accelerated atherogenesis and result in precocious coronary atherosclerosis. In addition, in susceptible persons with a compromised coronary circulation and in those with occult or overt established coronary heart disease, certain living habits appear to precipitate attacks and to affect survival once an attack occurs.

Modern technology has conspired to make it increasingly difficult to obtain, as part of daily routine living, an adequate amount of physical exercise. Muscle power has been replaced almost entirely by mechanical appliances, both in the home and at work. At the same time opportunities for obtaining a surfeit of food have been steadily increasing. Modern technology has also supplied a ready-made cigarette which has transformed the smoking habits away from non-inhaled cigar and pipe. These practices appear to have exacted a toll in cardiovascular mortality. As has been pointed out, both the obese and sedentary with an already compromised coronary circulation are especially prone to a fatal outcome either in the initial attack or in recurrences.

Diet
Evidence to date suggests that habitual diet is the single most important determinant of the level of blood lipids encountered in a population and a powerful contributor to the development of CHD. Except for animal experiments and metabolic studies in humans, most of the evidence is indirect. There is little direct prospective evidence which can be cited to show that persons under observation develop clinical manifestations of CHD in relation to the composition of their diet. Most prospective studies of free living population subgroups which have attempted to evaluate the role of diet in CHD have failed to demonstrate a relationship of what people eat to either their serum lipids or to their propensity to clinical CHD. Yet, it has been shown that specific alterations in the nutrient content of the diet can indeed produce rather predictable changes in the serum lipid content. In animals, atheromatous lesions can be produced by feeding experiments. This apparent paradox may be a consequence of a number of circumstances including: the relative homogeneity of dietary habits within the free living affluent population subgroups, the lack of a biologically important range of nutrient intakes within these populations, or methodologic difficulties in obtaining valid estimates of long-term nutrient intake. Most Western population samples studied have, in

general, been consuming a diet uniformly high in calories, saturated fat, cholesterol and refined carbohydrate. Only an insignificant proportion of these populations have been on intakes within the range observed in those geographic areas where low CHD prevalence has been reported or where low serum lipid values have been observed (table 5). Also, the range of nutrient intakes observed have been way above that level required to significantly alter serum lipid levels in metabolic studies.

Table 5. Mean values and ranges of some characteristics of the average daily intake of food, by sex, Framingham diet study.

| | 437 Men | | 475 Women | |
	Mean	Range	Mean	Range
		(10-90%)		(10-90%)
Calories				
Total	3156	2256-4056	2142	1423-2861
Per pound body weight	19	13.1-24.9	15.8	9.6-22.0
Fat (gm)				
Total	136	89-183	96	56-136
Animal	98	59-137	65	34-96
Vegetable	38	15-61	30	9-51
Percent calories from fat	39	32-46	40	33-47
Percent fat from animal sources	72	58-86	69	53-85
Cholesterol (mg)	704	421-987	492	274-710
P/s Ratio	0.41	0.24-0.58	0.42	0.25-0.59

Consequently, it is no surprise to find at Framingham that there was a rather poor correlation between reported intakes of foodstuffs and serum cholesterol values. In fact, all of the nutrients in the diet taken together in linear regression analysis could not account for more than 4% of the variance in serum cholesterol values in this population (table 6).

Table 6. Relation of multiple dietary components to serum cholesterol level (multiple linear regression analysis) 912 men and women in dietary subsample.

Measure	
Coefficient of multiple correlation	0.19
Proportion of serum cholesterol variance explained by the independent diet variables	3.7%

It may be that at these high levels of nutrient intake energy balance

is the controlling factor. An examination of the interrelationship between serum cholesterol and calories/lb of body weight, relative weight
and level of physical activity, strongly suggests that this may be the
case. As calories/lb increases, relative weights decrease along with the
cholesterol values while physical activity goes up proportional to
calories/lb consumed (table 7). Also, persons with pre-beta bands on
electrophoresis tended to be significantly heavier and to have gained
more weight after completion of musculo-skeletal growth than those
without this electrophoretic pattern.

Table 7. Relation of cholesterol, Framingham relative weight and physical activity to calories
per pound of body weight, Framingham diet study, men 30-59 at entry.

Cal./Lb.	Mean Chol.	Mean FRW	Mean P. A. Index
<13	253	108	30
14-15	247	106	31
16	243	102	32
17	236	108	32
18	236	101	33
19	231	100	33
20	241	101	34
21-22	229	99	33
23-25	228	93	38
26+	214	93	40

An examination of the reported nutrient intakes among those who
went on to develop CHD subsequent to dietary interview in comparison
with those who remained free of it revealed no differences for the fat,
carbohydrate, or calories. Some difference for total cholesterol may be
present (table 8).

Nevertheless, it is very likely that dietary habits are responsible in
large measure for the generally high serum lipids and for the high rate
of CHD observed in affluent populations. Over the past century agricul-
tural technology and the food industry have drastically altered the
composition of diets in western civilization. The resulting diet rich in
saturated fat, in cholesterol and in refined carbohydrate has reduced
nutritional deficiency dramatically in western civilization. A concomitant reduction in the demand for physical work as a consequence of
simultaneous advances in industrial technology, has helped to create a
problem of overnutrition to replace that of undernutrition. There is a

W. B. KANNEL

Table 8. Daily nutrient intake according to susceptibility to coronary heart disease, men 30-59 at entry: Framingham diet study.

Degree of susceptibility	Total no	Mean intake				% with low intake			
		Calorie	Sugar (tsp)	Fat (g)	Chol. (mg)	Calorie (≤2500)	Sugar (≤2 tsp)	Fat (% cal.≤35)	Chol. (≤550 mg)
No risk factors	64	3236	5.7	141	678	19	26	22	26
One or two factors	203	3172	4.8	136	707	15	34	25	25
Three or more factors	139	3127	4.3	132	713	19	45	27	25
CHD	25	3107	4.0	136	700	20	56	24	28
Total	431	3163	4.7	135	704	17	38	25	25

considerable body of evidence to suggest that this overnutrition is exacting a toll in cardiovascular disease that cannot be ignored. Whatever the type of hypercholesterolaemia or the lipoprotein pattern with which it is associated, a high blood cholesterol concentration has been shown to be associated with an increased risk of CHD, proportional to its level. However, there is some evidence to suggest that the determinants of high blood cholesterol content may differ depending on the associated lipoprotein pattern. More of those hypercholesterolemias associated with elevated pre-beta lipoprotein are apt to be sensitive to the carbohydrate content of the diet rather than the saturated fat and cholesterol content as is the case with hypercholesterolaemia associated with elevated beta-lipoprotein. To what extent these high cholesterol values and their associated lipoprotein patterns as seen in the general population are acquired through faulty living habits or reflect constitutional factors has not been completely resolved.

It seems likely, however, that the generally high lipid values observed in Western populations is to a great extent determined by the diet.

Dietary manipulation is more likely to be efficacious in young persons susceptible to CHD than in those with long-standing disease or those recovered from a myocardial infarction. The earlier fatty streak is a more reversible lesion than the later calcified fibrotic plaque. There is, however, some evidence to suggest that progression of advanced lesions and clotting characteristics of the blood may be influenced by dietary manipulation. Weight reduction diets in those with established disease should decrease the cardiac workload, reduce the blood pressure, improve carbohydrate tolerance, reduce serum lipids, increase exercise tolerance in those with angina or borderline cardiac decompensation and lessen the likelihood of sudden death.

In those with an already compromised coronary circulation, the cigarette habit can be extremely pernicious. While information on survival in those with established CHD who have given up cigarettes is not conclusive, the added risk of cigarette smoking in those who have stigmata of even occult CHD such as asymptomatic ECG abnormalities is formidable. There is much to suggest that the lethal effect of the cigarette habit is transient, non-cumulative, and reversible, so there is much to be gained in giving up the habit. Risk of every clinical manifestation of CHD is greater in the cigarette smoker with the possible exception of angina pectoris. While the risk is clearly related to the number of cigarettes consumed each day, it did not appear to be related to the duration of the habit even in heavy cigarette smokers. As might be expected from this, the ex-smoker had the same low risk as those who never smoked. It is also of interest that the pipe and cigar smoker had no increased risk (table 9).

Table 9. Risk of 'heart attacks' in 14 years according to tobacco habit on initial examination, men 30-62 at entry: Framingham study.

Tobacco habit	Pop. at risk	Observed	Expected	Morbidity ratio
Never smoked	288	29	33.3	87
Stopped smoking	208	15	26.0	58
Cigar and pipe	304	23	38.2	60
All cigarette smokers	1464	186	156.4	119
Heavy cigarette smokers (> 1 pkg/day)	483	69	49.0	141

'Heart attacks' = All coronary heart disease except angina pectoris.

The data suggest that the catecholamine stimulating effect of nicotine absorbed by inhaling tobacco smoke produces transient effects on circulatory dynamics, on myocardial irritability and possibly on clotting, which in a person with a compromised coronary circulation can trigger a lethal arrhythmia or coronary occlusion. There is little to

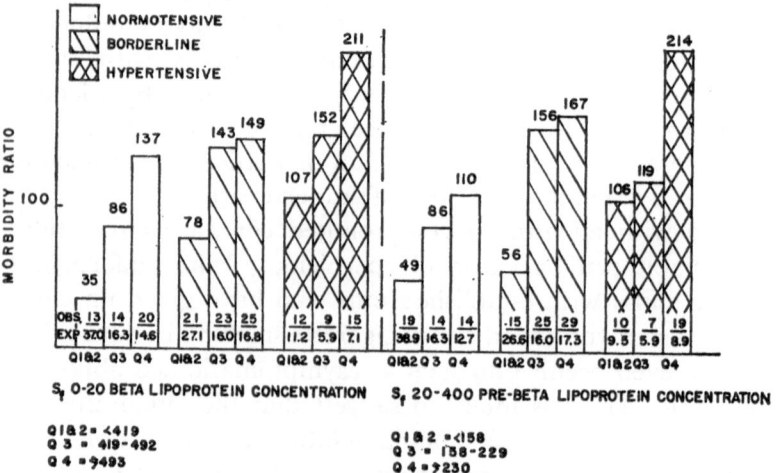

Fig. 15. Risk of 'heart attacks' (14 years) according to cigarette smoking habit and 'atherogenic' traits, men 30-62 at entry: Framingham heart study.

suggest that the cigarette habit accelerates atherogenesis since the effect is independent of atherogenic traits and at any level of blood pressure or serum lipid the cigarette smoker is at increased risk. In those predisposed by such atherogenic traits the habit is particularly pernicious further increasing the already enhanced risk (fig. 15). In discriminant function analysis the cigarette habit can be shown to exert a considerable net effect accounting for the multiple associated factors (table 10).

Table 10. Independent effect of factors of risk in CHD as indicated by discriminant function analysis, 10 year follow-up: men 30-59 at entry.

Factor of risk in development of CHD	Relative linear discriminant function weight
Age	1.00**
Cigarette smoking	0.67**
Systolic blood pressure	0.55**
Left ventricular hypertrophy (ECG)	0.50**
Serum cholesterol level	0.47*
Framingham relative weight	0.34*
Haemoglobin	—0.31*
S_f 0-12 B-lipoproteins	0.31
S_f 20-100 B-lipoproteins	0.30
Intraventricular block (ECG)	0.25
Phospholipids	—0.18
Nonspecific ECG abnormality	—0.10
Vital capacity	0.05

Significantly different from
Zero at: .01 Level**
.05 Level*

Coronary susceptibles and those with occult or symptomatic disease should no more be allowed to smoke a package of cigarettes per day than to receive the equivalent of 20 injections of epinephrine.

It is clear from the foregoing that in those who are highly vulnerable to CHD and in those who are already afflicted with a compromised coronary circulation and either asymptomatic or overt disease, certain modifications in living habits are prudent. These include discontinuance of the cigarette habit, a less rich diet and a less sedentary existence. Severe restriction of physical activity in recovered myocardial infarction victims or those with occult CHD may be unwise. When the attack recurs, it is more likely to be fatal. Sedentary persons with asymptomatic ECG abnormalities appear unusually susceptible to fatal attacks compared to their more active cohorts.

It is encouraging to note that not all prevalent habits enjoyed by the populace are harmful. Neither habitual coffee or alcohol consumption in moderation appeared to be associated with an increased propensity to CHD. Nor alas, was there any evidence that these practices were helpful. Neither were all personal traits associated with aging harbingers of CHD. Neither baldness nor premature greying of hair was associated with an increased risk of CHD.

IMPLICATIONS FOR PRACTICE

It is in the considerable latent period between the time of occurrence of a pathologic degree of involvement of the coronary arteries with atherosclerosis and the appearance of symptomatic disease that preventive measures must be implemented in this disease. Since the disease is one which characteristically strikes without warning, often presents with sudden death as its initial manifestation, and can damage the myocardium without producing symptoms, awaiting the onset of overt manifestations before intervening, can no longer be justified. The day is already here when the occurrence of a death in a hospitalized patient with an acute myocardial infarction is coming to be considered a medical failure. The day is not too distant when the occurrence of symptomatic CHD in persons under periodic medical surveillance must also come to be regarded as a medical failure. The current epidemic proportions of CHD are not an inevitable consequence of aging and genetics and there is every reason to believe that it can be substantially reduced as a contemporary health hazard.

An interruption of the chain of events leading to the occurrence of, and fatal outcome from, this disease as revealed by epidemiologic investigation should control this disease long before its fundamental 'cause' can be demonstrated. Coronary heart disease must at the present time be regarded as a multifactorial disease for which no essential cause can yet be specified. A profile of the likely coronary candidate can be constructed from readily measured characteristics of persons and the degree of vulnerability estimated over a thirtyfold range of risk (table 11).

From a preventive point of view the importance of the factors contributing to risk depends on their potency, the ease with which they can be detected and measured, the prevalence of the risk factors in

Table 11. 12 Year incidence of CHD according to decile of risk.

Decile of risk*	2187 Men		2669 Women	Observed
	Obs. cases	12 Year incid./1000	Obs. cases	12 Year incid./1000
10	82	375	54	202
9	44	201	23	86
8	31	142	21	79
7	33	151	14	52
6	22	101	5	19
5	20	91	6	22
4	13	59	2	7
3	10	46	0	0
2	3	14	3	11
1	0	0	1	4
Total	258	1180	129	483

* Deciles of risk according to: Age, SBP, Rel. Wt., Hb., No. Cigs.
  Level of all of following: – ECG ABN., Chol.
  (Using Multiple Logistic Function)

the general population and their amenability to control without undue hazard or cost. In the general population, the key factors appear to be the serum lipid content and the blood pressure. Persons with abnormalities of these deserve special attention, and since they are for decades completely asymptomatic abnormalities, they must be periodically sought after in apparently well persons. In those who also have occult myocardial involvement as revealed by ECG, the prognosis is so serious as to warrant the vigorous use of every reasonable means available to delay the onset of symptomatic disease. In such individuals prohibition of cigarettes, weight reduction, dietary manipulation and physical exercise should be prescribed. Should these hygienic measures fail, pharmacologic agents to lower blood pressure, to alter serum lipid content, and to correct impaired glucose tolerance would appear indicated whether symptoms are present or not.

Since susceptibility to CHD is almost universal, certain alterations in living habits in the general population must be seriously considered. It may be necessary to engineer physical activity back into daily work and leisure, to produce less rich foods with substitutes for refined sugar and saturated fat, and to breed more lean animal products. Denicotinized cigarettes may have to be promoted and advertising designed to motivate a change to non-inhaling smoking practices.

Field and clinical trials are urgently needed to demonstrate the efficacy of the preventive measures which seem indicated if we are to halt the appalling mortality from CHD. Meanwhile, prophylactic use of the indicated hygienic measures and pharmacologic agents for the purpose of delaying attacks and prolonging life would seem easily justified. In view of the gravity of the problem further temporizing would seem more difficult to defend unless one views coronary disease as the solution to the population explosion. The measures advocated are usually worthwhile per se and indicated for other reasons as well. Unless unforeseen hazards related to the long-term application of these measures in well persons appear, it is reasonable to assume that such measures will be more effective employed early rather than late in the disease process.

There is no assurance that primary prevention will achieve all that is expected but the potential for salvage is huge (fig. 16).

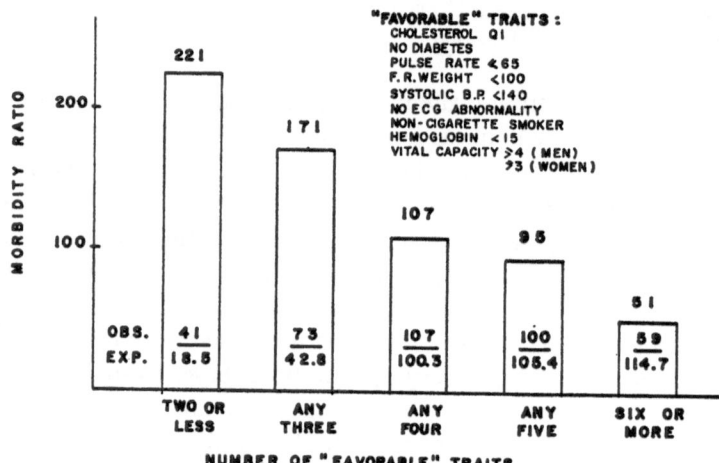

Fig. 16. Risk of coronary heart disease (12 years) according to number of 'favorable' traits, men and women 30-62 at entry: Framingham heart study.

The general hygienic measures indicated are not easy to implement. Both the patient and his physician would prefer a pill to counteract the bad habits which predispose, so that they may continue to enjoy them. We simply must be one means or another find a way to prevent sudden death, to detect unrecognized myocardial infarctions and other occult CHD, to delay recurrences and to detect and retard precocious atherosclerosis, if this principal killer of adults in the prime of life is to be conquered.

REFERENCES

1. Dawber, T. R., G. F. Meadors, F. E. Moore Jr., Epidemiological approaches to heart disease: The Framingham Study *Amer. J. Public Health*, 41, 279-286 (March 1951).

2. Dawber, T. R., F. E. Moore, Longitudinal study of heart disease in Framingham, Massachusetts: An interim report. *Research in Public Health*, papers presented at the 1951 Annual Conference of the Milbank Memorial Fund. New York, Milbank Memorial Fund, 241-247 (1952).

3. Gordon, T., F. E. Moore, D. Shurtleff, T. R. Dawber, Some methodologic problem in the long-term study of cardiovascular disease: observations on the Framingham Study. *J. Chron. Dis.* 103, 186-206 (Sept 1959).

4. Kahn, H. A., A method for analyzing longitudinal observations on individuals in the Framingham Heart Study. *Proceedings of the Social Statistics Section of the American Statistical Association*, (1961).

5. Kahn, Harold, Use of computers in analyzing Framingham data. *Circulation Research*, Vol. XI, (Sept. 1962).

6. Dawber, T. R., G. Pearson, P. Anderson, G. V. Mann, W. B. Kannel, D. Shurtleff, P. McNamara, Dietary assessment in the epidemiologic study of coronary heart disease. The Framingham Study. Amer. *J. Clinical Nutrition*, Vol. 11, (Sept. 1962).

7. Mann, G. V., G. Pearson, T. Gordon, T. R. Dawber, L. Lyell, D. Shurtleff, Diet and cardiovascular disease in the Framingham Study. *Amer. J. Clinical Nutrition*, Vol. 11, (Sept. 1962).

8. Dawber, T. R., W. B. Kannel, Computers in epidemiologic research: uses in the Framingham Study. *Circulation Research*, Vol. XI, (Sept. 1962).

9. Dawber, T. R., W. B. Kannel, G. D. Friedman, The use of computers in cardiovascular epidemiology. *Progress in Cardiovascular Diseases*, Vol. 5, No. 4, (Jan. 1963).

10. Dawber, T. R., W. B. Kannel, Coronary heart disease as an epidemiologic entity. *Amer. J. Public Health*, Vol. 53, No. 3, (Macrh. 1963).

11. Dawber, T. R., W. B. Kannel, L. Lyell, An approach to longitudinal studies in a community: The Framingham Study. *Ann. of N.Y. Academy of Sciences*, Vol. 107, 539-556 (May 1963).

12. Friedman, G. D., W. B. Kannel, T. R. Dawber, P. M. McNamara, Comparison of prevalence, case history and incidence data in assessing the potency of risk factors in coronary heart disease. *Amer. Jour. of Epidemiology*, Vol. 83, No. 2, (1966).

13. Friedman, G. D., W. B. Kannel, T. R. Dawber, P. M. McNamara, An evaluation of follow-up methods in the Framingham Heart Study *Amer. J. Pyblic Health* 57, 1015-1024 (June 1967).

14. Kannel, W. B., E. J. LeBauer, T. R. Dawber, P. M. McNamara, Relation of body weight to development of coronary heart disease: The Framingham Study. *Circulation* 35, 734-744 (April 1967).

15. Thomas, Jr., H. E., W. B. Kannel, T. R. Dawber, P. M. McNamara, Cholesterol-Phospholipid ratio in the prediction of coronary heart disease. *New Eng. Jour. of Medicine* 274, 701-705 (March 1966).

16. Kannel, W. B., T. R. Dawber, G. D. Friedman, W. E. Glennon, P. M. McNamara, Risk factors in coronary heart disease; an evaluation of several serum lipids as predictors of coronary heart disease. *Ann. Intern. Med.* 6, 888-899 (Nov. 1964).

17. Kannel, W. B., W. P. Castelli and P. M. McNamara, The coronary profile: 12-year follow-up in the Framingham Study. *J. Occup. Med.* 9, 611 (1967).

18. Kannel, W. B., T. R. Dawber, W. E. Glennon, M. C. Thorne, Preliminary report: the determinants and clinical significance of serum cholesterol. *Mass. J. Medical Technology*, Vol. IV, No. 3, (Fall 1962).

19. Cornfield, J., Joint dependence of risk of coronary heart disease on serum cholesterol

and systolic blood pressure. *Federation Proceedings*, Vol. 21, No. 4, Part II, July-August, 1962, Supplement No. 11, 58-61 (1962).

20. Cornfield, J., T. Gordon, W. W. Smith, Quantal response curves for experimentally uncontrolled variables. *Bulletin of the International Statustical Institute*, Tokyo, Vol. XXXVIII; Part III. 97-115 (1961).

21. Walker, S. H., D. B. Duncan, Estimation of the probability of an event as a function of several independent variables. *Biometrika* 54, 1 and 2, 167-179 (June 1967).

22. Truett, J., J. Cornfield, W. B. Kannel, A multivariate analysis of the risk of coronary heart disease in Framingham. *J. Chronic. Dis.* 20, 511-524 (July 1967).

23. Kagan, A., T. Gordon, W. B. Kannel, T. R. Dawber, Blood pressure and its relation to coronary heart disease in the Framingham Study. Hypertension: Drug Action, Epidemiology and Hemodynamics. Proceedings of the Council for High Blood Pressure Research, *American Heart Association*, (Nov. 1958).

24. Dawber, T. R., W. B. Kannel, Susceptibility to coronary heart disease, *Mod. Conc. Cardiov. Dis.* 30, 671-675 (July 1961).

25. Doyle, J. T., T. R. Dawber, W. B. Kannel, A. S. Heslin, H. A. Kahn, Cigarette smoking and coronary heart disease: combined experience of the Albany and Framingham Studies. *New England J. of Med.* 266, 796-801 (April 1962).

26. Kannel, W. B., A. Kagan, T. R. Dawber, N. Revotskie, Epidemiology of coronary heart disease: implications for the practicing physician. *Geriatrics*, Vol. 17, No. 10, 675 (Oct. 1962).

27. Kannel, W. B., T. R. Dawber, H. E. Thomas Jr., P. M. McNamara, Comparison of serum lipids in the prediction of coronary heart disease. *Rhode Island Med.* J. 48, 243-250 (May 1965).

28. Kannel, W. B., T. R. Dawber, P. M. McNamara, Detection of the coronary-prone adult. The Framingham Study. *Jour. of Iowa Med. Soc.* 26-34 (Jan. 1966).

29. Chapman, J. M., L. S. Goerke, W. Dixon, D. B. Loveland, E. Phillips, Measuring the risk of coronary heart disease in adult population groups: IV. The Clinical status of a population group in Los Angeles under observation for two to three years. *Amer. J. Public Health* 47 (Suppl., April 1957), 33 (1957).

30. Stamler, J., H. A. Lindberg, D. M. Berkson, A. Shaffer, W. Miller and A. Poindexter, Prevalence and incidence of coronary heart disease in strata of the labor force of a Chicago industrial corporation. *J. Chronic Dis.* 11, 405 (1960).

31. Keys, A., H. L. Taylor, H. Blackburn, J. Brozek, J. T. Anderson and E. Simonson, Coronary heart disease among Minnesota business and professional men followed fifteen years. *Circulation* 28, 381 (1963).

32. Paul, O., M. H. Lepper, W. H. Phelan, G. W. Dupertuis, A. MacMillan, H. McKean and H. Park, A longitudinal study of coronary heart disease. *Circulation* 28, 20 (1963).

33. Strong, J. P. and H. C. McGill Jr., The natural history of coronary atherosclerosis. *Amer. J. Path.* 40, 37 (1962).

34. Enos, W. F., R. H. Holmes, L. J. Beyer, Coronary disease among United States soldiers killed in action in Korea. *J.A.M.A.* 152, 1090 (1953).

35. Mason, J. K., Asymptomatic disease of coronary arteries in young men. *Brit. Med. J.* II, 1234 (1963).

36. Rigal, R. D., F. W. Lovell, J. M. Townsend, Pathological findings in the cardiovascular system of military flying personnel. *Amer. J. Cardiol.* 6, 19 (1960).

37. French, A. J. and W. Dock, Fatal coronary arteriosclerosis in young soldiers. *J.A.M.A.* 124, 1233 (1944).

38. Katz, L. N. and J. Stamler, *Experimental Atherosclerosis.* Charles C. Thomas, Springfield, III. (1953).

39. Fredrickson, D. S., R. I. Levy and R. S. Lees, *Fat transport in lipoproteins- an integrated approach to mechanisms and disorders.*

40. Wakerlin, G. E., W. G. Moss and J. P. Kiely, Effect of experimental renal hypertension on experimental thiouracilcholesterol atherosclerosis in dogs. *Circ. Res.* 5, 426 (1957).
41. Deming, Q. B., E. H. Mosbach, M. D. Bevans, M. M. Daly, L. L. Abell, E. Martin, L. M. Brun, E. Halpern and R. Kaplan, Blood pressure, cholesterol content of serum and tissues and atherogenesis in the rat. *J. Exp. Med.* 107, 581 (1958).
42. Bronte-Stewart, B. and R. H. Heptinstal, The relationship between experimental hypertension and cholesterol-induced atheroma in rabbits. *J. Path. Bact.* 68, 407 (1954).
43. Moses, C., Development of atherosclerosis in dogs with hypercholesterolemia and chronic hypertension. *Circ. Res.* 2, 243 (1954).
44. Nottiman, M. M. and S. Proger, Cephalins in the blood. Patients with coronary heart disease and patients with hyperlipemia. *J.A.M.A.* 179, 40-43 (1962).
45. Hatch, F. T., P. K. Russell, T. M. W. Poon-King, C. P. Canellos, R. S. Lees and L. M. Hagopian, A study of coronary heart disease in young men. Characteristics and metabolic studies of the patients and comparison with age-matched healthy men. *Circulation* 33, 679-703 (1966).
46. Sandler M. and G. H. Bourne, Some new observations on human aortic atheroma. The possible role of essential fatty acids in its development. *J.A.M.A.* 179, 43-45 (1962).
47. Gofman, J. W., W. Young and R. Tandy, Ischemic heart disease, atherosclerosis and longevity. *Circulation* 34, 679 (1966).
48. Albrink, M. J., J. W. Meigs and E. B. Man, Serum lipids, hypertension and coronary artery disease. *Amer. J. Med.* 31, 4-23 (1961).
49. Antonis, A. and I. Bersolin, Serum triglyceride levels in South African Europeans and Bantu and in ischemic heart disease. *Lancet* 1, 998 (1960).
50. Castelli, W. P., J. J. Nicherson, J. M. Newell and D. D. Rutstein, Serum NeFa following fat, carbohydrate and protein ingestion and during fasting as related to intracellular lipid deposition. *J. of Atherosclerosis Res.* 6, 328-341 (1966).
51. Ladd, A. T., A. Kellner and J. W. Correll, Intravenous detergents in experimental atherosclerosis, with special reference to possible role of phospholipids, *Federation Proc.* 8, 360 (1949).
52. Ahrens, Jr. E. H. and H. G. Kunkel, Stabilization of serum lipid emulsions by serum phospholipids. *J. Exper. Med.* 90, 409-424 (1949).
53. Gertler, M. M., S. M. Garn and J. Lerman, Interrelationships of serum cholesterol, cholesterol esters and phospholipids in health and in coronary artery disease. *Circulation* 2, 205-214 (1950).
54. Steiner, A., F. E. Kendall and J. A. L. Mathers, Abnormal serum lipid pattern in patients with coronary arteriosclerosis. *Circulation* 5, 605, 608 (1952).
55. Schlessinger, B. S., F. H. Wilson Jr. and L. J. Milch, Serum parameters as discriminators between normal and coronary groups. *Circulation* 19, 265-268 (1959).
56. Wurm, M., R. J. Kositchek and R. Straus, Lipoproteins quantitated by paper electrophoresis as index of atherosclerosis. *Circulation* 21, 526-537 (1960).
57. Straus, R., M. Wurm and R. J. Kositchek, Atherogenic indices: review and evaluation. *Am. J. Clin. Path.* 41, 352-365 (1964).
58. Cox, G. E., R. E. Trueheart, J. Kaplan and C. B. Taylor, Atherosclerosis in rhesus monkeys. IV Repair of arterial injury an important secondary atherogenic factor. *Arch. Path.* 76, 166 (1963).
59. Young, W., J. W. Gofman, R. Tandy, N. Malamud and E. S. Waters, The quantitation of atherosclerosis. I. Relationship to artery size. *Am. J. Cardiol.* 6, 288 (1960).
60. Texon, M., The hemodynamic concept. Concept of Atherosclerosis. *Am. J. Cardiol.* 5, 291 (1960).
61. Duguid, J. B., Thrombosis as a factor in the pathogenesis of coronary atherosclerosis. *J. Path. and Bact.* 58, 207 (1946).
62. Siperstein, M. D., I. L. Chaikoff and S. S. Chernick, Significance of endogenous

cholestercl in arteriosclerosis: synthesis in arterial tissue. *Science* 113, 747 (1951).

63. Zilversmit, D. B., E. L. McCandless, P. H. Jordan, W. S. Henly and R. F. Ackerman, The synthesis of phospholipid in human atheromatous lesions. *Circulation* 23, 370 (1961).

64. Paterson, J. C., T. Moffatt and J. Mills, Hemosiderin in early atherosclerotic plaques. *Arch. Path.* 61, 496 (1956).

65. Turpeinen, O., Diet and coronary events. *Jour. Amer. Dietitic Assoc.* 52, 209-213 (1968).

66. Sako, Y., Effects of turbulent blood flow and hypertension on experimental atherosclerosis. *J.A.M.A.* 179, 36-40 (Jan. 1962).

67. Freis, E. D., Veterans Administration Cooperative Study Group on Antihypertensive Agents. Effects of treatment on morbidity in hypertension. *J.A.M.A.* 202, 1028 (1967).

68. Wahlberg, F., The intravenous glucose tolerance test in atherosclerotic disease with special refrence to obesity, hypertension, diabetic heredity and cholesterol values. *Acta Med. Scand.* 171, 1 (1962).

69. Ostrander Jr., L. D, T. Francis Jr., N. S. Hayner, M. O. Kjelberg, F. H. Epstein, The relationship of cardiovascular disease to hyperglycemia. *Ann. Int. Med.* 62, 1188-1198 (June 1965).

70. Herman, M. V., R. Gorlin, Premature coronary artery disease and the preclinical diabetic state. *Amer. J. Med.* 38, 481-483 (April 1965).

71. Vallance-Owen, J., W. L. Ashton, Cardiac infarction and insulin antagonism. *Lancet* 1 1226, (1963).

72. Hall, A. P., P. E. Barry, T. R. Dawber, P. M. McNamara, Epidemiology of gout and hyperuricemia. A long-term population study. *Amer. J. Med.* 42, 27 (1967).

73. Mattingly, J. W., The post-exercise electrocardiogram. Its value in the diagnosis and prognosis of coronary arterial disease. *Amer. J. Cardiol.* 9, 395-409 (March 1962).

74. Brody, A. J., Master two-step exercise test in clinically unselected patients. *J.A.M.A.* 171, 1195 (Oct. 1959).

75. Rumball, A., E. D. Acheson, Latent coronary heart disease detected by electrocardiogram before and after exercise. *Brit. Med. J.* 5328, 423-428 (Feb. 1963).

PREVENTION OF ATHEROSCLEROTIC CORONARY HEART DISEASE BY CHANGE OF DIET AND MODE OF LIFE

J. STAMLER

EPIDEMIC PREMATURE CORONARY HEART DISEASE:

THE GREAT CONTEMPORARY CHALLENGE TO PREVENTIVE MEDICINE

The epidemic of premature coronary heart disease (CHD) continues to rage unabated in the economically developed countries. In fact, as our group's earlier presentation at this course noted, mortality rates are still rising in many countries – and none give evidence of a decline (1). In the words of the World Health Organization Executive Board's recent statement on, 'mankind's greatest epidemic':

'Ischaemic Heart Disease (IHD), or coronary heart disease, has reached enormous proportions, striking more and more at younger subjects. It will result in coming years in the greatest epidemic mankind has faced unless we are able to reverse the trend by concentrated research into its cause and prevention.' (2)

In the United States, for example, 600,000 deaths were recorded from this cause in 1965, about one-third of all fatilities. Of these 600,000 deaths, about 165,000 were in persons in the prime productive years of life, under age 65. And for every fatal episode, at least two nonfatal disabling events occur. The average apparently healthy American male has a 20 percent risk of developing clinical CHD before age 60. The female of the species is somewhat better off, but by no means immune. The threat of coronary heart disease is a major problem for her as well (3, 4).

One other aspect of this epidemic needs to be emphasized, if an effective strategy is to be developed to bring it under control: A cardinal characteristic of CHD is that it often leads to sudden death.

Thus, about 20 per cent of persons with first myocardial infarctions (the most frequent and important type of clinical CHD) die within 60 minutes of onset of symptoms, often before any medical care can be summoned or the patient can be hospitalized. Another 15 to 20 per cent die acutely usually during the first 24 to 72 hours – despite the best modern treatment in coronary care units.

The data of our group's long-term prospective epidemiologic study in the Chicago People's Gas Company are typical in regard to the problem of sudden death. Altogether, 82 men died from CHD in the first ten years of follow-up of the entire study cohort – 1,465 men age 40-59 in 1958. Of these 82 deaths (40.4% of all deaths), 41 were sudden deaths – precisely defined as death occuring within one hour of onset of symptoms. Thus, one half of all CHD deaths were sudden deaths, occurring out-of-hospital and too quickly to bring medical care to bear in most cases. Of the 41 sudden deaths, 18 (43.9%) were sudden and unexpected deaths, i.e. deaths with the very first illness, in men with no previous episode of clinical CHD.

Moreover, for the 60 to 65 per cent of middle-aged persons making a good recovery from an acute first episode of the so-called 'good risk' type, prognosis of dying in the next five years is about 20 per cent, five times that of persons free of a previous history of CHD (see also table 4 below). For persons with a history of two or more episodes, longterm prognosis is much worse (3).

These fundamental facts determine the strategy of the effort to control CHD. For any disease with this biology, *the main strategic thrust must be prevention, especially primary prevention* (i.e. treatment before illness to achieve prevention of first attacks), with the prophylactic effort focussed on high risk persons, beginning as early in life as possible. Nothing else has the potential for bringing about a sizeable downturn in the epidemic rate of premature CHD – not cardiac resuscitation, high-powered ambulance services, intensive care units, pacemakers, artificial hearts, cardiac transplantation, etc., important as all these recent advances are.

THE BASIC CAUSES OF THE EPIDEMIC OF PREMATURE CHD

The underlying disease process responsible for this epidemic of premature CHD is atherosclerosis of the coronary arteries – more precisely, severe atherosclerosis and its complications, particularly thrombosis. The challenge to medicine and public health inherent in the CHD epidemic, therefore, is in essence that of preventing and controlling severe atherosclerosis and its complications.

Study of the history of epidemic diseases, especially among adults – e.g. typhus, plague, cholera, tuberculosis, pellagra – compels a basic generalization most relevant for the CHD problem: Epidemic disease occurs only in those populations experiencing a confluence of multiple causes essential for the massive onslaught of sickness. Epidemic disease never has a single cause, not even when there is a clearcut single necessary cause for the given disease. Thus, the tuberculosis organism is indeed the necessary cause for TB, but it is not a sufficient cause for the development of the disease in epidemic proportions. Undoubtedly tuberculosis bacteria have been abroad among human populations for centuries and millenia. However, it was not until the 19th century that TB burst forth as epidemic disease, as the great white plague and major health problem of the era. The etiologic prerequisites for epidemic TB were the new social circumstances generated by the industrial revolution – rapid chaotic expansion of towns into cities, with inadequate housing, slums, mass overcrowding, poor sanitation, long hours of grueling dusty and dirty work, child labor, inadequate public health and medical care, etc. (5,6). These were the multiple factors – the confluence of several causes, together with the bacterium – producing epidemic tuberculosis.

Coronary heart disease has in the course of the 20th century replaced tuberculosis as the great epidemic disease of the era in the industrialized countries. CHD is the epidemic disease of mature, advanced industrial society, as TB was the epidemic disease of this society in its childhood and adolescence. Extensive evidence is available – from clinical-pathologic, epidemiologic and animal-experimental research – indicating that a confluence of socio-cultural circumstances is responsible for the emergence of CHD as the 20th century epidemic disease of economically advanced countries (1,3). One key circumstance is that the mass of the population in affluent countries has for the first time in history been able to enjoy a 'rich' diet high in animal products (meats, dairy foods) – to 'live off the fat of the land' like the 'lord of the manor' and the 'captain of industry', and not be restricted by harsh economic conditions to cheap starchy foods (bread, potatoes, pasta, oatmeal, cornmeal, etc.). This modern diet – excessive in calories in relation to energy expenditure, high in total fat, saturated fat, cholesterol, carbohydrate, sugar and salt – leads to high prevalence rates of hyperlipidemia (hypercholesterolaemia, hypertriglyceridaemia, hyper-beta-lipoproteinaemia) in the adult population. And sustained hypercholest-erolaemic hyperlipidaemia markedly increases risk of premature severe atherosclerotic disease and its clinical sequelae. This is generally true whether hyperlipidaemia is due to hereditary metabolic derangement of unknown cause, diabetes mellitus, hypothyroidism, nephrosis, or – as is most frequently the case in developed countries – habitual dietary habits. This interrelationship – among nutrition (especially dietary saturated fat and cholesterol), serum lipids (particularly cholesterol) and premature CHD – has been demonstrated repeatedly and consistently in several large-scale prospective epidemiologic studies, and has emerged as a fundamental finding from more than a half century of animal-experimental work on atherosclerosis in a wide range of species, including primates (3).

Important as this etiologic chain of events is, it is not the exclusive one involving diet in the pathogenesis and causation of the CHD epidemic. The modern 'rich' diet also contributes significantly to current high prevalence rates of obesity, and (largely as a consequence) of hypertension and diabetes – and all three of these are also important coronary risk factors (3). Thus diet is related to the CHD epidemic through at least four etiopathogenic mechanisms, and not just one – a fact all too often neglected because of preoccupation with serum lipids.

A second aspect of the 20th century way of life contributing powerfully to the CHD epidemic has been the development of mass consumption of cigarettes since World War I. As a result of several large-scale American and British studies, there is no longer any doubt that cigarette smoking is a major factor adding substantially to risk of CHD, at least among the populations of the advanced countries, with the nutritional-metabolic prerequisites for atherogenesis (3, 7-10).

A third circumstance, almost certainly, is the emergence of sedentary living as a mass phenomenon in the 20th century – as a result of greater and greater use of non-human energy in large-scale production, the motor car, television, etc., etc. Man no longer has to 'earn his bread in the sweat of his brow' – and he doesn't subsist chiefly on bread nowadays! Aside from any other negative effects, this change certainly contributes to chronic caloric imbalance and frequent obesity – e.g. prevalence rates of 20 and 50 per cent among teenagers and middle-aged adults respectively in the United States – with all the consequences. Although the evidence is not entirely airtight and consistent, there is good reason to believe that lack of exercise – habitual inactivity at work and leisure – is another important aspect of the modern mode of life increasing susceptibility to premature CHD (3).

Finally, data are available indicating that the stresses, tensions and conflicts of modern life in highly urbanized society, the pace, turmoil, mobility, change – and their effects on personality and behavior – act as 'insult added to injury' for sizeable segments of the populations of the advanced countries (3). These psycho-cultural factors too – along with the 'rich' diet, cigarette smoking, indolent living – seem to be playing an important role in the causation of the CHD epidemic in the developed countries.

THE CORONARY RISK FACTOR CONCEPT

The basic thesis summarized above is that socioeconomic and socio-cultural evolution in the 20th century has led to a way of life for tens and hundreds of millions in the advanced countries conducive to widespread premature coronary disease. Repeated reference has been made to coronary risk factors and their prevalence in populations. Coronary risk factors are those habits, traits and abnormalities associated with a sizeable (100% or more) increase in susceptibility to premature CHD. For example, persons with serum cholesterol levels of 250 mg/dl or greater have about twice the risk of developing CHD in middle-age, compared to individuals with levels less than 250. The same relationship prevails for blood pressure elevation, e.g., diastolic pressures of 90 mm Hg or greater, for cigarette smoking and for several other factors. The extensive documentation on this matter has recently been reviewed elsewhere, and need not be repeated here (3). However, two points – highly relevant to the matter of CHD prevention – merit brief reiteration.

First, high prevalence rates of coronary risk factors – repeatedly recorded at present in populations of the developed countries – are resultants of the contemporary mode of life. This is obvious in regard to diet, hyperlipidemia, obesity, hyperglycemia and hypertension (at least insofar as the latter two are diet related), cigarette smoking, sedentary and stressful living, impaired vital capacity. They are not 'bolts from the blue' mysteriously striking individuals. Nor are they, in most cases, chiefly genetic in origin. True, in a small per cent of the population severe hereditary metabolic dyscrasias are present, leading – for example – to severe hyperlipidemia, amenable only in a limited degree to dietary control. However, this is the exception rather than the rule. For most persons, hyperlipidemia (to continue the example) is in essence an acquired abnormality – a resultant primarily of a lifetime dieth high in calories, saturated fats and cholesterol (3, 11).

Actually, there is always a host factor, the phenomenon is never purely environmental in origin. This is evident from the fact that a small per cent of persons eating 'rich' diets maintain optimal low levels of all serum lipids throughout adulthood. The range of serum cholesterol and triglycerides in a given population – e.g., a standard deviation of about 40-50 mg/dl, about a mean of 230-240 for serum cholesterol for u.s. middleaged men – almost certainly is due in large measure to inborn differences in metabolism (presently unknown). Therefore, the distinction between acquired and genetic origin of risk factors is relative, not absolute. However, this conclusion in no way contradicts the inference that in terms of mass phenomena – the high prevalence rates of coronary risk factors in the adult populations of the developed countries – the fundamental cause is the mode of life.

This conclusion has important practical consequences: Change in diet and mode of life are not only essential to reduce risk in the adult population now. They are also vital prerequisites for rearing up-coming generations with new and better habits, instituted in infancy, childhood, and adolescence – to assure the disappearance of now wide-ly prevalent overeating, sedentary living, cigarette smoking and resultant hyperlipidemia, obesity, hypertension, hyperglycemia, hyper-uricemia, impaired vital capacity, etc. Only such a change – brought about by a steadily mounting, well planned, widespread social effort offers any hope of ending the upward spiral of the CHD epidemic and effecting a downturn (12).

The second major point about the coronary risk factors is that their effect on susceptibility to premature CHD is especially great when they are present in combination. Proneness is particularly high for persons with three or more factors. Tables 1 and 2 from our long-term pros-pective study in Chicago – present typical findings (3). This study in-volves a cohort of 1,594 men age 40-59 on January 1, 1958 – all the male employees of the Company on that date. Of the 1,594 men, 1,465 (91.3%) had complete research evaluation in 1958. Of the 1,465 men, 1,329 – free of definite CHD in 1958 – have been followed since, without systematic intervention.

Tables 1 and 2 deal with the relationship between original status in

Table 1. Status in 1958 with respect to three coronary risk factors* and ten year mortality from myocardial infarction and sudden death – 1,329 men age 40-59 in 1958, free of CHD and followed without systematic intervention, 1958-68 – Peoples Gas Company Study.

Risk factor status, 1958	No. of men	Ten year mortality			
		Myocardial no.	Infarction rate[4]	Sudden no.	Death rate
None high	284	1	3.0	0	0.0
Any one only high	621	23	35.7	12	18.4
Any two or all three high	420	22	50.0	16	36.6
All	1,325**	46	33.4	28	20.3

* Risk factors: Serum Cholesterol 250 mg/dl >
                Diastolic blood pressure 90 mm Hg >
                Smoking 10 > cigarettes per day
** No smoking data available for 4 of the 1,329 men.
[4] All rates are age-adjusted by 5 year age groups to the u.s. male population, 1960. Rates are per thousand.
t value: Myocardial infarction = 5.60
         Sudden Death   = 4.71

Table 2. Status in 1958 with respect to three coronary risk factors* and ten years mortality from all causes and all cardiovascular-renal diseases – 1,329 men, age 40-59 in 1958, free of CHD and followed without systematic intervention, 1958-68 – Peoples Gas Company Study.

Risk Factor Status, 1958	No. of men	Ten Year Mortality			
		All causes		All cardiovascular-renal diseases	
		No.	Rate[4]	No.	Rate
None High	284	13	42.6	4	11.9
Any One Only High	621	71	106.6	40	59.9
Any Two or All Three High	420	78	169.7	38	84.9
All	1,325**	162	113.1	82	57.5

* Risk factors: Serum cholesterol 250 mg/dl >
                Diastolic blood pressure 90 mm Hg >
                Smoking 10 > cigarettes per day
** No smoking data available for 4 of the 1,329 men.
[4] All rates are age-adjusted by 5 years age group to the u.s. male population, 1960. Rates are per thousand.
t value: All Causes = 5.87
         All CVR   = 5.99

1958 with respect to three major CHD risk factors – hypercholestero-lemia, hypertension, cigarette smoking – and ten year mortality rates. Only the single 1958 value for each risk factor has been utilized to classify the men. (Table 3 gives group mean values for four continuous variables, and prevalence rates for five risk factors.)

To avoid dividing the cohort into an excessive number of overly small groups, the men were classified as high or not-high for each of the three factors, using the cutting points specified in the footnotes of tables 1 and 2.

Despite the limitations (measurement error, normal variability, the simple dichomotization, possible treatment effects over the years), very marked and highly significant differences were delineated. Of the entire cohort (1, 329 men), 284 (21.4%) were classified not-high on all three factors. During ten years of follow-up (1958-68), no sudden deaths occurred in this group, only one fatal myocardial infarction, four cardiovascular-renal (CVR) deaths, 13 deaths from all causes. The ten year mortality rate from all causes was only 42.6 per 1,000 or about four per 1,000 per year – less than half the death rate of all U.S. males of this age. This low-risk group – unfortunately comprising only about 20 per cent of the Peoples Gas Company population under study – accounted for none of 22 sudden deaths, only one of 46 fatal myocardial infarctions (2.2%), only four of 82 CVR deaths (5.1%) only 13 of 162 deaths from all causes (8.0%).

Contrast the high mortality rates for the group of 420 men (31.7% of the population) with any two or all three risk factors. This group accounted for 57.1 per cent of sudden deaths, 47.8 per cent of fatal myocardial infarctions, 46.3 per cent of CVR deaths, 48.1 per cent of deaths from all causes. The ten year mortality rate from all causes for this group of 420 men with a median age of about 50 years in 1958 – 169.7 per 1,000 – indicates a risk of almost 20 per cent of dying before age 60, four times that of the low risk group (tables 1 and 2).

Of these 420 high-risk men, 67 – 5.0 per cent of the entire cohort – manifested all three risk factors. Their ten year age-adjusted mortality rate from myocardial infarction was 63.4 per 1,000 more than 20-times that of the low-risk group. Their death rate from all causes was 225.9 per 1,000, almost 6-times that of the low-risk group.

Note further that the sizeable group of 621 men with any one risk factor exhibited substantially higher mortality rates than the 20 per cent in the low-risk category, with no stigmata.

Table 3. Various risk factor categories, 1958 group means for continuous variables and percent with high level, men originally age 40-59 and free of coronary heart disease, Peoples Gas Company Study, 1958-68.

Risk factor category, 1958	No. of men	Group Means, 1958				Percent with High Levels				
		Serum cholesterol mg/dl	Relative weight*	Diast. BP mm Hg	Heart rate	Cholesterol 250>	Relative weight 1.15>	Diast. 90>	Heart rate 80>	10+ cigarettes per day
None high	284	208	1.18	77	67	0	60	0	9	0
Any one only high△	621	224	1.15	79	70	22	49	12	17	65
Any two or all three high	420	269	1.16	86	74	80	52	49	25	85
All	1,325**	235	1.16	81	71	36	52	21	18	57

△ Hypercholesterolemia (250 mg/dl), hypertension (diastolic 90> mm Hg), 10 + cigarettes per day.
* Ratio of observed to desirable weight, as defined in life insurance tables.
** No smoking data on 4 of the 1,329 men.

The challenge is obvious for preventive medicine and public health: Can high risk groups, constituting a majority of the adult population, be shifted to or toward low risk status by early identification and long-term treatment of risk factors?

Table 4. Status in 1958 with respect to coronary heart disease and ten year mortality rate from CHD and all causes, Peoples Gas Company Study, 1958-68.

1958 CHD Status	No. of men	Ten year mortality rate			
		All causes		Coronary heart disease	
		No.	Rate*	No.	Rate
Negative	1,199	138	109.6	48	38.5
Suspect[4]	196	36	158.7	13	58.5
Positive	70	28	300.7	21	229.9
All	1,465	202	126.6	82	52.0

* All rates are age-adjusted by 5 year age groups to the U.S. male population, 1960. Rates are per 1,000.
[4] Based chiefly on minor non-specific ST-T abnormalities on ECG, and/or suspect angina pectoris.

The need for primary prevention is further underscored by data on longterm prognosis of middle-aged persons with a history of CHD. The data of table 4 present the problem clearly. Again, they are fully in agreement with findings reported by other investigators (3). The 70 men originally positive for CHD may be viewed as persons with relatively 'mild' CHD, since they were working full-time, without marked incapacitation. Nonetheless, 30 per cent died in the ensuing ten years, chiefly from recurrent CHD. Their death rate was three times that of men free of evidence of CHD on initial examination. Clearly, the disease not only has a propensity for causing sudden death, and for killing acutely. For survivors of initial episodes, even under the best of circumstances (single uncomplicated attack in middle-age, no other major life-limiting diseases, good recovery, no frank disability), it grossly limits life expectancy.

The conclusion is inevitable: A strategy of primary prevention, for the whole population, beginning in childhood, to eliminate over the next decades the harmful living habits generating mass coronary proneness – with a pinpointed emphasis on high-risk persons. This strategy must be given first priority and made the main thrust of the overall social effort against the epidemic, if real progress is to be registered.

EARLY DETECTION OF CORONARY-PRONE PERSONS

In the United States, at least, the vast majority of young and middle-aged adults do not see personal physicians for evaluation of coronary proneness and long-term preventive care. Therefore, programs are being developed by voluntary and official health agencies for mass early detection – in the community and industry – of CHD risk. Our group has been increasingly engaged in such endeavors in recent years, through the Chicago Health Department and Chicago Heart

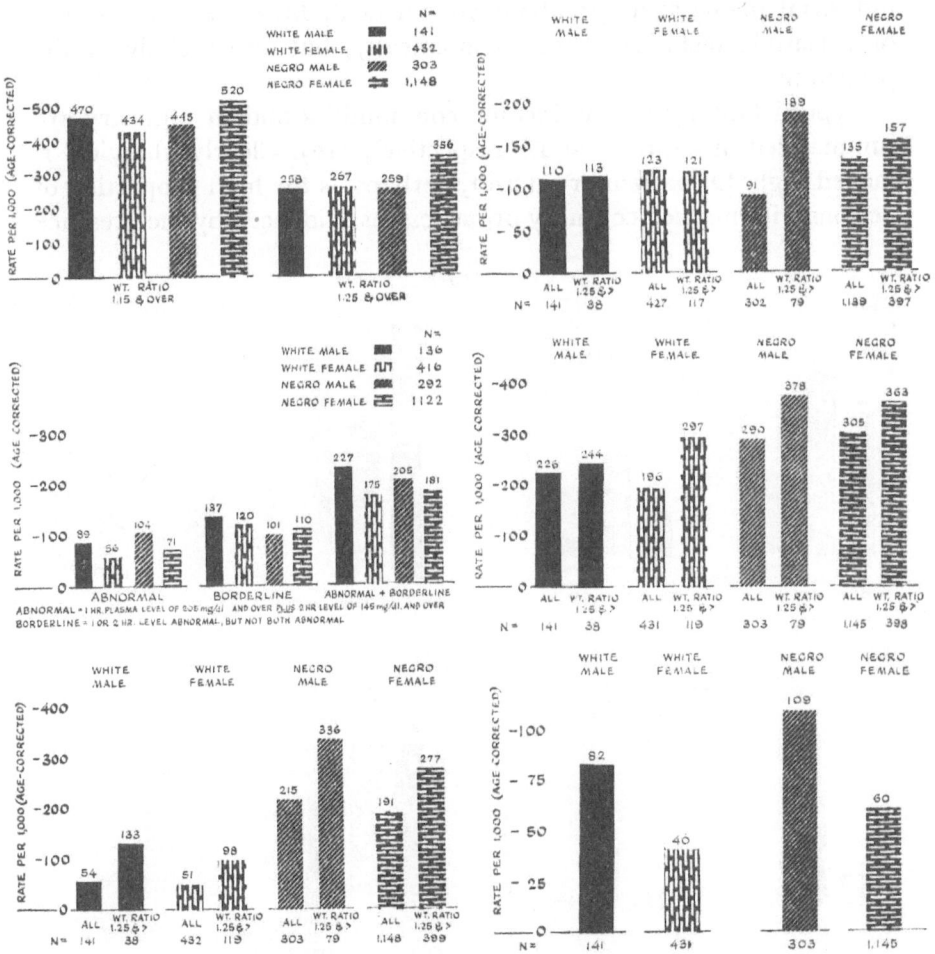

Fig. 1. Detection of cardiovascular abnormalities and risk factors in persons age 30-59, residing in low-income communities, Chicago, 1966.

Association. The procedure involves a battery of tests – simple, standardized, high-yield, meaningful and inexpensive, easily and reliably done by teams of trained clerks, technicians and nurses, without physicians on-site (13). A special-purpose portable computer is now being routinely used to obtain direct, immediate visual read-out to the technician of electrocardiographic findings (14). The response to screening has been uniformly good, based on a carefully planned, locally based publicity, educational and organizational effort, and assurance of data confidentiality. For example, volunteer rate in industrial plants averages about 70 per cent. Mass detection is not only feasible technically and economically, but also socially at the present time.

Typical findings in low income communities and in undustry are summarized in figures 1 and 2 respectively (13). Clearly, the yield is indeed high. Of particular interest, perhaps, is the high proportion of persons with marked coronary proneness, as evidenced by the presence

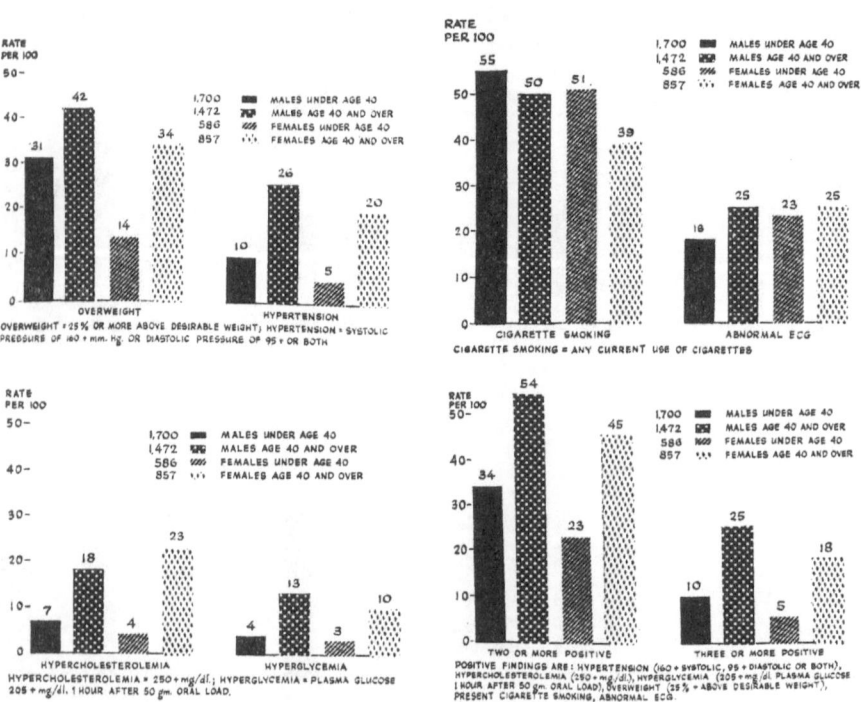

Fig. 2. Detection of cardiovascular abnormalities and risk factors in industry – first 4,615 volunteers, Chicago Heart Association, Detection Program, 1967-69.

of three or more risk factors – exhibited by 15.3 per cent of persons overall (see fig. 2 for age-sex specific rates).

Of course, screening is meaningful first of all if it detects abnormalities previously unknown to examinees. Therefore, for the survey in industry (see fig. 2), an analysis was made of previously unknown findings, plus the matter of status with regard to therapy for those previously aware of abnormalities. Of persons with screening findings indicative of hypertension or diabetes, 66.3 and 70.9 per cent respectively were unaware that they harbored these traits; 92.5 per cent of persons with abnormal ECG's gave no history of any prior cardiac positive findings. Moreover, of individuals giving a history of hypertension or diabetes, confirmed by screening findings, 56.2 and 81.0 per cent respectively were receiving no pharmacologic treatment. Thus, it is obvious that only a small minority of young and middle-aged adults with treatable CHD risk factors have been detected and brought under long-term preventive care.

These two sets of data indicate that screening has a two-pronged potential, i.e. to detect unknown traits and encourage persons with them to see their physicians for further diagnostic evaluation and possible care, and also to encourage persons with known findings to consult their physicians about instituting or re-instituting appropriate long-term care.

Obviously, detection is a means to an end, not an end in itself – as specified in the preceding paragraph. The key objective is to encourage persons with positive findings to see their physicians for further diagnostic evaluation and possible long-term care, for the control and management of risk factors, in order to attempt to realize the possibility of postponing and preventing premature catastrophic clinical cardiovascular disease (particularly heart attacks). Therefore it becomes of great concern to determine whether medical care does indeed result from the screening effort. As part of our evaluative work along these lines, last summer a special survey was organized, involving a sample of 213 persons referred to their physicians, among the approximately first 1,200 screenees seen from November, 1967 to March, 1968 in the Detection Project in Industry. Medical students interviewed the physicians named by these 213 individuals, and screenees were all re-surveyed by the same procedure and staff as previously. This repeat evaluation occurred on the average about six months after initial screening (13).

The great majority of those referred actually saw their physicians (79.3%), and in almost one half treatment was prescribed. On the other hand, the interview with the physician indicated that a further appointment was pending for only about one half of those treated, suggesting that truly long-term care was not being effected to a degree that could be regarded as satisfactory. This is a matter that is currently being pursued further.

The problem of cigarette smokers – and the role of mass detection in aiding them to end this dangerous habit – is of continuing concern.

Table 5. Results of referral – cigarette smokers detection project in industry, November, 1967-March, 1969 Special Survey, Summer 1968.

Group	No. of persons	Per cent		
		Of all referred smokers	Of referred smokers seen by MD	Of smokers advised to quit
Referred cigarette smokers	82	100.0	—	—
Referred cigarette smokers seen by MD	66	80.5	—	—
Not advised to quit	46	56.1	69.7	—
Advised to quit	20	24.4	30.3	—
Did quit	4	4.9	6.1	20.0

Referrals were for risk factors in addition to smoking.

Table 5 presents findings on cigarette smokers referred to their physicians. It should be understood that no one was referred for cigarette smoking per se. All 82 cigarette smokers were referred because one or more other risk factors were present. Of the 82 cigarette smokers referred, 66 did get to their doctors. However, only 20 were advised to quit smoking. These findings strongly suggest that physicians in the Chicago area are not yet being vigorous enough in counseling their patients – including patients with one or more other risk factors for premature heart attack – to quit smoking. Evidence is available from other sources indicating that this problem is not confined to Chicago. It would appear that many doctors are not yet transmitting their own example to their patients. (The estimate is that 100,000 physicians in the United States have quit smoking). It would seem that doctors need to be encouraged in this regard.

Of the 20 persons advised to quit, four apparently did. At first glance, this figure may seem disappointing. However, it may also be viewed positively as a step forward in the prolonged battle to change smoking habits. In this regard, it is noteworthy that of the 1,472 white males age 40 and over, 434 (29.5%) reported themselves to be past cigarette smokers, i.e. they had quit prior to being surveyed. Thus, these data confirm the information generally available for the nation as a whole, about the trend to cessation of cigarette smoking. Any 5, 10, 15 or 20 per cent addition to this trend contributed by the mass detection effort is a meaningful contribution, part of accelerating the positive long-term trend. This will be a long haul, and every achievement must be viewed in that light.

Limited information was collected in the special survey last summer concerning types of treatment prescribed by personal physicians for referred screenees for whom a positive diagnosis was made (13). They included medication (particularly for hypertension), diet (mainly for weight reduction), and advice to change sedentary living and smoking habits. Among patients given these recommendations, adherence was reported – in response to questionnaire – as 67.6 per cent to medication, 61.4 per cent to diet advice, 50.0 per cent to exercise recommendation and 20.0 per cent (as already noted) to admonition to quit cigarettes. At re-survey, objective data indicate modest group mean reductions in weight, serum cholesterol, plasma glucose and blood pressure. While these are all to the good, they indicate the need to develop new approaches – plus new resources and new types of manpower – to aid physicians and patients, and the community at large to effect and sustain changes in diet and living habits on a large scale (12).

The nature and scope of the problem is perhaps exemplified by the situation with respect to hypertension – in a sense a relatively easy CHD risk factor to bring under control, since pharmacologic therapy is frequently indicated (in addition to nutritional-hygienic treatment). It may be roughly estimated – from the data of the National Health Survey (3) – that there are about 20 million persons with hypertension in the United States at the present time. From several surveys, it may be further approximated that about half of these are undetected (1, 13, 15). Further, of the known hypertensives, only about half are under therapy. And of those being treated, only about a half have had their blood pressure normalized – a reasonable therapeutic goal for ambulatory, 'mild' hypertensives, who constitute the majority of cases. Thus, $\frac{1}{2} \times \frac{1}{2} \times \frac{1}{2} = \frac{1}{8}$th, i.e. about one-eighth of the hypertensives in the United States are under reasonably decent therapy, using the minimum criterion of normalization of blood pressure. If consideration is also given to need for treating concomitant hyperlipidemia, hyperglycemia, overweight, cigarette smoking – all factors adding further to risk of major cardiovascular complications for hypertensives – then the situation with respect to therapy for hypertensives is indeed even more unsatisfactory. Clearly the challenge is vast, the task ahead a big one. It will indeed take a well-planned, well-organized, well-financed long-term social effort – local, state and national, governmental and non-governmental – with progressive expansion over years and decades, until control is achieved (12). Undoubtedly other developed countries have a situation similar to that of the United States.

A start needs to be made now in this large-scale, long-range social endeavor to bridge the current gap between patients and doctors in relation to CHD prevention, and develop ever more widespread and effective early detection and enhancement of sustained care. At the same time greater efforts are needed to encourage men and women to present themselves to their physicians for periodic examinations, beginning in young adulthood. For physicians, the need is to incorporate tests for coronary risk factors (including the electrocardiogram) in their routine examinations, and to enhance their mastery of the nutritional, hygienic and pharmacologic methods for the long term treatment and control of these abnormalities.

RESEARCH STUDIES ON CORONARY PREVENTION INCLUDING THE CORONARY PREVENTION EVALUATION PROGRAM

The first prospective data from the Albany, Framingham and Los Angeles studies demonstrating relationships between serum cholesterol level, blood pressure, relative weight and CHD risk were presented to the American Public Health Association in October, 1956 and published the following April (16). This report – together with the mass of clinical, pathologic, animal-experimental and epidemiologic data available from other sources (17) – convinced our group in 1957 that the time had come to supplement descriptive-analytical epidemiologic studies on CHD with experimental epidemiologic studies. The fundamental objective was to explore problems involved in the effort to conduct mass field trials on the prevention of CHD – particularly primary prevention of premature clinical disease in coronary-prone middle-aged men. Other investigators independently came to a similar conclusion at more or less the same time (3, 18-22). In the latter half of 1959, Ivan D. Frantz, Irvine H. Page and the senior author independently recommended to the National Heart Institute, U.S. Public Health Service that a national co-operative study be undertaken on effect of diet change on CHD incidence. This led to the National Diet-Heart Study, a large-scale feasibility trial (23).

The inference from the findings available in 1957-8 was almost self-evident. Since risk of premature CHD is related to such factors as cholesterolemia, blood pressure and weight, then it might be possible to reduce risk of the disease and achieve its prevention by treating and controlling these abnormalities. Investigators were encouraged to explore this basic problem by research in the 1950s demonstrating that the atherosclerotic plaque is at least to a degree reversible, and that serum lipid levels can be lowered by nutritional means – particularly by decreasing intake of saturated fats and cholesterol (3, 17).

The question was: What are the problems involved in the testing of this hypothesis in mass field trials on man? Since correction of these risk factors related first and foremost to alteration of living habits, particularly patterns of eating, the problems might be formidable. In 1957-8, little or no information was available to serve as a guide line in this area. Would sizeable numbers of healthy middle-aged men volunteer to participate in such a study? If they volunteered, would they remain longterm as active participants? If they continued in the study, would they alter living habits sufficiently to effect sizeable reductions in cholesterolemia, blood pressure, weight? Would these alterations in risk factors, instituted beginning in middle age, have any impact on incidence and mortality from the disease? All these questions had to be clarified. Our group designed the Coronary Prevention Evaluation Program (CPEP) in 1957 to explore these matters. Since its experiences over the last decade extensively clarify the basic issues, they are detailed here, along with a brief review of other published work on primary prevention of CHD. (For a summary of secondary prevention studies see reference 3.)

Criteria for eligibility

The protocol of the Coronary Prevention Evaluation Program provided for participation in the study for at least five years of coronary prone men age 40-59, to be recruited as volunteers from the ranks of the general population in Chicago, particularly through their place of employment. Criteria for the high risk designation were:

1. Absence of organic heart disease, clinical atherosclerotic disease in other major arterial beds, diagnosed diabetes mellitus requiring drug treatment, other major life-limiting diseases.
2. Presence of severe hypercholesterolemia – 325 mg/dl or greater – as a single risk factor.
3. Presence of hypercholesterolemia (260 mg/dl or greater), overweight (15% or more above desirable weight), hypertension (95 mm Hg or greater diastolic pressure) – any 2 or all 3.
4. Presence of fixed minor non-specific T wave abnormalities in the ECG, plus at least one other risk factor.
5. Presence of cigarette smoking – 10 or more per day – plus at least one other risk factor.

Fixed minor T wave abnormalities were defined as low voltage, diphasic or flat T waves, present in repeat electrocardiograms and not attributable to extracardiac causes. Other ECG abnormalities required exclusion. Later in the study, with unequivocal demonstration of the role of cigarette smoking as a coronary risk factor, this trait plus at least one other of the foregoing risk factors became acceptable for entry into the study (criterion number 5).

Comprehensive baseline examination included: past medical history, family history, smoking history, review of weight change since young adulthood, previous diet therapy, physical activity pattern at work and leisure, young adult exercise and sports habits, physical examination, eye examination by an ophthalmologist with dilatation of pupils and retinal photography, 12-lead ECG, 14 × 17 P-A chest film, urinalysis, complete blood count, serology, fasting blood glucose, urea, uric acid, cholesterol, total protein, A/G ratio, cephalin flocculation, serum protein bound iodine (PBI) and endogenous creatinine clearance. To be eligible, volunteers had to be free of any form of organic heart disease or other major systemic illness influencing life expectancy. Clinical diabetes mellitus requiring drug treatment, grossly abnormal plasma glucose levels and marked hypertension (diastolic pressures of 110 mm Hg or greater) resulted in exclusion.

Forms of intervention

The protocol emphasized nutritional-hygienic means for the correction of five coronary risk factors – hypercholesterolemia, obesity, hypertension, cigarette smoking and physical inactivity. The deliberate decision was made to intervene against all these, with the view in mind of ultimately testing the general hypothesis that primary prevention of atherosclerotic coronary heart disease in high risk middle-aged men could be achieved by controlling major coronary risk factors. A nutritional-hygienic approach would be the cornerstone of the effort, in keeping with the basic theoretical conclusion that the CHD epidemic is a resultant of socioeconomic evolution leading to faulty living habits. If this thesis is correct, the key to prevention must be the effort to establish and maintain sound living habits, leading to correction and control of coronary risk factors. Drugs can only be adjuvant tools, not of central and decisive importance for mass prevention of disease – even as with tuberculosis.

Modification of nutritional habits was designated as of central importance, for the control primarily of hyperlipidemia and obesity, in addition to its role in the management of 'moderate' hypertension and hyperglycemia. The diets were to be moderate in calories, moderate (not low) in total fat, low in saturated fat and cholesterol, moderate (not high) in polyunsaturated fat (see below) (3, 11, 17). For obese hypertensive patients, the protocol provided that no recommendation be made with respect to pharmocologic treatment in the initial months of the program. The initial objective would be to assess ability to reduce blood pressure through weight reduction, with moderate salt restriction as a dietary adjuvant. It was further stipulated that for men who failed to respond to diet with blood pressure reduction during the first three to six months, consultation would proceed with their private physicians in regard to appropriate drug treatment. A similar approach was provided for control of mild impairment of glucose tolerance, in the absence of gross hyperglycemia, glycosuria, acidosis and clinical symptoms or signs of diabetes. (These required exclusion from the study.) In agreement with longstanding observations, it was postulated that nutrition management with weight reduction would result in rectification of mild carbohydrate intolerance in a sizeable proportion of obese persons. For those whose plasma glucose levels remained abnormal, consultation would proceed with private physicians concerning possible therapy with oral antidiabetic drugs or insulin.

The study would not assume responsibility for any pharmacologic treatment.

The cornerstone of the nutritional program would be emphasis on the concept of working for a permanent change in eating habits, in order to effect and maintain correction of hyperlipidemia and obesity. This approach would be stressed in preference to the idea of 'going on a diet'. A perspective would be developed of a change in eating habits to be achieved in two phases – a period of reduction of serum cholesterol and weight, followed by an indefinite period on a maintenance regimen, with longterm supervision and frequent consultation at least until the desired new habit pattern is fully established. During both phases, the dietary recommendations would be designed to achieve and maintain not only optimal weight and serum cholesterol, but also optimal levels of nutrition, blood pressure, glucose tolerance, etc. This approach precluded 'crash' and faddistic diets for weight reduction. It emphasized moderate caloric restriction and gradual weight loss, on a diet of mixed ordinary foodstuffs of low caloric density and of a composition calculated to maximize reduction in serum lipids during weight loss. In accordance with this overall approach, drugs for weight reduction would be avoided.

Correction of cigarette smoking was also set as one of the major objectives of the Program. Since experience of others had indicated the difficulty of simultaneously attempting to alter both eating and smoking habits, particularly when weight reduction is an objective, it was decided from the beginning to avoid this approach. Rather, the decision was made to tackle habits seriatim, with the first effort to achieve effective institution of a new dietary pattern, for purposes of correcting obesity and hyperlipidemia. By mutual consent, after full discussion of the longterm perspective and goal, the effort to control cigarette smoking would be postponed until the participant had 'gotten over the hump' in dietary alteration. Nonetheless, for all smokers of cigarettes, each and every interval visit would include a review of present smoking status, in addition to check on nutrition, exercise, interval illness, medication, etc. In this way, even during the period of deferred action on cigarette smoking, the matter would be kept clearly before the participant. At a certain point, a detailed discussion would be held and an effort made to arrive at a definitive decision on cessation of cigarette smoking. The alternatives would be to give up smoking altogether, or to switch to pipe or cigars in moderation, e.g. less than 5 cigars or less than 5 pipesfull per day, without inhaling. Detailed effort would be made during this period to assist the man in avoiding marked weight gain during the initial weeks off cigarettes. The participant would be encouraged to make frequent visits to consult with physician and nutritionist, in order to receive needed aid and support. Where indicated, medications (e.g., sedatives or tranquilizers) would be prescribed shortterm. For men electing to remain cigarette smokers, the point would be made that this matter would be rediscussed at intervals. The basic longterm objective would remain to break this habit. The fundamental approach would be one of maintaining 'friendly persuasion' and 'firm steady pressure' on this matter, without 'nagging' the participant. Since he is in a longterm program, with frequent repeat visits to the research center, the opportunity would present itself to pursue the effort in this way.

Since sedentary living had been implicated as a coronary risk factor, the protocol also provided for an effort to overcome this habit. The approach would be to examine the participant's daily living pattern in detail, as well as his past history with respect to exercise, in order to develop a practical approach to increasing physical activity as part of daily living. The emphasis would be on regular, moderate, frequent exercise of the type known to increase cardiopulmonary fitness – e.g. vigorous walking, bicycling, swimming, running.

Implementation and follow-up
Procedural details for the practical implementation of this protocol and for longterm follow-up of participants have been described in previous publications (3, 24, 25). Suffice it to note here that the emphasis from the beginning has been on close work with the participant – and his wife – by nutritionist and physician. Follow-up visits were provided for quarterly, more often if deemed advisable. At each visit, the man would be seen by both nutritionist and physician. Weight, pulse, blood pressure, serum cholesterol would be measured, a quarterly 7-day food record reviewed, interval medical history noted (including drug usage), smoking and exercise status recorded, and diet adherence reviewed. If necessary, he would be referred to his personal physician for follow-up of any significant medical complaint or finding. A comprehensive examination would be done annually. Data would be reviewed annually in an individual session with the participant and his wife.

As the study developed, additional measurements were added to the sizeable list in the original protocol – e.g. serum triglycerides, paper electrophoresis of lipoproteins, glucose tolerance test, image intensification fluoroscopy to detect coronary calcification, ergometric exercise test of fitness, skinfold thicknesses.

Based on accumulating experience in prospective studies, particularly our group's findings in the Peoples Gas Company Project, a subgroup of *very high risk men* was identified among the CPEP participants. These were men with three or all four risk factors (hypercholesterolemia, hypertension, cigarette smoking, overweight).

As the initial pilot phase of the CPEP effort developed successfully in 1958-9, and as increasing consideration was given to expanding the study and maintaining follow-up of participants for at least five years, the problem of controls became a key one. Originally, random assignment of high risk men recruited from industry into control and experimental groups had been proposed as part of the protocol. It was reluctantly abandoned, because management and labor in industry indicated uneasiness and disagreement with the approach of randomly assigning high risk men to a control group. Therefore, as an alternative method (although, it was recognized, not ideal) of dealing with this matter, large groups of men age 40-59 were identified – from the Albany civil servant, Framingham, Los Angeles civil servant, Minneapolis-St. Paul businessmen, Peoples Gas Company and Western Electric Company (Chicago) studies – to serve as comparison and control groups for the CPEP investigation (3, 4, 16, 26-31). With assistance from the National Co-operative Pooling Project established to pool data from the foregoing major U.S. prospective studies (and others eventually) (31), data tapes were obtained and men selected to match the CPEP participants, using the same medical and risk factor criteria.

Recruitment

Over the years, co-operation has been forthcoming from several Chicago employers and with their aid recruitment goals of the program have been fulfilled. These have included Armour and Company, the Chicago Health Department, the Illinois Bell Telephone Company, the Chicago office of the Internal Revenue Service, the Newspaper Division of the Field Enterprises, the Peoples Gas Light and Coke Company and the Standard Oil Company. The original protocol provided for accruing participants at a limited rate in the early years of the study, when the design was being tested and refined. Intensive recruitment was carried out during 1966 and 1967, to expand the study group to its goal of over 500 men. By mid-1968, recruitment was completed; 519 men meeting the criteria of the Program had been given a diet recommendation, e.i. had been enrolled as study participants. The median time of follow-up is now almost five years (see below).

This experience demonstrates ability to recruit sizeable numbers of middleaged healthy men for research endeavors of this type. It is in conformity with results in recent years of several other similar endeavours, e.g. the New York Anti-Coronary Club and the National Diet-Heart Study (18, 23). Unquestionably the public in the United States at the present time is deeply concerned with the problem of epidemic coronary heart disease, and is willing to join mass field trials on primary or secondary prevention. This question of ability to recruit participants for mass field trials, unanswerable based on experience as of 1957-8, can now be regarded as clarified in the affirmative.

Longterm participation
A key question requiring elucidation at the onset of this program concerned ability to maintain effective participation over a period of at least five years, estimated to be the minimum needed for a mass field trial on prevention of CHD. This too was an unknown in 1957-8. The original protocol of the study set a goal of keeping five year dropout rate under 50 per cent, since it was generally agreed that failure to attain this minimum objective would negate any possibility of an effective mass field trial.

Table 6. Cumulative dropout rate, Coronary Prevention Evaluation Program, as of March 31, 1969.

Year	No. of men at risk	No. of dropouts	Cumulative dropout rate per 1,000$^{\it \Delta}$
1	519	28	52.3
2	479	31	122.2
3	363	20	177.7
4	243	7	201.8
5	181	6	227.9
6	138	16	316.5
7	94	10	394.7
			($\pm$35.1)

$^{\it \Delta}$ Age-adjusted by five year age groups to the u.s. male population, 1960.

Each year, the program 'closes book' as of March 31, and makes a detailed evaluation of the status of all participants. Data as of March 31, 1969 reveal cumulative dropout rates (calculated by life table method) considerably less than 50 per cent at five years – i.e. only 22.8 per cent for the total group of 519 high risk men (table 6). Dropout rate is higher for current cigarette smokers than non-smokers. This finding is in accordance with the experience of the National Diet-Heart Study (23), and indicates that habitual cigarette smokers perform less satisfactorily in terms of continuation in long-term studies of this type, compared with men who never smoked or are ex-smokers. As shown by data on year-by-year dropout rates, a high proportion of dropouts occurring during the first 24 months. Thereafter, dropout rate was low, at least through the first years for which the volunteers originally committed themselves. During the eleven years the study has been in progress, therefore, it has become clear that it is possible to retain a substantial majority of high risk men in a program of this kind long term. Other studies – e.g. the New York Anti-Coronary Club and the National Diet-Heart Study – have in the intervening years had similar experience (18, 23). Therefore, this question of ability to carry out a long term study of this type – posed in the original protocol as one of the key matters requiring clarification – is now answerable in the affirmative.

Nutritional alterations

Men in the Coronary Prevention Evaluation Program keep a seven-day food record four times a year. Early in the study, considerable effort was expended in the development of a computer program to accomplish detailed interval analyses of the nutritional data derived from food records. These tabulations serve an additional purpose: They are excellent teaching and motivational tools for use in reviewing their status with participants.

Data on changes in daily nutrient intake have been previously reported (3). They indicate that the diets of the men were moderate in total calories (about 1,700 per day on the average during the early months of the study), with an estimated daily caloric deficit of about 500-800 calories, calculated to effect weight loss at a rate of about 1.0 to 1.5 pounds per week. They were moderate in carbohydrate (about 190-200 grams per day, 46 per cent of total calories) and moderate in total fat (about 55 to 60 grams per day, 30 per cent of total calories, rather than the usual American 40% or more), low in saturated fatty acids (less than 20 grams per day, 10% or less of total calories, rather than the usual 45 or more grams per day, 17% or more of total calories), low in cholesterol (300 mg per day or less, rather than the usual 600 mg or more) and moderate in unsaturated and polyunsaturated fatty acids. They were high in protein, 95 grams per day, 23 per cent of total calories. They were ample in all essential nutrients – amino acids, vitamins, minerals, polyunsaturated fatty acids – even during the early period of caloric restriction. As shown by correlated t tests, changes effected in intake of critical nutrients were highly significant statistically.

These changes in nutrient intake were accomplished by altering habits with regard to intake of all five of the major sources of saturated fat and cholesterol in the u.s. diet – meats, dairy products, commercial baked goods, eggs, table and cooking fats. A systematic and sustained process of education and motivation was carried out, emphasizing lean

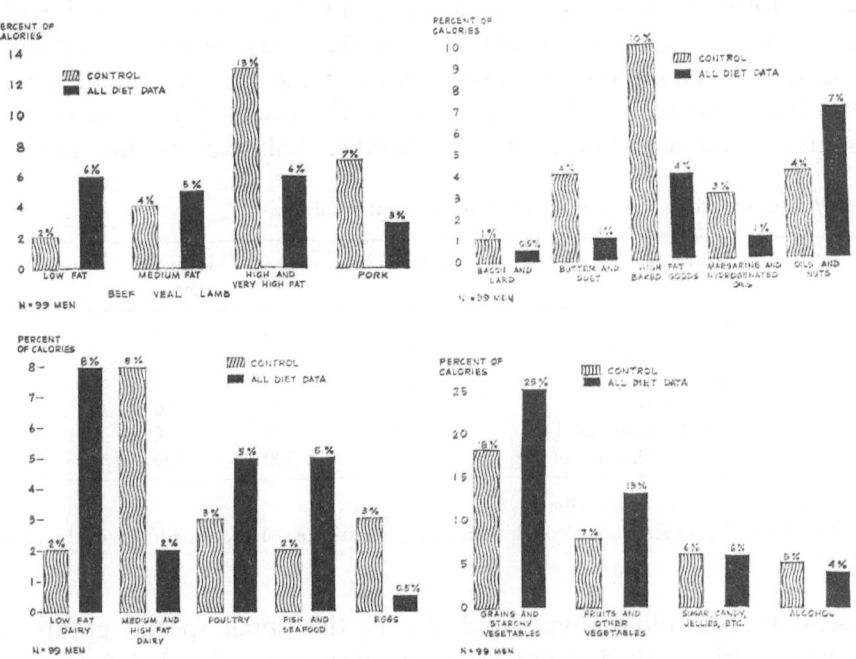

Fig. 3. Mean daily percent of calories from food groups, Coronary Prevention Evaluation Program.

cuts of beef, lamb, pork and veal, cooked to dispose of saturated fat, and eaten in moderate portion sizes; by de-emphasizing fat cuts of meat; by emphasizing low fat dairy products, and de-emphasizing fat-containing dairy products; by encouraging use of lean white meat of poultry, as well as fish and seafood; by de-emphasizing egg yolk, bacon, lard, butter, suet, high fat baked goods, hard margarines and hydro-genated shortenings; by emphasizing unsaturated oils, nuts and soft margarines (within limits of calorie control), grains, vegetables, legumes, fruits, jelly-jam-marmalade-honey as spreads (instead of butter or hard margarine), and moderation in alcohol intake (fig. 3).

For most active participants adhering satisfactorily to nutrient re-commendations, an essentially similar diet composition was maintained with shift to an isocaloric pattern after weight loss. Rarely, in an occasional man with marked familial hypertriglyceridemic hyper-lipidemia (hyperlipoproteinemia Type III or IV) (32), the general CPEP diet was not fully effective in preventing return of elevated serum lipid levels when isocaloric intake was restored. For these individuals, the pattern of nutrient intake has in recent years been modified, with marked reduction in carbohydrate intake, effected chiefly by sub-stituting vegetable oils for carbohydrate (table 7). This modification has been accomplished while retaining the essential features of low saturated fat and low cholesterol intake. This pattern has proved

Table 7. Comparison of dietary composition per cent of calories[4].

Nutrient	Control*	CPEP	Modified CPEP
Protein	18	23	23
Carbohydrate	39	47	30
Total fat	43	30	47
saturated	17	< 10	< 10
polyunsaturated	6	7	18
Dietary cholesterol (mg.)	627	< 300	< 300

* Similar to usual American diet.
[4] Exclusive of calories from alcohol, which may constitute 0-10% of calories in the CPEP diets.

useful in controlling hyperlipidemia in this small special group of persons with marked metabolic aberration of the familial type. For most participants – with moderately severe, non-familial, acquired hypercholesterolemic hyperlipidemia (with or without associated hypertriglyceridemia), resulting from habitual ingestion of the usual American diet – the CPEP diet in its unmodified form effects and maintains reduction of both hypercholesterolemia and hypertriglyc-eridemia (hyper-beta- and hyper-prebeta-lipoproteinemia) (see below).

Changes in serum lipids

As a result of the recommended nutritional alterations, men in the Coronary Prevention Evaluation Program experienced a highly signi-ficant decline in serum cholesterol concentration. Detailed findings as of March 31, 1968 have recently been reported (33). They are sum-marized in fig. 4 presenting data on hypercholesterolemic men with at least five years of consistent observation. (Two of these 63 men dropped out before completing five years in the Program). Fall aver-aged 15.4 per cent for the entire five years. A majority of these origi-nally hypercholesterolemic men had serum levels less than 260 mg/dl on CPEP diet. These falls were consistently associated with sizeable re-ductions in weight, in response to CPEP diet.

These data unequivocally demonstrate ability not only to achieve reductions in serum cholesterol with the CPEP diet, but also capacity to sustain this effect long-term, as long as adherence to this diet continues. For sizeable proportions of men, serum cholesterol levels were reduced well below the level for frank hypercholesterolemia (260 mg/dl or greater).

Since January, 1966, measurement has also been made of fasting serum triglycerides of CPEP participants. Findings to date are sum-marized in table 8. For 114 men with control and one year experimental data, mean serum triglycerides were reduced 17.3 per cent, serum cholesterol 12.1 per cent. Serum triglyceride response was marked – 21.6 and 29.9 per cent – in the two subgroups with elevated baseline levels (1.80 m.mol./l or greater*), whereas no fall occurred in normo-triglyceridemic men, whether or not they were hypercholesterolemic.

Data are now available for some of these men after two years in the Program. The overall findings to date for 37 men indicate that the fall in serum triglycerides induced by CPEP diet persists under isocaloric conditions, even in men with very marked hypertriglyceridemia (33).

Clearly the CPEP diet is highly effective in lowering elevated serum triglycerides. Undoubtedly weight reduction played a significant role

* 1.8 mM/l equals 5.4 m.eq./l and is approximately equal to 154 mg/dl, based on an estimated average molecular weight of serum triglycerides of 857.

Table 8. Effect of coronary prevention evaluation program on serum triglyceride groups divided by control levels of serum triglyceride and serum cholesterol.

Group Serum cholesterol mg/dl	Serum triglycerides m mol/l	No. of men	Mean serum cholesterol (mg/dl)			Mean serum triglyceride (m mol/l)			Mean weight (lbs)		
			control	one year	Percent change	Control	One year	Percent change	Control	One year	Percent change
< 260	< 1.80	29	214.8 ±32.4*	198.4 ±33.2	− 7.6	1.03 ±0.31	1.11 ±0.43	+ 7.8	201.6 ±28.3	192.1 ±29.7	− 4.7△
< 260	1.80 >	12	229.7 ±17.9	218.0 ±37.2	− 5.1	2.68 ±0.68	2.10 ±1.16	− 21.6#	194.9 ±32.0	191.5 ±36.3	− 1.7
260 >	< 1.80	35	293.8 ±30.2	263.1 ±45.7	− 10.4△	1.32 ±0.31	1.34 ±0.51	+ 1.5	181.9 ±20.2	170.9 18.7	− 6.0△
260 >	1.80 >	38	323.2 ±81.9	269.8 ±57.4	− 16.5△	3.01 ±1.81	2.11 ±1.25	− 29.9△	186.8 ±22.5	175.3 ±21.7	− 6.2△
All		114	276.7 ±69.3	243.2 ±56.3	− 12.1△	1.96 ±1.40	1.62 ±0.98	− 17.3△	189.9 ±25.4	179.9 ±26.3	− 5.3△

* Standard deviation of the mean
# p = 0.05
△ p = 0.01

in effecting this change, since hypertriglyceridemia of the usual types is known to be very sensitive to negative caloric balance (32, 33). It is appropriate to note further, however, that for most CPEP men weight loss occurs during the first three to six months of their participation. By the one year and two year visits, weight has usually been stable for months (if there has been no regaining!). Therefore, the CPEP diet is effective in sustaining reduction in serum triglycerides, when consumed isocalorically. Although modest reduction in per cent calories from total fat is often associated with modest increase in per cent calories from carbohydrate, the CPEP diet is moderate in carbohydrate, in terms of grams ingested per day. It is not a high carbohydrate diet. It does not result in so-called carbohydrate-induced hypertriglyceridemia when consumed isocalorically, except in a very small per cent of persons with severe lipid metabolic dyscrasia of the familial type. This conclusion from the CPEP diet is consistent with experience of other investigative groups (3, 17-23).

It is also worth emphasizing that reductions in serum lipids were effected by CPEP nutritional recommendations without utilizing jiggers of oil, special oil allotments or fat modified foods. Such dietary measures were not required to achieve the desired alterations in quantity and quality of ingested nutrients*. Ordinary foodstuffs generally sufficed, particularly since the main emphasis for most participants was not on achieving a high intake of unsaturated and polyunsaturated oils. Rather, it was on assuring a low saturated fat, low cholesterol intake, with consumption of polyunsaturated fats in moderate amounts as adjuvant.

Changes in weight

Overweight – a ratio of observed weight to desirable weight of 1.15 or greater – was one of the risk factors present in the overwhelming majority of men. A high proportion of them were markedly overweight, with relative weights of 1.25 or greater. Effects of participation in the Program on weight and relative weight have recently been reported in detail (33), and are summarized in table 8 and figure 5. Most of the weight loss occurred in the first months, although a modest additional loss was registered during the second year. Maximum average weight loss totalled about 13 pounds for the entire

---

* Availability of appropriate fat-modified foods would certainly be helpful, and must be realized for a mass public health preventive endeavor (12, 23).

cohort with control relative weight of 1.15 or greater (33). This amounted to about seven percent of original body weight. Although there was a tendency for some weight to be regained in later years in the program, the amount regained for continuing participants was small, so that the group tended to remain about 9 to 10 pounds below control weight (fig. 5).

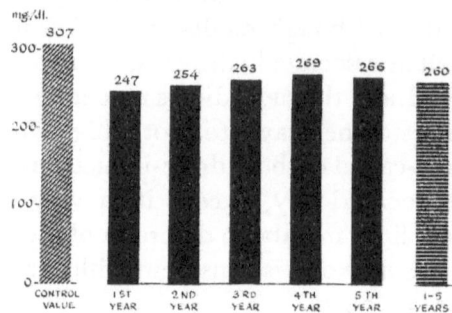

Fig. 4. Effect of Coronary Prevention Evaluation Program on mean serum cholesterol, 63 men with control values of 260 mg/dl or greater, in CPEP for at least 5 years, as of March 31, 1968.

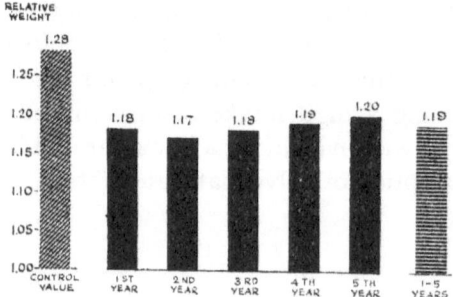

Fig. 5. Effect of coronary prevention evaluation program on relative weight, 63 men with control serum cholesterol values of 260 mg/dl or greater, in CPEP for at least 5 years, as of March 31, 1968.

Despite this achievement, a sizeable proportion of the men remained considerably above desirable weight, in the frankly overweight range. The effect of the Program may therefore be characterized for these men as blunting, rather than removing, this particular risk factor. However, it is possible that this degree of weight control may be beneficial, particularly when accompanied by control of hyperlipidemia, cigarette smoking, hypertension and physical inactivity.

Changes in blood pressure

For all men in the Program, a significant reduction in mean systolic pressure was recorded, maximum in the first year (7.9 mm Hg, from a control level of 137.3), and gradually decreasing thereafter. This time course of systolic pressure, in men exhibiting a sustained fall in weight over these years, may reflect the tendency of systolic blood pressure to rise with age. A significant fall in diastolic pressure was also recorded (5.6 mm Hg, from a control level of 88.5), and this appeared to persist with little increase throughout the five years of follow-up.

Effect of the Program on blood pressure for men with hypertension at onset is, of course, of particular concern. Long-term data on this matter are cigarette smokers in an effort to aid them in breaking this habit. Of the 176 cigarette smokers at entry, 90 were still active in the Program as of March 31, 1968, and 72 of these 90 had been participants for a year or longer. As noted earlier, cigarette smokers tended to have a higher dropout rate than non-cigarette smokers. Of 90 cigarette smokers still active in the Program, 33 (36.7%) had stopped smoking cigarettes as of March 31, 1968. Thirteen of these 33 had quit smoking within the last year, 20 had been off cigarettes for a year or longer. Of the 33 no longer smoking cigarettes, 22 had given up smoking altogether, 11 had switched to pipe or cigars. This choice had been recommended to the men at the time of entry into the Program.

Of 42 original cigarette smokers active in the Program for three years or longer, 18 (42.9%) had quit smoking, and 13 (31.0%) had been without a cigarette for a year or longer. Of 24 original cigarette smokers active for five years or longer, 12 (50.0%) had quit smoking cigarettes, and 11 of these 12 had been without a cigarette for a year or longer; 10 of these 12 had quit all tobacco usage.

Thus, in accordance with the approach of the Program, rate of cessation of smoking increased progressively with duration in the study, so that for longterm active participants effective cessation of smoking – defined as no usage of a cigarette for a year or longer – became the pattern achieved by almost a majority. These findings indicate the merit of a sustained approach to changing cigarette smoking habits among middle-aged coronary prone men, and the value of 'firm steady pressure' over months and years in aiding these men to break the habit.

It should also be noted, however, that – viewed overall – success in ending the cigarette smoking habit was achieved in only a minority of all men entering the Program as current smokers, and often success came late – in some cases only after recovery from an acute myocardial infarction.

Changes in exercise habits

Since the study has been limited to advising participants as to desirability and methodology of getting regular, frequent, moderate exercise, and supervised exercise is not part of the Program, valid assessment of change in exercise habit in these free-living men is difficult. Until 1967, the only approach to information in this area was by interview, at quarterly visits. In general, these data indicate that a majority of active participants had made a transition from an essentially sedentary living habit to one of habitual light activity.

Mortality

The Program 'closes book for inventory' of all participants annually on March 31. The staff then proceeds to establish the status of all men who have dropped out of the study. Insofar as possible, this is accomplished by re-examining them in our facility. When this is precluded, information is obtained from the man and/or his personal physician by telephone interview or letter. When all efforts lead to failure, and our staff cannot determine whether a man is dead or alive, follow-up is pursued with the assistance of a private detective agency. This last resort has been necessary for only two to four people annually.

As a result of these efforts, no man has been lost to follow-up. Death certificates, autopsy reports, hospital and personal physician records are obtained for all decedents. Data are also collected to evaluate all reported or suspected nonfatal illnesses. Since direct examination cannot be accomplished annually for all men who have dropped out of the Program, because of inadequate co-operation, information is less accurate on occurrence of nonfatal illnesses (e.g. clinical and silent myocardial infarction) for these men than for active participants. This is an important point apparently not fully appreciated until recently by investigators concerned with such studies, including our group. Thus, the truly 'hard' end-points for the total study group are coronary mortality, cardiovascular mortality and total mortality.

Upon completion of follow-up in April or May of each year, disease incidence and mortality analyses are accomplished, using a computer life table program. Incidence and mortality rates and their standard errors are generated for the 40-44, 45-49, 50-54 and 55-59 age groups, and for the 40-59 age group. For the latter, both raw rates and rates age-adjusted by five year age groups to the u.s. male population, 1960 are obtained. Rates are routinely generated for all participants, for non-dropouts and for dropouts. For all life table analyses for dropouts and nondropouts, a man is counted in one or the other of these categories, depending upon his status as of March 31, 1969. That is, if a man has dropped out of the study as of that date, he is classified exclusively as a dropout, and his entire experience over the years is dealt with exclusively as the experience of a dropout. This is based on the observation, in this investigation and the National Diet-Heart Study, that a man who becomes a dropout is generally an ineffective participant (i.e., a poor adherer) for much of the time preceding dropout.

Life tables are generated for the following major end points. CHD incidence (nonfatal plus fatal), CHD mortality, CVR mortality and total mortality. Special analyses for selected subgroups can also be accomplished at will – for men with specified combinations of risk factors; for all hypercholesterolemic men, all cigarette smokers, etc. (see below).

As indicated earlier in this paper, disease incidence and mortality experience in the Coronary Prevention Evaluation Program is being evaluated in comparison with findings for matched high risk men originally age 40-59, under long-term observation by six major prospective epidemiologic studies of CHD in the United States (3, 4, 16, 26-31). With assistance from the National Co-operative Pooling Project, data tapes were obtained and 3,243 men were identified (among almost 10,000) who met CPEP age, medical and risk factor criteria. Table 9 is a replica of the computer life table output, plus explanatory information (title, column numbers, footnotes). It should aid the reader in dealing with tables 10, 12-15, which presented abbreviated information from the life table computer output.

Number of persons at risk for each seven years of follow-up for four groups – Pooling Project, all CPEP participants, CPEP Non-Dropouts, CPEP Dropouts – are shown in table 10.

Although medical and risk factor criteria for selecting the Pooling Project men were identical with those required for participation in the CPEP study, it does not necessarily follow that the two groups are closely matched, in terms of specific constellations of risk factors. With the six risk factor criteria – serum cholesterol 260-324 mg/dl, serum cholesterol 325 or greater, diastolic pressure 95 mm Hg or greater, relative weight

Table 9. Sample of the computer output of life table data – for the 3,243 matching men of the Pooling Project – mortality from all causes△.

1 Intervals after entry*	2 Observed at start of interval	3 Terminated during interval△△	4 Effective number at risk	5 Events during interval	6 Events		7 Non-events		8 Standard error	9 Effective sample size
					p**	CUM p△△△	Q	CUM Q		
0 to 1	3243	1	3242.50	3	.0011	.0011	.9989	.9989	.000689	838.02
1 to 2	3239	3	3237.50	5	.0013	.0024	.9987	.9976	.000914	837.68
2 to 3	3231	24	3219.00	4	.0010	.0035	.9990	.9965	.001049	835.91
3 to 4	3203	3	3201.50	6	.0023	.0058	.9977	.9942	.001444	833.52
4 to 5	3194	80	3154.00	11	.0037	.0095	.9963	.9905	.001869	827.68
5 to 6	3103	123	3041.50	10	.0043	.0137	.9957	.9863	.002350	818.20
6 to 7	2970	363	2788.50	8	.0025	.0161	.9975	.9839	.002496	801.44
7 to 8	2599	72	2563.00	16	.0068	.0228	.9932	.9772	.003112	758.72
8 to 9	2511	92	2465.00	10	.0042	.0269	.9958	.9731	.003431	735.27
9 to 10	2409	22	2398.00	9	.0048	.0315	.9952	.9685	.003843	720.74
10 to 11	2378	2	2377.00	10	.0036	.0350	.9964	.9650	.003988	709.43
11 to 12	2366	343	2194.50	9	.0052	.0400	.9948	.9600	.004387	692.48
12 to 13	2014	446	1791.00	14	.0085	.0481	.9915	.9519	.004958	641.81
13 to 14	1554	28	1540.00	7	.0040	.0519	.9960	.9481	.005144	611.67
14 to 15	1519	18	1510.00	12	.0087	.0601	.9913	.9399	.005706	565.83
15 to 16	1489	12	1483.00	11	.0075	.0670	.9925	.9330	.006076	543.94
16 to 17	1466	25	1453.50	2	.0012	.0682	.9988	.9318	.006127	539.48
17 to 18	1439	19	1429.50	11	.0096	.0770	.9904	.9230	.006684	524.34
18 to 19	1409	30	1394.00	11	.0105	.0865	.9895	.9135	.007264	504.09
19 to 20	1368	72	1332.00	12	.0118	.0970	.9882	.9030	.007811	488.20
20 to 21	1284									

△ All rates are age-adjusted by 5-year age groups to U.S. male population, 1960.

* Each interval represents 6 months of exposure to risk.

△△ This column indicates the number of persons completing their total period of follow-up or observation during the specified time interval, without experiencing an event (in this case, death) (Column 5). Thus, a man in one of the six Pooling Project studies lost to follow-up in the fifth month of the first year after entry is terminated during the first interval. The number of persons observed at the start of any interval after the first (cf. Column 2), i.e. the number exposed to risk of an event during that interval, is equal to the number entering the previous interval minus the number terminating (Column 3) and minus the number experiencing an event (Column 5), e.g. for the second interval, 3243-1-3 = 3239.

** P is the proportion of events during the interval; to convert to rate per 1,000, multiply by 1,000.

△△ Cum P is the cumulative proportion of events, i.e. the sum of the event rate for each interval, from Column 6. The standard error (Column

Table 10. Number of men at risk for each of seven years of follow-up: Pooling Project men, all CPEP participants, CPEP non-dropouts, CPEP dropouts (CPEP at March 31, 1969).

		Number of men at risk[A]		
	Pooling project	CPEP		
Year		All	Non-dropouts	Dropouts
1	3,243	519	390	129
2	3,231	507	378	129
3	3,194	422	293	129
4	2,970	313	193	120
5	2,511	242	138	104
6	2,378	197	101	96
7	2,014	159	73	86

[A] From column 2 of the computer life table output (cf. table 9 and its footnotes).

1.15 or greater, cigarette smoking, minor ST-T abnormalities on ECG – 42 combinations are possible, consistent with eligibility for the study. In fact, the CPEP men were classified into 30 of these cells, the Pooling Project men into 37. The proportions of men classified into the major cells are shown in table 10, together with percentages of men in various cell combinations (e.g. all two factor groups plus serum cholesterol 325 or greater, all three factor groups). In addition, the last six lines of table 10 give data on the per cent of men exhibiting the single risk factors, irrespective of status.

From these latter data, it is first of all clear that proportions of men with hypertension, overweight, hypercholesterolemia, minor ECG abnormalities were higher for the CPEP than for the Pooling Project men (table 10). In contrast, per cent cigarette smokers was lower for the CPEP than for the Pooling Project group.

In terms of combinations of risk factors, the per cent with three or more factors – i.e. of very high risk men – was greater for the CPEP than for the Pooling Project cohort (table 11). Thus, the CPEP group as a whole may be characterized as slightly more coronary-prone than the Pooling Project group.

Most very high risk men were cigarette smokers in both cohorts. Overall, the proportion of very high risk men who were cigarette smokers – i.e. men with this habit plus two or more others factors – was very similar for the two cohorts (25.4 and 28.9% of all men respectively).

Number of deaths per year and age-adjusted cumulative mortality

Table 11. Percentage distribution in various risk categories, high risk men originally age 40-59 in Pooling Project and Coronary Prevention Evaluating Program.

Risk factor status	Pooling project 3,243 men	CPEP 519 men
All high risk	100.0%	100.0%
Very high risk	28.7	34.5
All 2 factor groups or cholesterol 325 >	69.8	60.3
Hypercholesterolemia + overweight	11.6	28.5
Hypertension + overweight	9.6	19.8
Hypercholesterolemia + smoking	13.6	1.5
Overweight + smoking	26.8	6.0
Hypertension + smoking	3.9	0.0
All Smoking + One other factor	44.7	7.7
All 3 factor groups	25.4	31.2
3, 4, 5 factor groups	30.1	39.7
All smoking + 2, 3, or 4 other factors	25.4	28.9
All hypertensive men	31.1	45.1
All overweight men	76.3	95.2
All hypercholesterolemic men	52.0	60.3
All hypercholesterolemic men – 325 mg/dl or >	10.7	9.6
All cigarette smokers	70.1	36.6
All ST-T DAC on ECG[a]	3.8	10.6

[a] DAC = definitely abnormal curve.

rates, calculated by life table method, are presented for CHD and all causes for the two cohorts in tables 12 and 13 respectively. Since numbers of CPEP men at risk were small beyond the seventh year of follow-up, data are presented only through this time period. For the Pooling Project and CPEP dropout groups, CHD deaths accounted for 47.5 per cent and 60.0 per cent respectively of all deaths (58 of 122, and 3 of 5 respectively). This high ratio of CHD to total mortality (compared to all U.S. men of this age, for example) was an expected finding, in view of the high risk status of these groups. The cumulative CHD mortality rate for the CPEP dropout group was similar to that for the Pooling Project men at seven years (table 12).

Table 12. Age-adjusted mortality rates from coronary heart disease in high risk men originally age 40-59, in Pooling Project and Coronary Prevention Evaluation Program (CPEP as of March 31, 1969).

			Annual number of deaths and cumulative mortality rate		
				CPEP	
Year	Pooling Project − 3, 443 men		All 519 men	Non-Dropouts − 390 men	Dropouts − 129 men
1	5+	1.7*	0 0.0	0 0.0	0 0.0
2	5	3.3	1 2.0	1 2.8	0 0.0
3	7	5.2	2 7.3	1 6.5	1 11.9
4	11	8.8	1 9.8	0 6.5	1 18.0
5	14	14.5	0 9.8	0 6.5	0 18.0
6	8	18.3	1 13.7	0 6.5	1 25.2
7	8	22.5	0 13.7	0 6.5	0 25.2
		(±3.2)ᴬ	(±6.2)	(±4.6)	(±14.8)

+ Number of deaths during the one year interval, from column one of the computer life table output (cf. table 9).
* Cumulative rate per thousand, age-adjusted by 5 year age groups to the U.S. male population, 1960; from column 7 of the computer life table output (cf. table 9).
ᴬ Standard error of the rate, from column 10 of the computer life table output (cf. table 9).

The findings for the critically important group of CPEP non-dropouts are intriguingly different from those of the foregoing two groups. First, only two of seven deaths (28.6%) were due to CHD. No CHD deaths occurred during years four through seven of follow-up. At the end of seven years, the cumulative CHD mortality rate for CPEP non-dropout men was only 28.9 per cent that of Pooling Project men, and the difference was statistically significant by conventional t test (see below) (table 12). Moreover, the lowest CHD mortality rate for any one of the six studies in the Pooling Project was 14.7 per 1,000 in seven years. Thus, the rate of 6.5 for the CPEP non-dropout group was less than half the lowest rate recorded among the six centers of the Pooling Project. As a result of the very low CHD mortality rate in the non-dropout group, the cumulative 7-year mortality rate for all CPEP men was only 60 per cent that of the Pooling Project men (13.7 vs. 22.5 per 1,000). However, the difference is not statistically significant at the 5 per cent level by t test.

Table 13. Age-adjusted mortality rates from all causes in high risk men originally age 40-59, in Pooling Project and Coronary Prevention Evaluation Program (CPEP as of March 31, 1969).

| | | Annual number of deaths and cumulative mortality rates | | |
| | | | CPEP | |
Year	Project − 3, 243 men	All 519 men	Non-dropouts − 390 men	Dropouts − 129 men
1	8 2.4*	2 4.1	2 5.7	0 0.0
2	10 5.8	3 10.7	3 15.1	0 0.0
3	21 13.7	5 25.5	2 24.8	3 27.5
4	24 22.8	1 27.9	0 24.8	1 33.4
5	19 31.5	0 27.9	0 24.8	0 33.4
6	19 40.0	1 31.8	0 24.8	1 40.5
7	21 51.9	0 31.8	0 24.8	0 40.5
	(±5.1)	(±9.3)	(±9.7)	(±18.3)

* Cumulative rate per thousand, age-adjusted by 5 year age groups to the U.S. male population, 1960.
Δ Standard error. See footnotes of table 12.

Cumulative mortality rate from all causes for the group of 390 CPEP non-dropouts – with no deaths during years 4-7 in the study – was one-half that of the Pooling Project cohort at seven years (24.8 vs. 51.9 per 1,000) (table 13). This difference is statistically significant by conventional t test. For all 519 CPEP men – non-dropouts plus dropouts – 7-year total mortality rate was almost 40 per cent less than for the Pooling Project men (31.8 vs. 51.9 per 1,000), but the difference is not statistically significant at the 5 per cent level. Nevertheless, the seven year age-adjusted cumulative mortality rate of 31.8 for the CPEP group is unusually low by any standard for men of this age. It is considerably lower than the rate for all U.S. males and all U.S. white males of this age (34). (This is probably to be expected, despite the high risk status of the CPEP men, since they were all free of life-limiting disease at the onset of the study.) Of greater importance, this rate is about one-half that reported for male standard life insurance risks of like age (35). Moreover, *this rate is almost identical with the calculated seven-year age-adjusted mortality rate from all causes for the 20 per cent of men of the same age at lowest risk – i.e. not high for serum cholesterol, blood pressure, cigarette smoking – in the People's Gas Company Study* (cf. table 2). Is this pure chance, or a true shift from high to low risk status of the CPEP active participants as a result of the prophylactic regimen?!

In order further to evaluate the possible impact of CPEP nutritional-hygienic measures on mortality, seven year age-adjusted cumulative mortality rates were also computed by life table method for subgroups of the two cohorts, based on original risk factor findings (tables 14 and 15). For CPEP men, no deaths have occurred over the seven years of participation – from CHD or other causes – in the first two subgroups evaluated, with the specified combinations of two risk factors only, hypercholesterolemia plus overweight, and hypertension plus over-

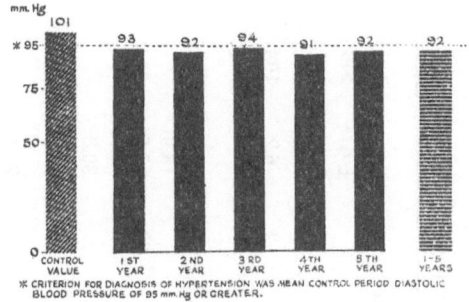

Fig. 6. Effect of participation in Coronary Evaluation Program on diastolic blood pressure of 27 hypertensive men, in CPEP for at least 5 years, as of March 31, 1968.

weight. For both of these subgroups, the differences in total mortality rate from the corresponding Pooling Project subgroups are significant by conventional t test.

With respect to the third set of subgroups – men with any two risk factors only, or original serum cholesterol level of 325 mg/dl or greater, numbering 2,325 men from the Pooling Project and 313 from CPEP – remarkably low mortality rates for both CHD and all causes

Table 14. Cumulative age-adjusted mortality rates from coronary heart disease in high risk men originally age 40-59, classified by risk factor findings at entry, Pooling Project and Coronary Prevention Evaluation Program (CPEP as of March 31, 1969) life table analysis.

Risk factor subgroup	Pooling Project			CPEP								
				All			Non-dropout			Dropout		
Hypercholesterolemia + overweight	312△	4*	14.6** ±7.7×	148	0	0.0	124	0	0.0	24	0	0.0
Hypertension + overweight	310	2	6.2 ±4.4	103	0	0.0	87	0	0.0	16	0	0.0
Any two factors Only or hypercholesterolemia 325 >	2,266	33	18.9 ±3.6	313	1	3.1 ±3.1	254	1	4.0 ±4.0	59	0	0.0
Any three, four or Five Factors	977	25	30.8 ±6.4	206	4	23.0 ±11.3	136	1	7.8 ±7.7	70	3	40.6 ±22.9
Very high risk	931	23	29.4 ±6.4	179	4	28.2 ±13.8	116	1	11.1 ±10.8	63	3	44.4 ±24.8

No. of men, no. of deaths and cumulative age-adjusted mortality rate per 1,000 at seven years

△ No. of men at entry.
* No. of deaths.
** Seven year age-adjusted mortality rate per 1,000.
× Standard error of the rate.
See footnotes of table 12.

Table 15. Cumulative age-adjusted mortality rates from all causes in high risk men originally age 40-59, classified by risk factor findings at entry, Pooling Project and Coronary Prevention Evaluation Program (CPEP as of March 31, 1969) life table analysis.

Risk factor subgroup	Pooling Project			No. of men, no. of deaths and cumulative age-adjusted mortality rate per 1,000 at seven years — CPEP								
				All			Non-dropout			Dropout		
	No. men	No. deaths	Rate	No. men	No. deaths	Rate	No. men	No. deaths	Rate	No. men	No. deaths	Rate
Hypercholesterolemia + overweight	312[Δ]	10[*]	42.9[**] ±15.2[x]	148	0	0.0	124	0	0.0	24	0	0.0
Hypertension + overweight	310	10	40.5 ±13.3	103	0	0.0	87	0	0.0	16	0	0.0
Any two factors only or hypercholesterolemia 325 >	2,266	77	46.5 ±5.8	313	1	3.1 ±3.1	254	1	4.0 ±4.0	59	0	0.0
Any three, four or Five factors	977	45	65.8 ±10.9	206	11	76.6 ±23.0	136	6	74.1 ±30.3	70	5	74.8 ±33.4
Very high risk	931	41	65.1 ±11.9	179	11	97.3 ±28.9	116	6	102.3 ±41.3	63	5	84.6 ±38.0

Δ No. of men at entry.
* No. of deaths.
** Seven year age-adjusted mortality rate per 1,000.
x Standard error of the rate.
See footnotes of table 12.

were registered. All differences between CPEP and Pooling Project rates, for both CHD and all causes, were significant statistically by usual t text.

Tables 14 and 15 also present 7-year cumulative age adjusted mortality rates for men with 3, 4 or 5 risk factors, and for the very similar subgroup designated very high risk (any 3 or all 4 of hyper-cholesterolemia, hypertension, cigarette smoking, overweight, irre-spective of ECG). For the CPEP non-dropouts of both these subgroups CHD mortality rates are only about one-third to one-fourth those of the corresponding Pooling Project men (7.8 vs. 30.8, and 11.1 vs. 29.4 per 1,000). For all CPEP men in these two subgroups, non-dropouts plus dropouts, CHD mortality rates are not significantly less than those of the Pooling Project men. Seven-year cumulative mortality rates from all causes for these two subgroups are higher – although not significantly so – for CPEP than for Pooling Project men (table 15).

Table 16, presenting detailed data on all deaths of CPEP men during the first seven years of follow-up, is informative with respect to the likely basis for this finding. As is evident, 11 of the 12 deaths occurred in men with three or more risk factors. In 10 of these 11, cigarette smoking was one of the risk factors. At least 8 of these 10 cigarette smokers persisted in this habit after entry into the CPEP, up to the time of their fatal illness. In all likelihood this was also true for the other two men, for whom no reliable information on smoking status was available, since they were both dropouts. Of these very high-risk continuing cigarette smokers, three (all non-dropouts) died of carcinoma (of lung, pancreas and liver respectively), four (one non-dropout, three dropouts) from CHD. Two other deaths were due attributed to hyper-tensive encephalopathy and auto accident respectively; evidence is available to indicate that alcoholism entered into the fatal outcome. The last of these ten deaths was a homicide.

These data suggest that for these very high risk men, both non-dropout and dropout, persistent cigarette smoking – despite efforts of the prevention program to bring about a change in habit – may have contributed significantly to their demise, at least in the majority dying of carcinoma or CHD. Of course, this cannot be proved, but the data strongly suggest this conclusion. In any case, this set of findings – together with the very low mortality rates in the non-smoking CPEP participants – lend further support to the mass of information already available that avoidance of or cessation of cigarette smoking is an

Table 16. Detailed data on twelve men dying during the first seven years of follow-up – Coronary Prevention Evaluation Program, total cohort 519 high risk men, as of March 31, 1969.

Participant No.	Age at Entry	Risk factors at entry△	Cigarette smoking status prior to death	Months between dropout and death	Months between entry and death	Cause of death
Non-Dropouts						
1045	59	C + W + S	Current smoker	—	18	Carcinoma of Lung
3202	51	C + H + W	*	—	9	Carcinoma of Stomach
5094	56	H + W + S	Current smoker	—	31	Carcinoma of Pancreas
6403	47	H + W + S	Current smoker	—	15	Homicide
6821	58	C + W + S	Current smoker	—	7	Carcinoma of Liver
1020	53	C + H + W + S	Current smoker	—	36	CHD
2971	47	C + H	Non-smoker	—	19	CHD
Dropouts						
0131	58	C + H + S	No information	12	33	Hypertensive Encephalopathy△△
1018	51	C2 + H + W + S	Current smoker	25	26	Auto Accident△△
1037	50	C2 + W + S	Current smoker	19	41	CHD
2117	53	H + W + S	Current smoker	57	65	CHD
3109	40	C + W + S	No information	8	29	CHD

△C is hypercholesterolemia 260-324 mg/dl, C2 – 325 mg/dl or >, W. is overweight, S is cigarette smoking, H is hypertension,
ECG is fixed minor nonspecific ST-T abnormalities on ECG.

* Current cigar smoker.

△△ Possibly complicated by alcoholism.

important part of the coronary prevention effort (fig. 7) (36).

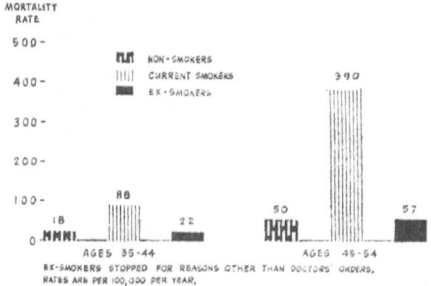

Fig. 7. Coronary heart disease mortality rates of non-smokers, current smokers of 20-39 cigarettes per day, and ex-smokers, age 35-54 and 45-54, u.s. Veterans Study, 1954-1962 (36).

In summary, the mortality data to date – viewed overall – indicate a highly favorable effect of the Coronary Prevention Evaluation Program multifactor prophylactic regimen on these 519 high risk men. Obviously, this conclusion is tentative, first of all because several years of additional experience are required to complete long-term of follow-up for most men. Moreover, the limitations in design of this study must not be overlooked in evaluating its findings, i.e. the relatively small sample size, the lack of a randomized control group, and therefore the special problem of evaluating whether lower mortality rates reflect special characteristics of volunteers, unrelated to the CPEP regimen, or are really due to the changes in risk factors it has effected (23, 37). Finally, as has become clear recently, particularly through the work of the National Co-operative Coronary Drug Project in the United States, conventional statistical methods for evaluating siginifinance have serious inadequacies when used periodically to evaluate data trends, as is being done in the CPEP study.

Therefore, our overall evaluation – that the data to date in the CPEP study are apparently indicative of a positive prophylactic effect on mortality – is presented as preliminary, tentative and guarded.

OTHER LONG-TERM RESEARCH STUDIES ON PRIMARY PREVEN-
TION OF CHD
All other long-term studies on coronary prevention have concerned themselves almost exclusively with assessing effect of reducing serum lipids, by nutritional or pharmacologic means (18-23). The New York Anti-Coronary Club study routinely prescribed diets for correction of

both obesity and hyperlipidemia (18). All studies have demonstrated ability to effect and maintain fall in serum cholesterol. Findings in this regard have been reviewed previously (3, 33).

In October, 1964 the New York Anti-Coronary Club presented a report on its seven years' experience, including data on coronary incidence (18). Recently, these results were up-dated through November 30, 1967 (38). This report dealt with 941 men accruing 3,954 person-years of experience as active participants in the study, 432 men with 3,207 person-years of exposure, after becoming inactive (dropouts), and 457 controls with 3,122 person-years of exposure. All men were age 40-59 at onset of observation and free of CHD. Confirmed new events numbered 17, 24 and 32 respectively in the three groups. Incidence rates were 4.3, 7.5 and 10.3 per 1,000 per year respectively. Thus, the active experimental group continues to have an unusually low rate, particularly in view of its risk factor status (18, 39), compared both to inactive and control groups, and to similar groups in long-term prospective studies (3).

Recently reports have also become available from the primary prevention study in progress since 1958 in two mental hospitals in Finland (22, 40, 41). This investigation has involved male patients originally age 34-64, 327 in the hospital serving for six years as the experimental institution, 254 in the hospital serving for six years as the control. (In March, 1965, dietary patterns in the two hospitals were reversed, with corresponding reversal of serum lipid levels, and the study is continuing according to this crossover design.) In the experimental hospital, diet was changed by replacing most milk fat by soybean oil, whereas the other hospital was kept as control, without any intentional dietary change. On the average, serum cholesterol level was 51 mg/dl lower in the experimental than in the control hospital. Serum triglycerides and phospholipids were also lower in the former. Incidence of ECG patterns indicative of CHD was markedly and significantly lower in the experimental hospital. Coronary mortality also appeared to be lower, but number of deaths was too small for statistically valid conclusions. Lower incidence in the experimental group was ascribed primarily to protective effect of the cholesterol-lowering special diet. The second phase of this study, after crossover, is continuing, with initially promising results (41).

At the end of 1968, a summary report on end-of-study data was published for the long-term Los Angeles Veterans Administration

Domiciliary Center Study (20, 42). This double-blind study of elderly men recorded a significant reduction in incidence of sudden death and definite myocardial infarction (its primary end point) in the experimental group fed a fat-modified diet, compared with controls. Further, for the subgroups of men under age 65 on entry into the study, the controls had an eight year combined incidence of myocardial infarction, sudden death, and cerebral infarction of about 41 per cent, whereas the rate was only about 22 per cent for the men on fat-modified diet over eight years. No positive effect was recorded for the experimental subgroup age 65 and over. Finally, for the entire cohort, irrespective of age, death rate from atherosclerotic events was lower for the experimental group, compared with the controls. However, death rate from all causes was not, due to a small excess of accidental and neoplastic deaths in the experimental group.

Thus, four 'first-generation' studies (37) – the Chicago Coronary Prevention Evaluation Program, the New York Anti-Coronary Club, the Finnish Mental Hospital Study, and the Los Angeles Veterans Administration Domiciliary Center Study – have presented findings indicating that change in living habits, particularly diet, with reduction especially of serum lipids is associated with decreased incidence and/or mortality from CHD. None of these studies is foolproof or perfect in design, methodology or results. All are limited by small sample sizes. Each has one or another additional flaw, e.g. high dropout rate, absence of control group set up simultaneously with experimental group on the basis of randomized assignment of participants to the two groups, lack of double blind design, imperfection of statistical evaluation. Therefore, their suggestive positive results have not settled the issue of ability to achieve primary prevention of CHD. Nevertheless, their similar findings are encouraging, assume added significance in view of their consistency, and certainly cannot be dismissed or ignored.

The National Diet-Heart Study was carried out to test feasibility of a truly mass field trial on primary prevention of CHD by modifying dietary saturated fat, polyunsaturated fat and cholesterol content in middle-aged men (23). It was deliberately designed to assess ability – through a large-scale national co-operative research effort of 'tight' design – to overcome shortcomings inherent in the pioneering smaller local studies, and it drew greatly upon their experience. It did not attempt to acquire data on the end point of final concern, effect on CHD rates. Its extensive positive findings, recently published, led to recommendations for definitive large-scale mass field trials on both primary and secondary prevention by nutritional means in both free-living and institutionalized populations (11, 23). Initial efforts in mental hospital patients are already in progress (43). Hopefully, additional undertakings to implement these recommendations can be launched soon (37).

Another major study on primary prevention is currently in progress in Edinburgh, Budapest and Prague, assessing effects of longterm treatment with clofibrate (Atromid-S®, CPIB), particularly in hypercholesterolemic men (44). A British study on effects of cessation of cigarette smoking is also in progress (45). Co-operative investigations on feasibility of trials on prophylactic effects of exercise are in progress in the United States, with at least one counterpart in Helsinki (46, 47).

Studies on secondary prevention are reviewed elsewhere (3, 33).

Finally, no review of CHD prevention can be regarded as complete without reference to very important recent findings on the therapeutic value of adequate treatment of hypertension. Emphasis on this matter is necessary, for several reasons: the high proportion of hypertensive persons either still undetected, under no medical management, or inadequately treated; still current tendencies among physicians to underestimate the serious prognostic significance of so-called 'mild' 'benign' hypertension; lingering attitudes of therapeutic nihilism with regard to hypertension; narrow focus on diet and serum lipids, to the neglect of hypertension and its control as a key aspect of the coronary prevention effort. Against this background, the significance cannot be overestimated of the positive results recorded in the excellently designed study of the U.S. Veterans Administration co-operative group on drug treatment for 'moderately severe' hypertension (48). Hopefully, a report will be forthcoming shortly on this group's findings on effects of therapy for 'mild' hypertension.

IMPLICATIONS FOR MEDICAL PRACTICE AND PUBLIC HEALTH

Clearly great advances have been registered in research on the primary prevention of CHD. A pattern of positive results has emerged, but the findings are not without their flaws and inconsistencies. The work is still in progress, and – given the problems of sound mass field trials on CHD – will be so for another decade.

However, practitioners of preventive and therapeutic medicine cannot – should not – 'sit on their hands' in the interim, especially in the face of the CHD epidemic confronting them. Wisdom and responsibility call for widespread implementation of the approach taken by the American Heart Association; the Council on Foods and Nutrition, American Medical Association; the President's Commission on Heart Disease, Cancer and Stroke; the u.s. Second National Conference on Cardiovascular Diseases; and particularly the Medical Boards of Norway, Sweden and Finland (3, 49). All of these responsible groups have urged early mass detection and long-term effective care of coronary-prone adults, to attempt to realize the possibility of prevention. The Medical Boards of the Scandinavian countries jointly elaborated and issued recommendations for prophylactic dietary modification for their entire populations.

The challenge to medical practice, public health and society-at-large was succinctly stated in the Report on Smoking and Health, by the Advisory Committee to the Surgeon General (7):

'It is established that male cigarette smokers have a higher death rate from coronary disease than non-smoking males. ...If cigarette smoking actually caused the higher death rate from coronary disease, it would on this account be responsible for many deaths of middle-aged and elderly males in the United States. Other factors such as high blood pressure, high serum cholesterol, and excessive obesity are also known to be associated with an unusually high death rate from coronary disease. The causative role of these other factors in coronary disease, though not proven, is suspected strongly enough to be a major reason for taking countermeasures against them. It is also more prudent to assume that the established association between cigarette smoking and coronary disease has causative meaning than to suspend judgment until no uncertainty remains.'

ACKNOWLEDGEMENTS

It is a pleasure to acknowledge the co-operation and support of Eric Oldberg, M. D., President, Chicago Board of Health and Chairman, Chicago Health Research Foundation. It is also gratifying to pay tribute to our colleagues and associates co-operating in the research of our group presented in this paper – particularly Linda Andersen, R. N., George Barr, Ph. D., Alyce Booker, Stevie Catchings, R. N., Roberta Crawford, Nancy Dalton, Helen Dean, Wanda Drake, Celene Epstein, George Farah, M. D., Edith Fitzhugh, Elizabeth Frazier, Eleanor W. Hicks, R. T., Betty Humbert, Virginia C. Jauch, M. S.,

Dana T. King, William MacIntyre, M. D., William McAtee, Wilda A. Miller, M. P. H., Dorothy Moss, M. S., Joy Nelson, R. N., Gail Pacelli, Frances Petersen, Peggy Powell, Laura Radford, Geraldine Rennhack, B. S., Raymond R. Restivo, Margie Shores, Wesley E. Sime, M. S., Eva Smolin, Adele Stamler, Elizabeth L. Stevens, R. N., David Stewart, Michael Thompson, Thomas J. Tokich, Ika Tomaschewsky, June M. Wallace, R. T., Ira T. Whipple, M. A, Carol Zehnle, M. S.. We are also grateful to Paul Meier, Ph. D., Professor, Department of Statistics and Biological Sciences Computation Center, University of Chicago and to Richard B. Remington, Ph. D., Associate Dean for Research, School of Public Health, University of Texas for invaluable statistical advice and consultation. It is a further pleasure to acknowledge the splendid long-term co-operation in research of the Medical Department and the Executive Leadership of the Peoples Gas Light and Coke Company, particularly Remick McDowell, Chairman, and Leslie A. Brandt, President; the Newspaper Division of the Field Enterprises, particularly Wilbur Munnecke, formerly Vice-president and General Manager, John G. Trezevant, Vice-president and General Manager, and Jacques Smith, M. D., Medical Director; the Medical Department of the American Oil Company, particularly Gilbeart Collings, M. D. and John Malia, M. D.; Armour and Company, particularly William Wood Prince, Chairman of the Board; Marshall Field and Company, particularly Joseph A. Burnham, Vice-president; Illionois Bell Telephone Company and its Medical Director, Robert R. J. Hilker, M. D., Internal Revenue Service in Chicago and its Medical Director, Michael W. Langello, M. D.; and Mr. Donald J. Erickson of Arthur Andersen and Company. We also gratefully acknowledge the co-operation of Dr. James A. Schoenberger, Medical Director, Louis de Boer, Executive Director and our other colleagues in the Chicago Heart Association Heart Disease Detection Project in Industry. We are also most grateful to the principle investigators of the Albany civil servant, Framingham, Los Angeles Civil Servant, Minneapolis-St. Paul business men, and Western Electric Company (Chicago) studies, and the co-ordinators of the national co-operative Pooling Project for making data available from these major u.s. prospective studies for comparison with findings of the Coronary Prevention Evaluation Program. It is a pleasure to acknowledge this co-operation and aid of our colleagues in this endeavor – Drs. John M. Chapman, Thomas R. Dawber, Joseph T. Doyle, Frederik H. Epstein,

William B. Kannel, Ancel Keys, Felix J. Moore and Oglesby Paul.

The research of our group presented in this paper was made possible by grants from the American Heart Association, Chicago Heart Association, Corn Products Institute of Nutrition, National Dairy Council, National Heart Institute, National Institutes of Health, United States Public Health Service (HE 04197 and HE 09426) and Wesson Fund for Medical Research.

REFERENCES

1. Stamler, J., Regional Differences in Mortality, Prevalence and Incidence of Ischaemic Heart Disease. *Boerhaave Course on Ischaemic Heart Disease*, Leiden, The Netherlands, in press. (1969).
2. Executive Board, World Health Organization. *Mankind's Greatest Epidemic: Heart Disease.* Resolution and Press Release, World Health Organization, Division of Public Information, Geneva, Switzerland, 27 Feb. 1969.
3. Stamler, J. *Lectures on Preventive Cardiology*, Grune and Stratton, New York, N.Y., (1967).
4. Dawber, T. R., W. B. Kannel and P. M. McNamara, The Prediction of Coronary Heart Disease. Trans. Ass. Life Insur. *Med. Dir. Amer.* 47, 70 (1964).
5. Dubos, R. and J. Dubos, *The White Plague – Tuberculosos, Man and Society*. Little Brown, Boston, Mass., (1952).
6. Brockington, C. F., *A Short History of Public Health.* 2nd ed., J. and A. Churchill, London, England, (1966).
7. *Smoking and Health* – Report of the Advisory Committee to the Surgeon General of the Public Health Service, U.S. Department of Health, Education, and Welfare, Public Health Service, Washington, D.C., (1964).
8. *The Health Consequences of Smoking* – A Public Health Service Review: 1967. US Dept. of Health, Education, and Welfare, Public Health Service, Washington, D.C., Public Health Service Publication No. 1696, (1967).
9. Goodman, H. A., Ed., *World Conference on Smoking and Health*, September 11, 1967 – A Summary of the Proceedings, National Interagency Council on Smoking and Health, New York, N.Y., (1968).
10. Stamler, J. Cigarette Smoking and Atherosclerotic Coronary Heart Disease. *Bull. N.Y. Acad. Med.*, 44, 1476 (1968).
11. Page, I.H. and J. Stamler. Diet and Coronary Heart Disease. *Mod. Conc. Cardiov. Disease*, 37, 119 and 125 (Sept. and Oct. 1968).
12. Stamler, J., O. W. Anderson, L. Breslow, L. de Boer, V. A. Getting, M. Lepper and M. H. Stiles, Atherosclerosis – Community Services. In: Andrus, E. C. and C. H. Maxwell, Eds., *The Heart and Circulation* – Second National Conference on Cardiovascular Diseases, Postprint Reports, Vol. II, Community Services and Education, Federation of American Societies for Experimental Biology, Washington, D. C., 748 (1965).
13. Stamler, J., J. A. Schoenberger, H. A. Lindberg, R. Shekelle, J. M. Stokes, M. B. Epstein, L. de Boer, R. Stamler, R. Restivo, D. Gray and W. Cain, Detection of Coronary Proneness. *Bull. of the N.Y. Acad. of Med.*, in press.
14. Berkson, D. M., J. Stamler, E. Stevens, R. Soyugenc and E. Smooth, The Electro-Cardio Analyzer, *Proceedings of the Fourth Asian-Pacific Congress of Cardiology*, in press.
15. Wilber, J. A., Detection and Control of Hypertensive Disease in Georgia, U.S.A. In:

Stamler, J., R. Stamler and T. N. Pullman, Eds., *The Epidemiology of Hypertension*, Grune and Stratton, New York, N.Y., 439 (1967).

16. Measuring the Risk of Coronary Heart Disease in Adult Population Groups – A Symposium. *Amer. J. Public Health*, 47, No. 4, Part 2, (April, 1957).

17. Katz, L. N., J. Stamler and R. Pick, *Nutrition and Atherosclerosis*. Lea and Febiger, Philadelphia, Pa., (1958).

18. Christakis, G., S. H. Rinzler, M. Archer, G. Winslow, S. Jampel, J. Stephenson, G. Friedman, H. Fein, A. Kraus and G. Hames, The Anti-Coronary Club: A Dietary Approach to the Prevention of Coronary Disease. A seven year report. *Amer. J. Public Health*, 56, 299 (1966).

19. Green, J. G., H. B. Brown, A. P. Meredith and I. H. Page, Use of Fat-Modified Foods for Serum Cholesterol Reduction. *J.A.M.A.*, 183, 5 (1963).

20. Dayton, S., M. L. Pearce, B. S. Hashimoto, L. J. Fakler, E. Hiscock and W. J. Dixon, A Controlled Clinical Trial of a Diet High in Unsaturated Fat – Preliminary Observations. *New Eng. J. Med.*, 266, 1017 (1962).

21. Ollendorf, P., T. Geill, T. Astrup and E. Lund, The Influence of Diets Containing Certain Animal and Vegetable Fats on the Initiation of Blood Coagulation. *Acta. Med. Scand.*, 170, 351 (1961).

22. Turpeinen, O., P. Roine, M. Pekkarinen, M. J. Karvonen, Y. Rautanen, J. Runeberg and P. Alivirta, Effect on Serum Cholesterol Level of Replacement of Dietary Milk Fed by Soy Bean Oil. *Lancet*, 1, 196 (1960).

23. National Diet-Heart Study Research Group. The National Diet-Heart Study Final Report. *Circulation*, 33, Suppl. 1, (1968).

24. Stamler, J. Current Status of the Dietary Prevention and Treatment of Atherosclerotic Coronary Heart Disease. *Prog. Cardiov. Dis.*, 3, 56 (1960).

25. Stamler, J., D. M. Berkson, H. A. Lindberg, Y. Hall, W. Miller, L. Mojonnier, D. B. Cohen and Q. D. Young, Coronary Risk Factors – Their Impact and Their Therapy in the Prevention of Coronary Heart Disease. *Med. Clin. No. Amer.* 50, 229 (1966).

26. Doyle, J. T. Risk Factors in Coronary Heart Disease. *New York State J. Med.*, 63, 1317 (1963).

27. Keys, A., H. L. Taylor, H. Blackburn, J. Brozek, J. T. Anderson and H. H. White, Coronary Heart Disease among Minnesota Business and Professional Men Followed Fifteen Years. *Circulation*, 28, 381 (1963).

28. Paul, O., M. H. Lepper, W. H. Phelan, G. W. Dupertuis, A. MacMillan, H. McKean and H. Park, A Longitudinal Study of Coronary Heart Disease. *Circulation*, 28, 20 (1963).

29. Chapman, J. M. and F. J. Massey, The Interrelationship of Serum Cholesterol, Hypertension, Body Weight, and Risk of Coronary Disease. Results of the First Ten Years Follow-up in the Los Angeles Heart Study. *J. Chron. Dis.*, 17, 933 (1964).

30. Weinstein, B. J., F. H. Epstein, H. Blackburn, L. P. Cook, J. T. Doyle, S. P. Ehrlich Jr., H. A. Kahn, F. E. Moore, O. Paul, D. M. Spain, J. Stamler, P. W. Willis. III and W. J. Zukel, (Working Subcommittee on Criteria and Methods, Committee on Epidemiological Studies, American Heart Association). Comparability of Criteria and Methods in the Epidemiology of Cardiovascular Disease. Report of a Survey. *Circulation*, 30, 643 (1964).

31. Epstein, F. H. and F. Moore, Personal Communication on the Progress Report to the National Heart Institute on the National Co-operative Pooling Project .

32. Fredrickson, D. S., R. I. Levy and R. S. Lees, Fat Transport in Lipoproteins – An Integrated Approach to Mechanisms and Disorders. *New Eng. J. Med.*, 276, 34, 94, 148, 215 (1967).

33. Stamler, J., Prevention of Atherosclerotic Coronary Heart Disease, in Jones, M., Ed., *Modern Trends in Cardiology* 2, Butterworth, London, (1969).

34. Moriyama, I. M., J. Stamler, D. E. Krueger, *The Major Cardiovascular Diseases* – An

Epidemiologic Analysis. *Am. Pub. H. Assoc.*, New York, N.Y., in press.

35. Lew E. A., Blood Pressure and Mortality – Life Insurance Experience. In: Stamler, J., R. Stamler and T. N. Pullman eds. *The Epidemiology of Hypertension*, Grune and Stratton, New York, N.Y., 293 (1967).
36. Kahn, H. A., The Dorn Study of Smoking and Mortality Among u.s. Veterans: Report on 8½ Years of Observation. In Haenszel, W., ed., *Epidemiological Approaches to the Study of Cancer and Other Diseases*, National Cancer Institute, usphs., Bethesda, Md., Monograph No. 19, 1-125 (1966).
37. Stamler, J., et al., *Mass Field Trials on the Prevention of Coronary Heart Disease: Perspectives and Tasks* – Report of an International Working Meeting, Privately Printed, Chicago, Illinois, (1969).
38. Rinzler, S. H., Primary Prevention of Coronary Heart Disease by Diet. *Bull. N.Y. Acad. Med.*, 44, 936 (1968).
39. Christakis, G., S. H. Rinzler, M. Archer and A. Kraus, The Effect of the Anti-Coronary Club Program on Coronary Heart Disease Risk-Factor Status. *J.A.M.A.*, 198, 596 (1966).
40. Turpeinen, O., M. Miettinen, M. J. Karvonen, P. Roine, M. Pekkarinen, E. J. Lehtosuo and P. Alivirta, Dietary Prevention of Coronary Heart Disease. Long-Term Experiment. I. Observations on Male Subjects. *Amer. J. Clin. Nutr.*, 21, 255 (1968).
41. Turpeinen, O., *A Controlled Study on the Effects of Diet Modification on Blood Lipids and Primary Coronary Events.* Paper presented at the Minnesota Symposium on Prevention in Cardiology, May 2-3, 1968, Minn. Med., in press.
42. Dayton, S., M. L. Pearce, H., Goldman, A. Harnish, D. Plotkin, M. Shickman, M. Winfield, A. Zager and W. Dixon, Controlled Trial of a Diet High in Unsaturated Fat for Prevention of Atherosclerotic Complications. *Lancet*, 2, 1060 (1968).
43. Frantz, I. D., Personal Communication.
44. Oliver, M. F. and J. A. Heady, *Preventive Trials in Ischaemic Heart Disease – Primary Prevention. I. Reduction of Hyperlipidemia by Drugs.* Paper presented at the British Atherosclerosis Discussion Group, Dec. 8-9, 1967, London.
45. Rose, G. and D. Reid, Personal Communication.
46. Stamler, J., D. M. Berkson, H. A. Lindberg, I. T. Whipple, W. Miller, L. Mojonnier, Y. F. Hall, R. Soyugenc, M. J. Levinson and A. Andelman, *Long-Term Epidemiologic Studies on the Possible Role of Physical Activity and Physical Fitness in the Prevention of Premature Clinical Coronary Heart Disease.* Presented at the International Symposium on Physical Activity and Aging, Oct., 24-26, 1966, Tel Aviv, Israel, in press.
47. Taylor, H. Personal Communication.
48. Veterans Administration Co-operative Study Group on Anti-Hypertensive Agents. Effects of Treatment on Morbidity in Hypertension. *J.A.M.A.*, 202, 1028 (1967).
49. Keys, A., Official Collective Recommendation on Diet in the Scandinavian Countries. *Nutrition Revs.*, 26, 259 (1968).

PANEL DISCUSSION ON EPIDEMIOLOGY AND PRIMARY PREVENTION

MODERATOR: L. WERKÖ

Werkö: What is primary prevention? What do we mean by risk factors? Are risk factors signs of the disease or are they possibly only related to the disease?

Kannel: Primary prevention denotes an effort to avoid symptomatic disease by intervention while the person is still in good health.

Werkö: I wonder if Dr. Rose could give us the British definition.

Rose: I would prefer an operational or perhaps administrative definition of the term. In practice this would be more useful. Therefore, I would say that primary prevention is prevention before a person is under medical care.

Groen: Primary prevention are those steps taken to prevent symptoms and signs of disease in an individual or group. It secondly prevents people from needing medical care.

Werkö: Do you really mean the last statement? Most of the preventive methods require him to see a doctor. It is really a question of what we are trying to prevent: atherosclerosis, vascular disease, or ischaemic heart disease.

Stamler: If illness resulted from just atherosclerosis in general, i.e. any atherosclerosis (slight, moderate, or marked), then 95 per cent or more of the people in this room would be ill. For all of us have a good deal of atherosclerosis, as autopsy studies of young people have shown, particularly autopsy studies in economically developed societies. Fortunately, there is a good deal of biological reserve in the key arterial beds, and clinical illness is almost always due to *severe advanced* athero-sclerosis and its complications (thrombosis, embolism, etc.). Therefore, our goal – the objective of primary prevention – is to delay and prevent development of severe atherosclerosis and its complications, or to retard and prevent further progression of the pathologic process in people who already have it but who are asymptomatic – and even to achieve reversal, at least partial reversal, of the process.

Oliver: It is difficult to answer the question what is primary prevention. There are very many people who have extensive atherosclerosis in their sixties or seventies, who have never had ischaemic heart disease. Equally there are quite a number of young people who die from abrupt and sudden death, presumably arrhythmic death, who have minimal atherosclerosis. Strictly, primary prevention means prevention of atherosclerosis but it might also be extended to include prevention of arrhythmic death.

Werkö: Let us now continue by defining risk factor.

Kannel: A risk factor is a factor that one interprets as contributing to the development of the disease in its clinical state or to the underlying process. Whether this is directly causal or not is always going to be a matter of some dispute. It is a contributing factor which is associated with a high probability of developing clinical disease.

Werkö: That is more or less a statistical relationship. We can divide the risk factors that have been discussed into laboratory values and mode of life on one side and definite disease on the other side. Hyper-tension and diabetes are diseases by definition while high uric acid and blood cholesterol levels are not diseases.

Kannel: I do not know where normal blood pressure leaves off and hypertension begins. This is an entirely arbitrary designation as it is currently used. We need different concepts of 'normality' in biochem-ical or physiologic phenomena. Blood pressure is a physiological variable. At what point does it become hypertension? It is like fever. It is a finding that may indicate a whole host of underlying phenomena. Risk of its cardiovascular consequences is proportional to its level with no 'critical' value discernible.

Groen: We can divide risk factors into those factors within the individual like high serum cholesterol, and environmental risk factors like being a member of certain professions or leading a certain way of life. It is very interesting that in the epidemiology of coronary heart disease we have been much more succesful in defining the risk factors within the individual like hypertension and hypercholesterolemia than the environmental factors that lead to these conditions.

Rose: A risk factor is a characteristic that identifies a person with an increased risk of disease. It enables us to make statements about associations that do not commit us in any way to saying whether they are causal or coincidental.

Werkö: We must recognize that risk factors are something that identifies the individual but does not permit you to say whether or not he has disease at a particular time.

We have heard about the following risk factors today: high blood lipids, smoking, overweight, hypertension and inactivity. Elevated uric acid and diabetes or hyperglycaemia could perhaps be added to this list. As suggested by Dr. Stamler, we should narrow this list down as much as possible. One additional factor which has not been discussed but which is mentioned occassionally, is psychological stress. Is it really a risk factor? Can we measure it?

Stamler: In the Western Electric Study, where certain efforts were made to assess psychological factors and their role through use of the Minnesota Multiphasic Personality Inventory and other tests, generally negative results were obtained. However, other types of assessment were made in that study, with positive results, supporting the broad hypothesis that incongruities in social status are associated with increased risk of premature CHD. For example, men married to women higher up on the social ladder were at greater risk of developing coronary disease, compared to men marrying women on the same or lower rangs of the social ladder. Another interesting effort in this area is the work of the Western Collaborative Study in the United States, where the so-called Type A and Type B personality-behavior patterns and their relationship to risk of premature coronary disease are being studied prospectively. The 'high-drive', time-stressed, driven-by-deadlines, overextended person is the epitome of Type A. Type A personality-behavior pattern is obviously to a considerable degree a product of modern life in competitive industrial society. Data to date from the study indicate that – independent of serum cholesterol, blood pressure, smoking status, relative weight and other usual risk factors – the Type A personality-behavior pattern is associated with a greater risk of coronary disease. Data from the study of North Dakota rural residents also indicate that certain psycho-social stresses may be coronary risk factors. Unfortunately, none of these intriguing findings has been subjected to verification in replicate studies. Obviously, that must be done for these presumed risk factors, just as it has been done for others. This is a basic rule of science. Until that has been done, the positive findings must be viewed as tentative.

Oliver: As I understand it, we are talking about the primary prevention of clinical disease. We are also talking about the association with this disease of various factors which may or may not be causally related. There is one factor which triggers the disease, and that is thrombosis. We need to be able to measure a thrombogenic tendency. I suggest that those interested in the disease should look much more closely to see whether or not we cannot derive simple indices indicating when a patient or high risk individual is likely to develop a thrombosis.

Werkö: Age and sex are factors about which we cannot or will not do anything about. Family history is also something about which you can do nothing. These factors certainly help us to define the individual, however. Let us now return to the psychological stress factor.

Groen: We have tried to measure not only serum cholesterol, smoking habits, hypertension etc., but have also tried to quantitate some of these so-called psycho-social factors in a group in which we did some prevalence studies in Israel. We compared the frequency of the disease among the Jewish port workers of Haifa, among a group of Arab villagers and among Bedouins, the Arab nomads of the Negev desert.

In unskilled and skilled labourers the prevalence of both myocardial infarction and angina pectoris (together total coronary heart disease) was very low (0.4%). In white collar workers and in the free professions the figures for myocardial infarction and total coronary heart disease were 4.1 and 11 per cent respectively, far above the expected values (table 1). There were differences in blood cholesterol levels and in activity between the groups (table 2a and b). Our questionnaire contained a number of items which indicated that those with high job responsibility had a higher prevalence of myocardial infarction and total coronary heart disease than those workers with low job responsibility. The difficulty of assigning risk factors comes in here. Is it the responsibility or is it the lack of exercise which is the causative factor of the higher prevalence of the white collar workers?

As the level of education increases from the elementary school level to university level, we also see an increase in the prevalence of coronary heart disease (table 3).

We further asked the workers if they had any serious work problems in the past. Among those who answered many, there was a 5.3 per cent prevalence myocardial infarction and 12.9 per cent of coronary heart disease. Those workers who only had a few or no work problems had prevalences of 1.4 and 4.9 per cent for myocardial infarction and total coronary heart disease respectively (table 4).

Only a 2.2 per cent prevalence occurred in workers who were liked by there co-workers but 4.1 per cent among those who answered that they were not liked (table 5).

Those who had had many work problems and who felt that they were unliked had a prevalence of 7.3 per cent of myocardial infarction and of 24.4 per cent of coronary heart disease. Those who had had no or few work problems and who were liked by their fellow workers had only a 0.8 per cent prevalence of myocardial infarction and 3.7 per cent prevalence of total coronary heart disease. The last figures are almost similar to those found in the Bedouins who have so little infarctions (table 6).

We have tried to show that by the use of psycho-sociological techniques, certain of these psycho-social risk factors can indeed be measured. By further developing and perfecting our techniques we may hope that in the future we can add to our knowledge of these and other risk factors. We have since begun to apply similar techniques to our incidence studies.

Kannel: Psychological and social data are very difficult to interpret in general and they are even more difficult to interpret when they are prevalence data. Obviously, if you have had a myocardial infarction, you may begin to feel quite insecure simply as a result of your illness. We also tend to be influenced by what we are doing lately in obtaining

Table 1. Myocardial infarction and coronary heart disease by type of occupation (Haifa male port workers).

Type of occupation	Total	Myocardial infarction			Coronary heart disease		
		Abs. no.	(Exp. no.)	%	Abs. no.	(Exp. no.)	%
Unskilled worker	114	1	(2.8)	0.9	4	(7.6)	3.5
Skilled worker	230	1	(5.5)	0.4	7	(15.1)	3.0
Custom, police, foreman	113	2	(2.8)	1.8	6	(7.6)	5.4
White collar worker store keepers, free profession	285	14	(6.9)	4.1	31	(18.6)	11.0
Does not work	2				1	(0.1)	
All males	744	18		2.4	49		6.6

Table 1a. Myocardial infarction and coronary heart disease by serum cholesterol level in three ethnic groups (males only).

Serum cholesterol (mg %)	Bedouin			Arab villagers			Jewish port workers		
	Total	MI (%)	CHD (%*)	Total	MI (%)	CHD (%)	Total	MI (%)	CHD (%)
-150	270	0.4		91	1.2	2.2	56	—	—
150-199	167	—		108	0.9	6.5	339	2.1	6.0
200-269	36	—		33	—	6.4	311	3.0	8.1
270+	—	—		1	—	—	35	5.7	11.3
No blood obtained	37	—		21	—	—	3	—	—
Total	510	0.2	*?	254	1.1	4.7	744	2.4	6.6

* No figures available because the data about angina pectoris among the Bedouin are unreliable.

Table 1b. Physical activity among the Bedouin (0.2%) MI and the Jewish port workers (2.4% MI.) What is your usual means of transportation? (in %).

	Bedouin		Port workers	
	males	females	males	females
By cart or car	1	—	3	2
By bus or tender	17	6	80	82
Motor cycle or scooter	—	—	3	2
Bicycle	0.2	—	6	2
Horse, donkey or camel	38	20	—	—
Walking	44	74	8	12

Table 3. Myocardial infarction, coronary heart disease and educational level (Haifa port workers).

Educational level	Myocardial infarction			Coronary heart disease			Total
	Abs. no.	Exp. no.	%	Abs. no.	Exp. no.	%	
Illiterate	—	(0.4)		—	(0.80)		12
Religious school	—	(0.4)		1	(1.2)	5.6	18
Elementary	3	(5.9)	1.2	8	(16.3)	3.2	247
Secondary/Vocational	10	(9.4)	2.5	31	(26.0)	7.8	396
University	5	(1.9)	7.0	9	(4.7)	12.7	71
All Haifa males	18			49			744

Table 4. Myocardial infarction and coronary heart disease and work problems in the past (Haifa port workers).

	Total	Myocardial infarction			Coronary heart disease		
		Abs. no.	Exp.* no.	%	Abs. no.	Exp.* no.	%
Very many or many	171	10	4.1	5.3	22	11.3	12.9
Some or none	573	8	13.9	1.4	27	37.7	4.9
All	744	18		2.4	49		6.6

* Exp. No. = Number of cases to expected if the frequency would have been independent of having had troubles during work.

Table 5. Myocardial infarction and coronary heart disease and attitude of coworkers (Haifa male port workers).

Liked by coworkers	Total	Myocardial infarction			Coronary heart disease		
		Abs. no.	(Exp. no.)	%	Abs. no.	(Exp. no.)	%
Very much and fairly	666	15	(16.3)	2.2	37	(43.8)	5.5
Indifferent or not liked	74	3	(1.7)	4.1	12	(5.2)	16.2
No coworkers	4						
All males	744	18		2.4	49		6.6

Table 6. Myocardial infarction and coronary heart disease among Jewish port workers by age. Work problems and attitude of coworkers (males only).

Age group	Work problems + unliked			Work problems + liked			No work problems + unliked			No work problems + liked		
	MI (%)	CHD (%)	Total	MI (%)	CHD (%)	Total	MI (%)	CHD (%)	Total	MI (%)	CHD (%)	Total
Under 49	—	2 (9.1)	22	3 (1.7)	7 (4.0)	176	—	1 (4.3)	23	3 (1.1)	6 (2.3)	262
50-69	3 (15.8)	8 (42.1)	19	9 (9.4)	15 (15.6)	96	—	1 (10)	10	—	9 (6.7)	136
All males	3 (7.3)	10 (24.4)	41	12 (4.4)	22 (8.1)	272	—	2 (6.1)	33	3 (0.8)	15 (3.7)	398

histories intended to reflect past activities. We have looked at this problem in a semi-objective way and we are still analyzing this puzzling area. We have looked into the effect of the loss of a spouse. This revealed *no* differences in the rate of coronary disease compared to steadfastly married people. Also, disease rates were no different in school drop-outs, and persons who failed to complete courses of study. We saw *no* relationship of disease incidence to family size, which often creates social stress. This is a very difficult area and it deserves and needs further study. We need better methods for assessing the phenomena and we need better definitions of them before we can make sizeable strides in delineating the effect of this particular parameter.

Morrison: In relation to the Type A, Type B story, isn't it felt to be interesting that this has been associated with the raised blood pressure? The finding in that study was that raised blood pressure only turned out to be a risk factor in the type A people and that there is in this case a relationship between the psycho-social factor and the biological messurements. A few speakers have mentioned individuals, but we are really always considering group relationships. There is no direct applicability to an individual. It is simply that if you take a group of people with higher blood pressure, then the group rate is higher than for people with a lower blood pressure. What one is always trying to do is to narrow this down until we can get it to almost an individual basis.

Werkö: That is the same point that we made when we discussed exercise electrocardiograms. They are predictive of coronary disease in groups but not necessarily in individuals.

Kannel: I do not think that this distinction between individuals and groups is a very useful concept. Every piece of information that we have in medicine is properly based on information derived from groups. It is not possible to do any kind of analysis of a single case of anything. When you say to a diabetic patient that he must take care of his feet or else he will develop gangrene, this is not based on the experience of a single case. You are saying that if the patient behaves like a hundred diabetics, he may have trouble with gangrenous toes. You do not base your management on one case. This particular patient may never have trouble with his circulation, but you must assume that the will behave as most diabetics do and therefore you treat him on that basis.

Rose: I have not had much personal experience with working on psycho-social factors because there are so few tools to measure them that have been adequately validated. My only contribution is to suggest that we have not really given sufficient thought to the use that we might make of findings. It is *not* very helpful if one merely finds that a particular personality type is coronary prone, except that those of us who are Type B can feel a little happier. It is desirable that we should have more exploration of the relation between psychological and social characteristics and those habits and patterns of practical physical behaviour which we believe to be related to the causation of the disease.

Werkö: As of today, the most important risk factors related to the development of cardiovascular disease are smoking, raised blood pressure, raised blood lipids, and physical inactivity.

Stamler: I would add hyperglycaemia. It too is probably an important independent risk factor. For a couple of decades, at least, it has been evident that clinical diabetes is associated with increased risk of premature severe atherosclerotic disease. This is what kills most diabetics nowadays, at least in the economically developed countries. Based on the findings to date of the Framingham, Peoples Gas Company, and Tecumseh studies, it is now possible to go a step further, beyond the old dimension of clinical diabetes. It is likely that asymptomatic hyperglycaemia – subclinical or chemical diabetes – is probably also a risk factor. Based on measurement of random blood glucose, the Framingham study has obtained data to this effect on incidence of atherosclerotic coronary, cerebral and peripheral vascular disease. The study of the Tecumseh, Michigan population measured blood glucose one hour after a 100 gram oral load in their first round of examinations. Analysis of the prevalence data indicated an association between glucose level and atherosclerotic disease in both men and women, independent of – and additive to – serum cholesterol and blood pressure. In our group's study of middle-aged men employed by the Peoples Gas Company in Chicago – a study begun in 1958 – plasma glucose one hour after a 50 gram oral load was measured for the first time only in 1965. Therefore, only limited data are available to date – on 940 of the original cohort of 1,329 men free of clinical coronary disease at entry in 1958. The findings indicate a more than twofold greater mortality rate from coronary disease for men with plasma glucose levels ≥ 205 mg/dl, compared with men exhibiting levels < 205. However, the latter group had lower mean levels of serum cholesterol, blood pressure and relative weight, and lower prevalence rates of hypercholesterolemia, hypertension and obesity. Thus, the association between glycemia and mortality may be significantly confounded. In fact, data to date from the prospective studies are not entirely consistent on the role of glycemia as a risk factor, in the absence of hypertension. Data that will become available in the next few years should resolve this matter. For the present, it seems reasonable to regard chemical diabetes (hyperglycemia) as a probable risk factor.

A similar situation exists with respect to hyperuricemia. In our Peoples Gas Company study, for example, men with serum uric acid levels ≥ 7.0 mg/dl had coronary mortality rates more than double those of men with values < 7.0 – but again, the latter group had lower mean blood pressures and relative weights, and lower prevalence rates of hypertension and obesity. Moreover, uric acid and serum fasting triglyceride levels have been shown to correlate significantly. Therefore, further work is necessary to determine whether uric acid contributes *independently* to risk of coronary disease. At present, it appears useful to use measurement of uric acid in assessment of risk.

Family history is also relevant in risk assessment, particularly when two or more members of the family have developed the disease prematurely, e.g. before age 60. One practical conclusion from this is that all members of the immediate family should be assessed for risk factor status when one is stigmatized – either by premature coronary disease or by a major risk factor. This is a valid and relevent approach, since the mechanisms of the familial tendency are no mystery. Data currently available indicate that about 80 per cent of positive family history of premature coronary disease can be accounted for by familial tendencies to hyperlipidemia, hypertension, hyperglycemia, obesity and cigarette smoking. Since these are all more or less amenable to treatment, no matter what the genetic component of the familial tendency, the earlier they are detected, the better, in all likelihood.

Finally, the impact of a risk factor is worth emphasizing. The American Heart Association in its definition has called a risk factor any habit, trait, characteristic or abnormality associated with at least a doubling of risk, compared to risk of an otherwise similar individual who lacks the stipulated trait. This is a sizeable difference. Moreover, differences of this order exist even with simple dichotomization of the data – e.g. comparing persons based on a serum cholesterol cutting point of 250 mg%, a diastolic blood pressure of 90 mm Hg. Actually, for all these continuous variables, dichotomous cuts are highly artificial, since risk is a continuous function of level, and a curvilinear (rather than a linear) function at that. Thus, when a population is divided into quartiles or quintiles, risk ratios for each of the factors are in the order of three or four to one (rather than two to one) for the highest versus the lowest group.

Werkö: You are attempting to diminish the number of risk factors under consideration in your large trials. Which three would you consider to the most important?

Stamler: The three factors which are best documented are hypertension, cigarette smoking, and hypercholesterolemia. All are frequently present in young and middle-aged adults, at least in the usa. Of course, in evaluating the individual patient, a physician appreciates that the most important trait is the one present, and when two or all three are coexistent, risk rises markedly, as I showed in my paper. I agree with Dr. Kannel completely and disagree with Dr. Morrison. There *is* '...direct applicability to the individual'. What the prospective epidemiologic studies on risk factors for CHD have shown is completely in keeping conceptually and methodologically with basic principles and approaches of clinical medicine. Consider the process of differential diagnosis carried out by the physician evaluating a patient. The reasoning process involves the application of probability information painstakingly amassed in the course of experience with legions of patients who came before. Thus, when three or four findings are present, the doctor infers from his storehouse of knowledge that – on a probability basis – the most likely diagnosis is disease *a*. He also considers diseases *b*, *c*, and *d*, as less likely probabilities, given the available facts and circumstances.

The risk factors can and must be utilized in essentially the same way by physicians dealing with individual patients. Given a person with a certain set of characteristics, he is – for example – ten times as likely to develop frank clinical coronary disease in the next five or ten years as a person without such characteristics. He may be one of the lucky ones who will escape this probability, this actuarial risk. But no physician can assure his patient that he will escape. I wish we could predictively distinguish those with the factors who will not and those who will become ill. I know no way of doing this. Therefore the need is to treat and remove risk factors – for preventive purposes.

Werkö: You still have the old American idea that inactivity is not one of the main risk factors. Do you have any comments on this point, Dr. de Haas?

De Haas: I would like to put some more general questions to our Scottish and American friends. If hypercholesterolemia, hyper-lipidemia, excessive smoking, hypertension, inactivity and perhaps mental stress are really risk factors, we should try to reconstruct their 'levels' over a certain period of time, since we definitely know that age-specific mortality rates in coronary disease are much higher than a few decades ago, at least in men. We should not ignore the trend in coronary heart disease. In America and in Anglo-Saxon countries one has seen an increase in the last three to five decades and in most European countries for at least in the last two decades. I would there-fore like to ask if it is absolutely certain that hypertension and hyper-cholesterolemia are more prevalent now than twenty or thirty years ago? There is no doubt that cigarette smoking has increased tremen-dously in that time. The same holds true for physical inactivity.

Oliver: Dr. de Haas has asked a very important question which I would suggest to all members of the panel is unanswerable. We do *not* know anything, in fact, about cholesterol levels 25 to 40 years ago. The same really applies to blood pressure levels. In those days, the pro-fession did not address itself to population studies. We have *no* infor-mation upon which to answer your question. This is not so, however for coronary heart disease. I would remind the audience, that if they care to look up the publication by Heberden exactly two-hundred years ago, they will find an account of one hundred cases of angina pectoris. If you study these case histories, you will find 50-60 have symptoms of myocardial infarction. This disease was certainly common two-hundred years ago.

Werkö: Some of these were in young males. Many of his patients were not very old. Dr. Stamler has emphasized earlier that the time has now come to implement the public health activity to interfere with the risk factors. Do you think that this is true?

Rose: The evidence that we could benefit the incidence of coronary disease by changing risk factors is probably a good deal stronger than was the evidence 50 years ago that we could benefit tuberculosis by the then available means of treatment. The campaigns for the mass detection of tuberculosis and the treatment of patients discovered were nevertheless considered justified.

It is very difficult to know why we view this problem of coronary disease control differently from the way that tuberculosis prevention was viewed. Partly, it is that science has advanced and quite rightly we like our medical advice to be founded on better evidence. Partly, perhaps there are other reasons connected with our particular emotional response as doctors to prevention, which we still do not regard in some way as proper concern for doctors – as opposed to the treatment of cases, which we feel is why we are here. We cannot wait until we are certain that coronary disease can be prevented by this or that measure, because we shall never be certain. The question is what level of evidence, what level of probability is required that will be sufficient for particular kinds of action. Here, we have to balance the hopes of what can be gained against the risks of what may be lost. The level of probability required is different when we are concerned with individual patients, the man who has had a myocardial infarction, or individuals known to be at special risk who come to us for advice, from the situation where we are considering the advice to be given to the mass of the public where a higher level of evidence is required. We know enough to advise the public at large to give up cigarettes and to avoid overweight. It may be argued whether we know enough to advise them to be physically more active or to change the fat constitution of their diet. With regard to individual high-risk subjects, we know enough to include those last two factors in our advice.

Kannel: I concur with almost everything that Dr. Rose said and in the way it was said. I think that if we as physicians demand absolute proof of efficacy before we treated a patient, we would in most cases be reduced to therapeutic nihilism. You have to act on the basis of the best evidence available and you must weigh the possible hazards against the possible benefits. I do find a little troublesome, the sanctimonious attitude many have towards coronary prevention. What is being advocated seems to me something we can justify whether or not it prevents a single case of coronary disease. Nobody can argue that it is healthy to inhale smoke so why be apologetic about advocating cessation of the cigarette habit? Nobody can argue logically that it is a bad idea to maintain a slender, pleasing figure and physical fitness, or to eat a less rich diet, or to have diabetes or hypertension treated. It seems to me that we are being overly cautious.

Oliver: Our advice to nations and the public should be regarded in a different light from that which we ought to give as physicians and cardiologists to the individual. It is perfectly acceptable for us to advise our patients to stop smoking, to alter their diet so that they do not get obese, and to be more physically active. This we appear to be agree upon. But are we agreed that an individual, whether he has or has not yet got an infarct, should lower his cholesterol? Over a five year period, only 1 in 5 men in his forties with high cholesterol levels will get the disease. We therefore have to consider what we are asking this man with his high cholesterol to do in the next five years. We are suggesting that he should alter his way of living to prevent a disease which he may never get. What are the repercussions of this? How is this man going to react?

Again, Stamler talked about the man with high blood pressure. He told us that about 80 percent were unaware that they had high blood pressure. Maybe that is a good thing.

De Haas: To change the way of life and daily habits of older people will be difficult. As Dr. Oliver has said, it will be even more difficult if you cannot tell them definitely that they will not get the disease. If we really want to change one's way of life, we should begin in early life. We should try to influence mothers and housewives who have a greater deal of influence on daily diet and the education of children than husbands or fathers have. We have a good example in terms of child health. The fact that infant mortality decreased rapidly is not only due to medical and to preventive measures, but also because mothers have been educated and know how to handle their children. If these same mothers in the future know how to handle the food and nutrition in their households and how to educate their children, to advise them against smoking, to urge them to get physical exercise, we will have better results than if we only try to influence adult people.

Werkö: I wonder if we can really influence the way that young people live. We are constantly being told by students that we are too old, that we do not understand what is going on with the young people. It is much easier to get public health measures adhered to by people who are 65, 70, or 75 because they are closer to death and they are becoming worried. The young people do not care about what you are trying to do.

Groen: Irrespective from where we started out, from the prevention of organic diseases like carcinoma of the lung, or coronary heart disease, or obesity we came to the conclusion that we needed for that prevention to bring about important changes in their way of life which we could not obtain by simply telling people to change. Look at ourselves. We have unanimously come to the conclusion that one must eat less, that one must eat less satured fat, and that one must take more exercise. And yet we have been for the past two days sitting and talking, and we have been excellently entertained with food which was definitely high in satured fatty acids. Why did not we change our way of life? Because these habits are engraved not only in our 'intellectual', 'logic' behaviour patterns but they are 'traditions' engraved in our emotional ways of life. The development of modern scientific medicine leads us to the necessity of studying how one can change the emotional roots of behavior in men.

One can do that firstly by the study of behavior in animals. But there is also room and even need, for experiments in this respect in humans. In a preventive program for the prevention of ischaemic heart disease one has to investigate this difficult problem of psycho-biological relationships of human behavior, particularly addiction, food and exercise habits. We must also investigate ways of changing these habits.

Some work has been done in this area. One of our most helpful results was the observation that if you want a man to stop smoking, you must have the co-operation of his wife. A similar fact has also been observed by the Alcoholics Anonymous. They found that wives, if properly instructed and supported can be much more efficient than doctors or clergymen in changing the habits of their husbands. Therefore, it appears as if we shall have to introduce the whole family unit into your approach when you want to change an individual's way of life.

Werkö: The question raised by Dr. Oliver is a good one. There is one thing about the Framingham data that disturbs me. Even in the group without any risk factors at all there were many cases of sudden death or new events of cardiovascular disease. How do you explain that Dr. Kannel?

Kannel: The information on the natural history of coronary disease is certainly far from complete. While we can predict the probability of events over a thirty-fold range of risk we cannot be 100 percent accurate. In fact, using all of the factors currently identified, we can only explain about 25 percent of the variance in the incidence of coronary disease. So there may still be other hidden factors.

There is one major problem that handicaps us here. We are in a position equivalent to trying to study typhoid fever in a population where everybody has typhoid fever and everybody is drinking dirty water. This is very difficult to do. Everybody in our populations have high lipid values. What we call 'low' is not necessarily so. This is the nature of the problem. We can none the less, estimate probability over a very wide range of risk based on the identified risk factors.

Vergroesen: I agree with Dr. Oliver when he warns against advocating to the general public to use agents reducing blood lipids especially if we want to use pharmalogical means to do so. The side effects of the drugs up to now known to reduce blood lipids are quite well known. We should of course evaluate the favourable against the unfavourable effects of such therapy.

I should like to raise the following points. Several years ago Dr. Thomassen et al. published the results of two long-term experiments with rabbits fed a non-atherogenic diet. The effects of a low-fat rice diet were compared to those diets with 40 calorie – percent of fat, the satured coconut oil or the poly-unsaturated soybean oil. Low blood lipid levels and a low incidence of atherosclerotic lesions were observed in the high fat soybean oil diet. Extremely high blood lipid levels and atherosclerotic lesions were observed in the coconut oil diet. The low fat diet occupied an intermediate position and induced more atheros-clerotic lesions and higher blood lipid concentrations than the soybean oil diet. To test the human response to comparable diets, we recently investigated the effects of three different dietary fats given at three caloric levels as liquid formula diets as developed by Dr. Ahrens on volunteer Trappist monks living in three monasteries. The participants were matched for age and cholesterol level within each monastery. The effect of the diets was followed for six weeks. The three dietary fats which were given were the highly saturated glyceryl tri-laurate, mixed with 10 percent safflower seed oil to provide the essential fatty acids, the mono-unsaturated olive oil, and the highly di-unsaturated safflower seed oil. The fat content of the diets were 20, 35, or 50 percent of the calories. The amount of food consumed during this six week period was also recorded. Although the subjects who consumed the 20 calorie-percent fat diet had to eat twice the amount of food compared to those eating the 50 calorie-percent fat diet, the mean caloric intake was quite comparable between all of the groups. Weight reduction occurred only during the first week of the study and was probably due to the low salt content of the diet. For the rest of the study, the diet was isocaloric.

It appeared that the 20 calorie-percent fat diet induced the smallest changes in the blood lipid level. To obtain the lowest blood lipid levels, we had to give 35 or 50 calorie- percent of the highly di-unsaturated safflower seed oil.

I would therefore recommend a diet with a high (at least 35 cal % fat) concentration of di-unsaturated fat to achieve the maximum effect of dietary modification with respect to blood lipid lowering effect and to prevent the development and progression of atherosclerosis. This should be started early in life before the lesions have progressed to a recognizable disease.

Stamler: I cannot concur in detail. It is not that I believe Dr. Vergroesen to be wrong. What concerns me here – and he and I have talked about this – is what concerned Dr. Keys and me when we similarly disagreed with Dr. Kinsell in the discussions of the design of the National Diet-Heart Study. That disagreement ended in the Diet-Heart Study with a compromise – a design for a three group project, i.e. a control and two experimental groups, one of Dr. Vergroesen's type and one (if you will permit) of our type. This latter was not a group on a low fat diet, but on a moderate fat diet with about 30 percent of total calories from fat, with a moderate – but not a large – amount of polyunsaturates.

There were three important reasons behind this disagreement. First, it was argued – Dr. Keys and I disagreed – that Americans would not accept a diet of reduced fat content, i.e. with 30 percent of total calories from fat, rather than their usual 40 percent. Second, it was argued – again Dr. Keys and I disagreed – that high intake of polyunsaturated fat was vital to get good reductions of serum cholesterol. We were skeptical about both these hypotheses, and felt that at least equal success in both adherence and cholesterol-lowering could be achieved with a diet moderate in total fat and polyunsaturated fat – provided it is low in saturates and dietary cholesterol. Our third concern stemmed from our knowledge as epidemiologists. Looking out around the world, we knew of no populations that have subsisted for generations on a diet high in polyunsaturated fats, e.g. with 15 or 20 percent of total calories from this source. The actual maximum is about 9 percent. Most populations are in the range 3 to 7 percent, including those with low coronary rates compared to ours (see the data of my formal paper). We were – and remain – wary and concerned about ultimate problems of safety. We prefer – deem it discrete and wise – to recommend diets based not only on animal experiments, metabolic ward studies and the trials to date (all relatively small and short term), but also based on widespread population experience with human nutrition over generations. With this approach, diets can only be recommended based on Mediterranean culture, Far-Eastern culture, etc., i.e. diets moderate in total fat, with moderate (not large) amounts of oil, with no more than 9 or 10 percent of calories from polyunsaturates. Before we push polyunsaturates up to 15 or 20 percent of total calories, we need to be sure that there are no dangers. The National Diet-Heart Study also confirmed our view that with good control of saturated fat and cholesterol intake, high polyunsaturated fat (as distinct from moderate polyunsaturated fat) intake is not at all important in lowering serum lipids. It also verified that moderate reduction of total fat intake is as acceptable to Americans as their present diet or a high polyunsaturated fat diet.

Werkö: I would like to have the WHO-view on when we will have enough evidence to act and what can we do?

Pisa: Public Health information and recommendations are different on the national and international level from what they are on group level or on the individual level. Such recommendations to change diets or to introduce drugs will certainly have a great impact on the society and on the organizations of the health services. Therefore, the case which is presented in support of such recommendations must be very, very strong. I do not feel that we have such a strong case at this time. We still must go further in our studies before we can make any final conclusions and recommendations.

Werkö: Do you favour mass screening at this time to detect new cases of cardiovascular disease?

Rose: Unless we can identify coronary subjects before they become diseased we can never control the problem. Whether this potential can be realized, we do not know at the present time. There is a widespread feeling among doctors that the discovery of unrecognized dangers has to have some justification in that we can reduce those dangers. At the present time, I would personally think that screening programs should not be recommended on an all-comers service basis but they should be gone ahead with very enthusiastically on a research basis combined with evaluation.

Groen: We could, or should do a great many things in our fight against coronary heart disease. But what should have priority? Which approach offers, at present, the most hopeful outlook in our fight and which will give us the necessary data to evaluate the results the quickest? As Dr. Rose has already said, if we screen the whole population for either risk factors or early signs of coronary heart disease, the following question will be: So what? What can we advise, what can we do for these individuals that we have detected? I feel therefore that priority over just early detection drives, should be given to another type of epidemiological study, like that which was indicated by Dr. Kannel and other speakers, namely, a preventive trial. We could localize certain populations, and I am thinking about the civil servants in a particular city. They are a homogeneous, sessile population. We can screen them, and after having followed them up for two years in a prospective study like the Framingham study, we could then try on them on a larger scale some of those measures which Dr. Stamler and the Coronary Club have tried on small groups. By comparing the results with another city, where the civil servants would not be exposed to such measures, we might then find out in, say five years whether such preventive measures are successful or not. We would attain two aims. Firstly, we would have accumulated data about the actual results, and secondly we would know how far we stand in the efficiency of our methods of prevention. I am, therefore, not against screening procedures, but I would give priority to such preventive, well controlled trials.

Kannel: I would be against population screening until we have the means for the physician to implement an effective preventive program. If one sets the screening level at identifying persons with a two-fold increased risk, it would result in sending a quarter of the entire population to the physician. He is going to be asked to implement a program of prevention that requires losing weight, changing diet, giving up the cigarette habit, all of which are very difficult to accomplish successfully. Prevention is most effectively and efficiently accomplished by getting the source of the problem. If one is convinced that diet is an important factor in coronary disease, then change the diet of the population. Do not attempt to motivate people to give up things they like for some future benefit. I do not know of any diseases that have been prevented in that way.

Stamler: Dr. Pisa has put his finger on one important reason for the slow and reluctant development – the implications of a vigorous preventive approach for the work of the health services. I feel this has not been discussed enough here. I learned from reading Professor C. E. A. Winslow of Yale University that we must always be alert to this problem. He noted in the 1920's that for all the common diseases of the 20th century, there will be major social obstacles to overcoming them. Level of scientific knowledge and technique will not be the sole or even the main problem. There will be a social problem. Specifically with respect to the current CHD epidemic in the developed countries, a social policy decision to do nothing now either in mass detection or mass preventive intervention, until mass field trials are completed, is a postponement for 10 years at least of control efforts. Frankly, I regard this as injudicious – not judicious – neglect, as a dereliction of duty on the part of the medical profession and public health in the face of the choices before us. The choices are to do nothing, justifiable only if one explicitly concludes that everything is as good as we can get it at this time, or – alternately – to do something on the high probability that almost certainly matters can be improved (e.g. better diets are available), the risks are negligible and the possibilities of prevention are real and substantial. Medicine has always acted on that basis. If the risks are low and the possibilities are real, it is better to act than to do nothing. If we can find 20 percent of men and women who are very high risk, get a sizeable proportion to give up smoking, to change their eating habits and thereby lower their elevated weight, lipids, glucose levels, blood pressure, etc., it is likely that we can reduce the epidemic substantially. This would be an achievement. Is not an effort in this direction a wiser commitment than leaving things as they are now?! Of course, the budgets of the health service would have to expand to do the job, although over the years the likely prophylactic achievement against premature CHD among productive people in the prime of life would more than make up the social cost. Therefore, I cannot accept the alternative of doing nothing now as the best choice, and I demand of everyone who says 'do nothing now' to be logical and explicitly state that he regards this as the best thing for our populations for the next 10 years or more, until mass field trials are completed.

Of course, the mass field trials should also proceed, as rapidly and efficiently as possible. It is entirely possible both to mount them and the public health control effort. As many of you know, several of us in the United States are doing all we can there to move both these endeavors forward.

Pisa: Mass screening campaigns create certain pressures. I agree with Dr. Kannel, that we have to be aware of what it means to detect 20 percent of the population. Having done so, what do we do next? Are the medical services prepared to deal with these patients? Are the people prepared to accept our recommendations? We are well aware of the poor results of health education up to now. We must go on here, but we must be aware of the impact of our decision.

Oliver: We in Britain learn in our schools to debate and we are not always impressed by rhetoric. It is easy for Dr. Stamler to produce a little applause from the audience, but I do not know if that necessarily means that the case is made. I certainly do not consider that we should now start mass screening programs. People who think this way should take into account the enormous impact that this is going to make on medical resources, already grossly depleted in most countries. We have not discussed this at all. One also must take into account the grave and possibly serious psychological effects that mass screening may induce on many healthy people.

Werkö: The majority of the panel favours preventive trials in order to know what recommendation to make.

CHAPTER VI

TREATMENT AND SECONDARY PREVENTION

PREVENTION OF EARLY DEATH DURING CARDIAC INFARCTION

M. F. OLIVER

INTRODUCTION

There are four particular problems concerning the prevention of early death during acute myocardial infarction which require individual consideration and will form the basis of this paper. These are:

1. The causes and timing of early deaths
2. The causes of delay in admission to hospital
3. The accurate identification of the most vulnerable patients
4. Pre-infarct symptoms and signs

For the purposes of this paper, early death will be defined as death occurring within 24 hours of the onset of symptoms suggestive of acute myocardial infarction.

The causes and timing of early deaths

The majority of observed deaths in the first six hours are due to serious ventricular arrhythmias, shock and complete pump failure. Deaths which occur after the first 24 hours are more frequently due to a further episode of cardiac ischaemia or infarction, ventricular rupture, cardiac failure or one of the complications of infarction such as pulmonary embolism.

Perhaps it is still not fully appreciated that coronary care units are really 'anti-arrhythmia units'. The majority of patients with acute myocardial infarction develop some form of arrhythmia and it is the early recognition and the prevention of progression of these arrhythmias that have led to reduction in mortality in the coronary care units (1, 2). During the last three years, more than 2,000 patients have been admitted to the Coronary Care Unit of the Royal Infirmary of Edinburgh and in the region of 1500 of these have had a proven myocardial infarct. This has provided us with a vast experience of the management of arrhythmias and of cardiogenic shock. The mortality in this unit is

17% in all patients under 70 years, while it is 11% in patients under 50 years and 23% in patients between 60-69 years. The mortality in the same hospital before the opening of the Coronary Care Unit was probably in the region of 24-25% but, of course, it is very difficult to assess this with accuracy since the establishment of a coronary care unit in any hospital leads to a very different experience both with regard to the type and numbers of coronary patients admitted to the hospital. The reduction in mortality of approximately one quarter is a figure which has now been reported from many of the high grade coronary care units (3).

It is probably about all that can be expected since the remainder of the early deaths are mostly due to cardiogenic shock. We are not satisfied that we have been able to make any appreciable impact on this mortality and consider that a number of those patients with cardiogenic shock who have survived have probably done so in spite and not because of our management of them! The extent of myocardial damage in these patients is very considerable. From a consecutive series of 86 post-mortems on patients who died of cardiogenic shock, we have found that 79 had a previous myocardial infarct even although there may not have been any history of even electrocardiographic evidence of this, and 70 of these 86 patients had in the region of two-thirds of their left ventricle infarcted. This may mean, of course, that the degree of damage in most patients with cardiogenic shock is so extensive that no therapy is possible. On the other hand, the picture may not be quite so depressing because there is the possibility that some of these very extensive infarcts are a result of slowly extending infarction during the last few hours of life. We do not know, for example, to what extent an occlusion of a fairly major artery can cause reduced flow and pressure in the immediate surrounding collateral vessels and lead to relative stasis and late thrombus formation. There is evidence that this mechanism operates in some patients and it makes the situation a little more cheerful therapeutically, since it might be possible to intervene before the thrombus has extended. Indeed, claims have been made for beneficial effects of thrombolytic treatment at this stage.

From the Edinburgh Community Study of Acute Coronary Disease (4), it has been possible to determine the time relationship of death during the first four weeks after infarction. This study was conducted for a year in the City of Edinburgh which consists of a population of 500,000. During this time, 1298 patients suspected of having acute myocardial infarction were notified by family doctors: 543 of these died and from these deaths it has been possible to derive the curve illustrated in fig. 1.

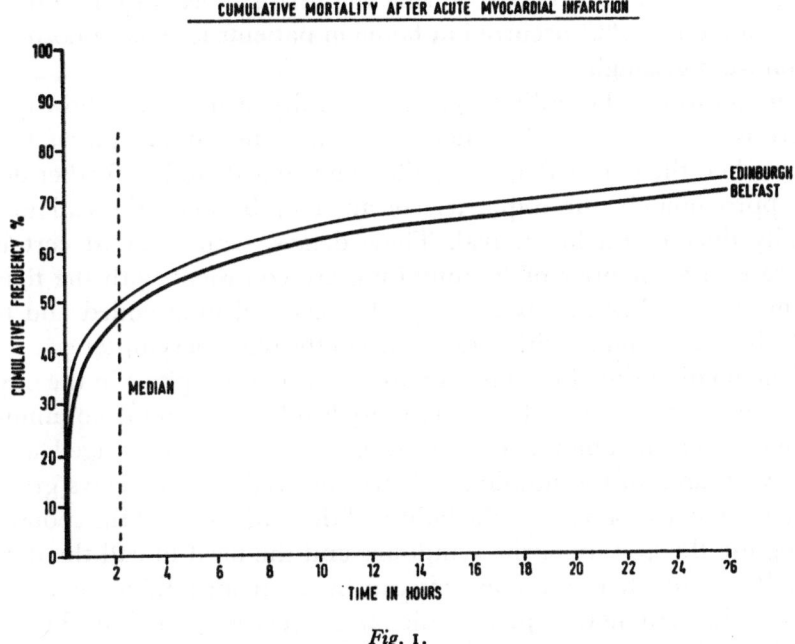

Fig. 1.

This has been contrasted with the experience reported from Belfast by McNeilly and Pemberton (5), who studied the time relationship between the onset of symptoms and death in 998 patients who died. The similarity between these two reports is close, and the most important finding is that the median time of death is approximately 2 hours. Further, 58% in Edinburgh of the deaths over the four week period had occurred within the first 24 hours.

These figures have been compared with those from other reports and it can be stated that about 25% of all patients with myocardial infarction die within the first hour of the onset of symptoms and that 30-40% die within the first 24 hours (6).

Delay in admission
The figures outlined in the preceding paragraph and in fig. 1. indicate that there is very little time of act. From the same Community Study, information has been gained concerning the circumstances surrounding these deaths. In 63%, death occurred when the patients were

unattended; 6% of the deaths occurred while patients were waiting for an ambulance, during transit to hospital or on arrival in the hospital; 24% of the deaths occurred during the first 4 weeks in hospital; and the remainder (7%) occurred at home in patients for whom hospitalisation was not sought.

In addition, the Edinburgh Community Study has shown that there is a delay of nearly 2 hours from the onset of symptoms to the time when the family doctor is called and that there is a further delay of approximately three quarters of an hour between the call to the family doctor and his arrival. These delays, which almost certainly operate in a majority of communities, are consistent with the figures mentioned earlier that 60% of deaths occurred unattended and that 50% had taken place within two hours of the onset of symptoms.

The median time for admission to the various hospitals in the city of patients notified under the Community Study was 4 hours 30 minutes. While a certain amount of improvement could be envisaged at the receiving area in the hospital, this will not reduce the delays greatly. The main cause of delay is the failure of the patient, or of the spouse, to recognise the gravity of the symptoms and the need to call the doctor (7). It is difficult to see how this can be overcome. Education of the public through newspapers, radio and television, so that they will quicker the symptoms of acute myocardial infarction would help, but there will be a heavy price to pay for this education in terms of the numbers of patients who do not have true ischaemic pain calling their doctors and referring themselves to hospital. However, the Belfast group (8) have shown that a certain amount can be achieved by publishing the value of mobile coronary services. This has undoubtedly made it possible to retrieve some patients who collapse at their work. Attempts at resuscitation of these patients are of no value, if there is no means of bringing expert treatment to the place where they have collapsed or of transporting them to a coronary care unit. These mobile coronary services cannot, however, be expected to make much impact on early death because the majority of sudden collapses occur when the patient is unattended by anybody trained to recognise the gravity of the event or trained to start resuscitation. They will be most effective when the patient collapses in a factory where there is already some form of first aid service and least effective when the collapse occurs at home. The widespread establishment of mobile coronary services cannot be encouraged because they will mostly operate after the median time of death (fig. 1), and the organisation and cost required is not inconsiderable.

The identification of those most vulnerable

It would be a great advance if it were possible to determine with accuracy, the immediate prognosis of every patient who has acute myocardial infarction. Ideally, we should aim at being able to do this when the patient is first seen by the family doctor. This would enable him to institute the appropriate therapy and to decide which patient is likely to benefit from transference to a Coronary Care Unit and which patient might be made worse by a long and hurried journey and be best treated initially at home.

There have been various attempts to derive prognostic indices. Existing clinical and biochemical indices are not satisfactory, and the best available is probably continuous electrocardiographic monitoring of the cardiac rhythm.

The clinical prognostic indices (9, 10, 11) can be criticised on several grounds. They do not take into account the relation of arrhythmias or conduction defects to the final outcome, or give them a very low rating. They do not take into account the duration of time between the onset of symptoms and the time when the patient is first seen, or admitted to hospital; the longer the delay, the better the prognosis since most of the arrhythmic deaths will have already occurred. They do not allow for change in the first hours: it is notoriously difficult to predict from clinical symptoms and signs the progress during the next few hours. It is essential also if any of these prognostic indices are to be used widely that some sort of continuing assessment score should be built into them, and this would be hard to do on a numerical system.

Various biochemical measurements have been used in an attempt to derive prognostic indices but because it usually takes an appreciable time before the results of these measurements are available, they have little or no value. This comment applies, for example, to estimations of noradrenaline and cortisol — both of which have been shown to be elevated after acute myocardial infarction (12, 13). The same criticism is true for estimations of aspartate-aminotransferase (GOT) and any of the lactic dehydrogenases, since they are usually raised 24-48 hours after acute infarction which is a long time past the point when an accurate prognostic index is most needed. Creatine kinase (14) is of more value, since its peak usually occurs between 12-16 hours. The degree to which it is raised above the normal values 6 hours after the onset of symptoms is greater than that for other enzymes and it has recently been suggested that the creatine kinase levels at 6 hours are of considerable prognostic importance (15), but again the estimation of this enzyme takes time.

The possibility that estimations of serum free fatty acids might be of value is under exploration in Edinburgh. A positive correlation has been shown between elevated serum free fatty acids and serious arrhythmias and death (16), but again the same criticism can be applied since it takes 2 hours on average for the results of routine estimations to be available.

Studies have been made of central venous oxygen saturation and PaO_2 in relation to prognosis after myocardial infarction (17). While the estimations of these indices of oxygen saturation are quick, they are only disturbed in failure and shock and the clinical features of these conditions are usually self-evident. They have not been found to be of prognostic value in patients without complications after myocardial infarction.

Continuous electrocardiographic monitoring of cardiac rhythm will usually reveal a transient and prodromal arrhythmia, but often this occurs only a few minutes before the onset of a serious and irreversible arrhythmia and such monitoring is seldom possible at the time when it is most required – namely in the first 2 to 3 hours.

In short, we are as yet unable to estimate the immediate prognosis in a patient suspected of having myocardial infarction.

Symptoms and signs before myocardial infarction
Remarkably little is known about the incidence of prodromal features occurring before the onset of acute myocardial infarction. Similarly, very little is known about the natural history and significance of recent-onset angina. Figures (18) concerning the percentage of patients with recent onset angina that proceed to sudden death, to classical acute myocardial infarction, to develop minor electrocardiographic changes with subsidence of pain or even to disappearance of all symptoms, are inevitably based on those patients who present to a doctor. It is almost certain that a large number of such patients never report to a doctor, probably because they do not recognise the gravity of their symptoms.

Further, additional information is required concerning the frequency and nature and significance of transient arrhythmias occurring before the onset of infarction. Monitoring of rhythm in ambulant individuals has suggested that patients who die suddenly have more transient arrhythmias than those who do not (19, 20). It is to be hoped that careful study of these patients may give additional information concerning the circumstances surrounding the onset of arrhythmias. Laboratory studies to elucidate the mechanism of onset of arrhythmias are urgently needed and are complementary to any community study.

While there is some evidence that sudden death is more common in cigarette smokers (21) we do not really yet know the type of patient who dies suddenly. It is not certain whether the chances of sudden death are aggregated more in categories of increased risk e.g. hypertension, hypercholesterolaemia or cigarette smokers, or whether the chance of sudden death is equally distributed among individuals with high and low risks of developing ischaemic heart disease. This information should soon be available from large community studies, such as that in progress in Tecumseh, Michigan.

CONCLUSION

The prevention of early death during myocardial infarction is a major therapeutic challenge. However successful primary prevention trials may be during the next ten to twenty years, many people will continue to get acute myocardial infarction and die from it within the first few hours of symptoms. We should be aiming not only at identifying those most at risk but also in developing new methods of treatment which could be given to such individuals to prevent the onset of serious arrhythmias if and when they develop acute myocardial hypoxia. To this end, more research should be carried out into the mechanism of onset of arrhythmias and more attention should be paid to all the circumstances surrounding the onset of acute ischaemia and infarction.

REFERENCES

1. Lawrie, D. M., T. W. Greenwood, M. D. Goddard, A. C., Harvey, K. W. Donald, D. G. Julian and M. F. Oliver, A coronary care unit in the routine management of acute myocardial infarction. *Lancet* 2, 109 (1967).
2. Lown, B., A. M. Fakhro, W. B. Hood and G. W. Thorn, The coronary care unit, new perspectives and directions. *J. Amer. Med. Ass.* 199, 188 (1967).
3. Julian, D. G. and M. F. Oliver, *Acute myocardial infarction*, E & S. Livingstone, Edinburgh (1968).
4. Armstrong, A. In: *Acute Myocardial Infarction*. Ed. by Julian, D. G. and M. F. Oliver. E & S. Livingstone, Edinburgh. (1968).
5. McNeilly, R. H. and J. Pemberton, Duration of the last attack in 998 fatal cases of coronary artery disease and its relation to possible cardiac resuscitation. *Brit. Med. J.* 3, 139 (1968).
6. Fulton, M., D. G. Julian and M. F. Oliver, Sudden death and acute myocardial infarction. *Circulation*. In press (1969).
7. Adgey, J., P. G. Nelson, M. E. Scott, J. S. Geddes, J. D. Allen, S. A. Zaidi and J. F. Pantridge, Management of ventricular fibrillation outside hospital. *Lancet* 1, 1169 (1969).
8. Oliver, M. F., The place of the coronary care unit. *J. Roy. Coll. Phycns.* Lond. 3, 47 (1968).
9. Peel, A. A. F., T. Semple, I. Wang, W. M. Lancaster and J. L. G. Dall, A coronary prognostic index for grading the severity of infarction. *Brit. Heart J.* 24, 745 (1962).
10. Hughes, W. L., J. M. Kalbfleisch, E. N. Brandt and J. P. Costiloe, Myocardial infarction prognosis by discriminant analysis. *Arch. Int. Med.* III, 338 (1963).
11. Norris, R. M., P. W. T. Brandt, D. E. Caughey, A. J. Lee and P. J. Scott, A new coronary prognostic index. *Lancet*, 1, 274 (1969).
12. Valori, C., M. Thomas and J. P. Shillingford, Free noradrenaline and adrenaline excretion in relation to clinical syndromes following myocardial infarction. *Amer. J. Cardiol.* 2, 605 (1967).
13. Logan, R. W. and W. R. Murdoch, Blood levels of hydrocortisone transaminases and cholesterol after myocardial infarction. *Lancet* 2, 521 (1966).
14. Smith, A. F., Diagnostic value of serum-creatine-kinase in a coronary care unit. *Lancet*, 2, 178 (1967).
15. Freisinger, G. C., Personal communication (1969).
16. Oliver, M. F., V. A. Kurien and T. W. Greenwood, Serum free fatty acids and arrhythmia and death after acute myocardial infarction. *Lancet* 1, 710 (1968).
17. Goldman, R. H., M. Klughaupt, T. Metcalf, A. P. Spivack and D. C. Harrison, Measurement of central venous oxygen saturation in patients with acute myocardial infarction. *Circulation* 38, 941 (1968).
18. Levy, H., The natural history of changing patterns of angina pectoris. *Ann. Int. Med.* 44, 1123 (1956).
19. Hinkle, L. E., Personal communication (1969).
20. Chiang, B. N., L. V. Perlman, L. D. Ostrander and F. H. Epstein, Relationship of premature systoles to coronary heart disease and sudden death in the Tecumseh Epidemiologic Study. *Ann. Int. Med.* In press, (1969).
21. U.S. Public Health Service. *The health consequences of smoking.* 59 (1967).

THE DILEMMA OF ANTICOAGULANT THERAPY IN CORONARY HEART DISEASE

E. A. LOELIGER

'While still several hundred yards away, a motorcyclist was observed by the driver of an oncoming motor car to be 'asleep'. The driver stopped, and waited helplessly while the motorcycle ran into his car.' This episode was reported in the daily press under the headline: 'The Dead Motor Cyclist Rode On'.

Such an accident dramatically illustrates one of the most frequent causes of death, the acute stand-still of the heart due to ischaemic heart disease; it is described in 'The Incubation Period of Coronary Thrombosis' written by Osborn in the early 1960s (1). Not only Osborn's anatomical study of coronary arteries obtained from individuals of all ages, most of whom had died in accidents or of diseases other than atherosclerosis, but also the work on coronary heart disease patients published by Fischer in 1963, (2) have shown very clearly that coronary heart disease has a life-long history and must be considered as the result mainly of thrombosis developing repeatedly at sites of endothelial damage, most extensively when there is intimal bleeding. At the annual meeting of the International College of Angiology held in London in 1965, French reviewed the series of papers published since Rokitanski, representing an accumulation of evidence in favour of the thrombogenic hypothesis of coronary heart disease. Finally, Mitchell and Schwartz in 1965 (3) and Harland and Holburn in 1966 (4) have irrefutably demonstrated that more than 90 per cent of the terminal coronary occlusions resulting in acute myocardial infarction are thrombothic in origin. On the basis of all these findings, thrombolytic and anticoagulant therapy may be expected to abolish and prevent occlusions.

Thrombolytic agents such as streptokinase and urokinase are assumed to remove thrombi by means of enzymatic dissolution of their fibrin network. Indeed, coagulation thrombi are very rapidly lysed *in vitro*;

and experimental venous thrombi have been succesfully eliminated in volunteers. Arterial thrombi, on the other hand, most of which belong to the classical white thrombi, are much more resistant to thrombolytic agents. In addition, the circulatory stand-still at the site of the thrombotic occlusion of a coronary artery makes it difficult for the drug to reach its victim. As a matter of fact, there is still no proof that the prognosis of patients suffering from acute myocardial infarction is improved by streptokinase. Urokinase, a similarly powerful but non-antigenic thrombolytic agent prepared from human urine, is under investigation in the USA and in the Netherlands as well as other European countries, but it is too early to judge the results.

More familiar to most of us are the *anticoagulants* of the coumarin and heparin types. These drugs have been proven to be powerful weapons in the battle against venous as well as intracardial thrombosis. Thrombus formation and growth are both retarded by these drugs, probably through inhibition of thrombin-dependent platelet aggregation (Poller, 1969) (5), platelet viscous metamorphosis, and secondary blood coagulation. There is no reason whatsoever to suppose that these drugs do not exert a similarly powerful antithrombotic action in arterial thrombosis. We must bear in mind, however, that white thrombi – which, despite impaired blood coagulation, continue to develop, albeit to a lesser extent – rather soon become occlusive, especially in case of a narrowed lumen of the coronary artery. Fischer (2) has shown that in patients treated with anticoagulants on a long-term basis, thrombotic deposits are less extensive and not multifocal, as compared to the findings in untreated patients.

This situation explains why we look at the reports of clinicians with the greatest interest. Our expectations, however, are often disappointed by the conflicting results in the literature. To detect the reason for this confusion, we must read the papers very carefully; it then proves to originate from a lack of rigour in experimental design as well from insufficient clinical and pharmacological knowledge. The two most recent examples of such confusing papers are to be found in the current volumes of two reputable periodicals, the first in the British Medical Journal (February 29th; Assessment of Short-term Anticoagulant Administration after Cardiac Infarction, performed by the Medical Research Council (16) and the second in the New England Journal of Medicine (March 27th; Treatment of Chronic Arterial Occlusions with Streptokinase, reported by Poliwoda c.s.) (7).

To comment on the first example: the Working Party on Antico-agulant Therapy in Coronary Thrombosis of the British Medical Research Council, while evincing an excellent grasp of biostatics – a high- and low-dosage group were compared – failed to take important clinical and pharmacological aspects sufficiently into account: many cases with a duration of more than 7 to 10 days after the acute infarc-tion were included in the study. In this stage of the disease, the risk of thromboembolic complications originating from the heart and peripheral veins is high; and since these complications are not imme-diately prevented by the institution of anticoagulant treatment, they bias the results unfavourably for the high dosage group. In addition, the first 48 hours following the acute infarction were not considered separately from the later stages, even though it is known that the death rate is highest in the first two days and that these early deaths, because they are caused by electrodynamic or myodynamic insufficiency and surrender, are extremely unlikely to be prevented by anticoagulants. Even more deplorable is the use of the designation 'high-dosage group', which suggests a group of patients adequately treated with anticoagulants. As a matter of fact, this so-called 'high-dosage group' displayed grossly inadequate anticoagulation.

The second example concerns Poliwoda's report of a study of 27 peripheral atherothrombosis patients who were treated with strepto-kinase and coumarin. Not to be forgiven at present is the use of results obtained without controls, to suggest a possible favourable effect of streptokinase; this objection holds particularly for cases of complete ob-struction of a peripheral artery, which, as we know, may disappear spontaneously.

Table 1. This table illustrates the slight but significant difference in mortality and the highly significant difference in thromboembolic episodes observed in two comparable groups of patients who had survived the first 48 hours after an acute infarction, one treated with dicoumarol, the other with placebo. The figures are clearly in favour of patients treated with anticoagulants.

	anticoagulant	placebo	P
Deaths	10.8%	20.8%	0.02 -0.05
Thrombo embolic episodes	2.6%	10%	0.001-0.01

In sharp contrast to these and many other confusing reports, a small series of carefully designed and meticulously performed studies is to be found in the literature.

To begin with short-term anticoagulant administration after cardiac infarction, we wish to mention a recent, carefully controlled Danish study (8). The results of this work show that anticoagulants do not alter the mortality during the first 48 hours, whereas during the following four weeks the mortality is significantly lowered by adequate anticoagulation.

This excellent study corroborates our experience that anticoagulant drugs should be administered in acute myocardial infarction mainly in order to prevent thromboembolic complications.

After the acute period has passed, long-term treatment must be considered. Meuwissen and co-workers at Utrecht were in fact the first to demonstrate with a double-blind trial – phenprocoumon versus placebo – that coumarin-treated coronary heart disease patients benefit from long-term anticoagulant therapy during the first year after its institution, as judged from a significantly lower mortality (9). The Meuwissen study was performed under the exceptionally favourable conditions offered by a Netherlands Thrombosis Service, (10) which probably explains the large difference in mortality between the two groups. The recent Danish report (8) already mentioned has corroborated these findings, although the difference in mortality is less spectacular.

Table 2. This table shows the results obtained in the same patients as those of the preceding table, but now for the period of two years after acute infarction, excluding the first month of treatment.

	anticoagulant	placebo	P
Deaths	9.5%	19.1%	0.1-0.05
Recurrences	6.5%	20%	<0.001

We investigated the possibility of benefit after at least two years of long-term anticoagulant treatment, again under the conditions of a double-blind trial and the tight organization of the Netherlands Thrombosis Service (11). As judged from the morbidity, our results were unexpectedly favourable, particularly with respect to the recurrency rate.

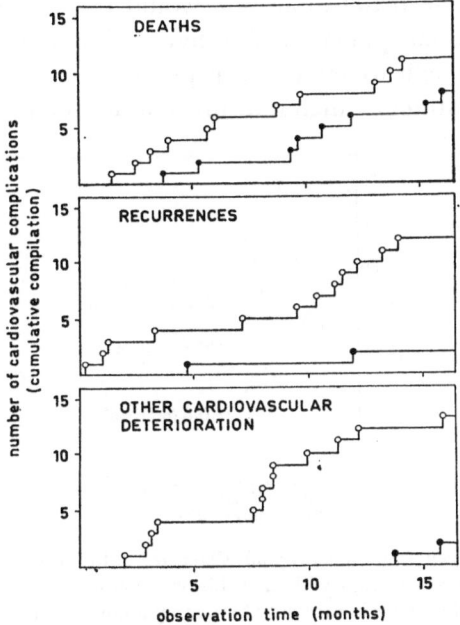

Fig. 1. This figure shows our results, compiled and indicated cumulatively on the y-axis, for the observation period indicated in months on the x-axis. White and black spots refer to placebo and phenprocoumon-patients, respectively. The difference in the number of deaths after 16 months of observation is far from significant, but taken together with the results obtained from a parallel trial performed under the same conditions in patients suffering from peripheral sclerosis, the death rate has become significantly different (10 deaths in the coumarin groups as against 19 deaths in the placebo groups) (11a). The differences for recurrences (2:12) and other cardiovascular complications (2:13) are highly significant. Patients under the age of 65 appeared to have been benefitted most.

Also with respect to long-term treatment after infarction has occurred, the recent final report of the Veterans Administration Cooperative Study of Long-Term Anticoagulant Therapy after Myocardial Infarction has confirmed several of the results just mentioned and also indicates that patients who have suffered more than one infarction before institution of anticoagulation may benefit most, as judged from survivorship (12). This study, too, was performed under close supervision of the patient and with adequate anticoagulation (using human brain thromboplastin for the coagulation check), both of which are rather exceptional for the USA.

A discussion of the results obtained from long-term anticoagulant treatment *after* myocardial infarction would not be complete without mention of the recent paper by Borchgrevink c.s. (13) in which it is shown that the benefit to females is as great as that to males, but with an intensity of treatment which is insufficient for men.

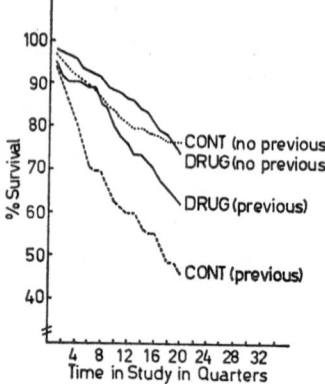

Fig. 2. This figure, taken from the original Veterans' Administration paper, shows the survivorship for patients with and without a history of myocardial infarction before the qualifying event. The difference in mortality between patients with no previous infarction in favour of the treated group is lost after about 5 years, whereas in those with previous infarctions it is still highly significant after 5 years of treatment.

To conclude with a brief consideration of patients suffering from *angina pectoris*, it may be said that equally good results have been obtained in these patients (14):

Table 3. These figures on the death and infarction rates pertain to a well-controlled study by Borchgrevink. The differences are highly significant in favour of the high dosage group.

	high dosage	low dosage
Death rate	0.9%	7.4%
Infarction rate	1.9%	11.0%

This study on angina pectoris, unlike Borchgrevink's just-mentioned investigation in women, was performed on the basis of an intensity of treatment known to be effective in men.

CONCLUDING REMARKS

Anticoagulant treatment appears to develop antithrombotic action in coronary artery thrombosis as judged from anatomical as well clinical studies. But it by no means offers a panacea for the prophylaxis and treatment of ischaemic heart disease. Anticoagulant treatment makes only a minor contribution to longer and better survival of patients suffering from atherothrombosis. For acute myocardial infarction, the benefit lies in an order of magnitude comparable to that of cardiac units (15), and with long-term anticoagulant treatment it is certainly larger than that so far obtained by dietary measures (16, 17, 18). The main condition for successful anticoagulation, however, remains: adequate hypocoagulability. In terms of assay procedures, the following ranges of hypocoagulability should be aimed at:

Table 4.

Thrombotest (Owren)	5-10
P & P (Owren)	10-20
Prothrombin time (Quick) thromboplastin:	
human brain	
Roche	15-30
Geigy	
Simplastin, Dade, Ortho	20-40

ADDENDUM

Relevant references not mentioned in the text (according to subject)
General aspects of thrombosis in coronary heart disease (19).
Long-term anticoagulant treatment (20, 21, 23).
Results of anticoagulant therapy in Norway (22).
Examples and discussion of negative results in cases of insufficient hypocoagulability (24, 25).
Comparability of prothrombin times and the influence of PIVKA (26, 27).
The use of heparin in acute myocardial infarction (28, 29).
Long-acting versus short-acting coumarins (30).

REFERENCES

1. Osborn, G. R., *The incubation period of coronary thrombosis.* Butterworths, London (1963).
2. Fischer, S., *Pathology of coronary occlusion with special reference to anticoagulant medication.* Thesis Copenhagen (1963).
3. Mitchell, J. R. A., C. J. Schwartz, Arterial disease. Blackwell, London (1965).
4. Harland, W. A., A. M. Holburn, Coronary thrombosis and myocardial infarction. *Lancet*, II, 1158 (1966).
5. Poller, L., J. M. Thomson, C. M. Priest, Coumarin therapy and platelet aggregation. *Brit. Med. J.* I, 474 (1969).
6. Report of the Working Party on Anticoagulant Treatment in Coronary Thrombosis to the Medical Research Council: Assessment of short-term anticoagulant administration after cardiac infarction. *Brit. Med. J.* 1, 335 (1969).

7. Poliwoda, H., K. Alexander, V. Buhl, D. Holsten, H. H. Wagner, Treatment of chronic arterial occlusions with streptokinase. *New Engl. J. Med.* 280, 689 (1969).
8. Sørensen, O. H., T. Friis, A. W. Jørgensen, M. B. Jørgensen, N. I. Nissen,Anticoagulant treatment of acute coronary thrombosis. *Acta Med. Scand.* 185, 65 (1969).
9. Meuwissen, O. J. A. Th., M. C. Vervoorn, O. Cohen, F. A. Nelemans, A double-blind trial on long-term anticoagulant treatment after myocardial infarction. *Acta Med. Scand.* 186, 361-368 (1969).
10. Jordan, F. L. J., Organization of the 'Thrombosis Service' in the Netherlands. *Thrombos. Diathes. haemorrh.* 2, 527 (1958).
11. Loeliger, E. A., A. Hensen, F. Kroes, L. M. van Dijk, N. Fekkes, H. de Jonge, H. C. Hemker, A double-blind trial of long-term anticoagulant treatment after myocardial infarction. *Acta Med. Scand.* 182, 49 (1967).
12. Ebert, R. V., C. W. Borden, H. R. Hipp, D. Holzman, A. F. Lyon, H. Schnaper, Long-term anticoagulant therapy after myocardial infarction. *J. Amer. Med. Ass.* 207, 2263 (1969).
13. Borchgrevink, C. F., C. Bjerkelund, A. M. Abrahamsen, G. Bay, P. Borgen, B. Grande, I. Helle, H.Kjörstad, A. M. Petersen, T. Rörvik, R. Thorsen, A. Odegaard, Long-term anticoagulant therapy after myocardial infarction in women. *Brit. Med. J.* 3, 571 (1968).
14. Borchgrevink, C. F., Long-term anticoagulant therapy in angina pectoris and myocardial infarction. *Acta Med. Scand.* Suppl. 359 (1960).
15. Nager, F., R. Rösli, H. Albert, P. Lichtlen, A. Bühlmann, Behandlung des akuten Myokardinfarktes in einer Koronar-Wachstation. Erfahrungen mit 260 Patienten. *Schweiz. med. Wschr.* 99, 309 (1969).
16. Leren, P., The effect of plasma cholesterol lowering diet in male survivors of myocardial infarction. *Acta Med. Scand.* Suppl. 466 (1966).
17. Report of a Research Committee to the Medical Research Council: Controlled trial of soya-been oil in myocardial infarction. *Lancet*, II, 693 (1968).
18. Turpeinen, O.,M. Miettinen, M. J. Karvonen, P. Roine, M. Pekkarinen, E. J. Lehtosuo, P. Alivirta, Dietary prevention of coronary heart disease: long-term experiment. *Amer. J. Clin. Nutr.* 21, 255 (1968).
19. McDonald, L., Thrombosis in coronary heart disease. *Brit. Heart J.* 30, 151 (1968).
20. Borchgrevink, C. F., Anticoagulant therapy in coronary heart disease (review 1964). *Thrombos. Diathes. haemorrh.* 15, 610 (1966).
21. Douglas, A. S., Anticoagulant therapy in coronary artery disease. *Conf. Thrombos. Washington* (1967). In press.
22. Wright, I. S., Anticoagulants after myocardial infarction. *Brit. Med. J.* II, 188 (1969).
23. Owren, P. A., The results of anticoagulant therapy in Norway. *Arch. Int. Med.* 111, 240 (1963).
24. Ritland, S., T. Lygren, Comparison of efficacy of 3 and 12 months' anticoagulant therapy after myocardial infarction. A controlled clinical trial. *Lancet*, I, 122 (1969).
25. Seaman, A. J., H. E. Griswold, R. B. Reaume, L. W. Ritzman, Prophylactic anticoagulant therapy for coronary artery disease. A seven-year controlled study. *J. Amer. Med. Ass.* 189, 183 (1964).
26. Biggs, R., Standardization of the one-stage prothrombin time for the control of anticoagulant therapy. *Brit. Med. J.* 1, 84 (1967).
27. Hemker, H. C., E. A. Loeliger, Kinetic aspects of the interaction of blood clotting enzymes. III. Demonstration of an inhibitor of prothrombin conversion in vitamin K deficiency. *Thrombos. Diathes. haemorrh.* 19, 346 (1968).
28. Aarseth, S., H. F. Lange, The influence of anticoagulant therapy on the occurrence of cardiac rupture and hemopericardium following heart infarction. I. A study of 89 cases of hemopericardium (81 of them cardiac ruptures). *Amer. Heart J.* 56, 250 (1958).
29. Enger, E., A. C. Julsrud, K. Kirkeby, Initial heparin therapy as a supplement to

peroral anticoagulants in acute myocardial infarction. *Acta Med. Scand.* Suppl. 397 (1963).

30. Fekkes, N., J. J. Veltkamp, R. Bieger, E. A. Loeliger, *The value of the short-acting acenocoumarin and long-acting phenprocoumon in long-term anticoagulant treatment.* A comparative study. To be published.
31. French, J. E., Thrombosis as a factor in atherosclerosis. *Angiology*, 17, 590 (1966).
32. Hamming, J. J., A. Hensen, E. A. Loeliger, *The value of long-term coumarin treatment in peripheral sclerosis* (a clinical trial). To be published.
33. Seaman, A. L., H. E. Griswold, R. B. Baume, L. W. Ritzman, Long-term anticoagulant prephylayis after myocardial infarction. *New Eng. J. Med.* 381, 115 (1960).

EXERCISE THERAPY IN CORONARY DISEASE

REHABILITATION AND SECONDARY PREVENTION

H. K. HELLERSTEIN

The invitation to participate in this Boerhaave Course on the Prevention of Ischaemic Heart Disease at the University of Leiden is a high honor which I truly appreciate and hope to be worthy thereof. The locale of the Course is also gratifying, since it has provided me with an opportunity to visit the city of Leiden, home of so many historical personages and scientific events; to mention a few:

Professor Boerhaave, the great clinician; the discovery of the condenser (the Leyden jar); Professor Einthoven and his string galvanometer, which ushered in the modern era of electrocardiography.

Rehabilitation has been defined as the process which *restores* and *maintains* the individual at his optimal physiologic, psychologic, emotional, social and vocational status (1). It includes institution of measures to *prevent* the progression of the underlying disease process. In the forthcoming presentation, I will present the thesis that exercise therapy has a valuable place in the restoration and the maintenance of the coronary subject, and in the secondary prevention of the effects of atherosclerosis. Like all potent therapeutic measures, exercise therapy must be properly prescribed, or proscribed when indicated, and supervised. Periodically its value must be reassessed.

The attitude of the medical profession toward the patient with coronary artery disease (ischaemic heart disease) is changing rapidly, due in large part to the advances of the past several decades. Individuals have been identified for susceptibility to develop coronary artery disease prematurely; methods have been developed to characterize the structure of the heart by special x-ray techniques, angiograms, etc.; and the function of the heart can be evaluated more precisely by effort tests and metabolic studies. Fortunately function often can be enhanced by drug therapy, direct coronary surgery in some cases, and as recently demonstrated by physical conditioning. The distinction between the known coronary patient and the precoronary individual has been shown to be only one of time. The coronary prone subject in reality has already started down the same pathway worn so deeply by the coronary stricken. The relative significance of the various risk factors has been validated by prospective epidemiologic studies. Efforts are currently in progress to attempt to modify these factors, by control of the lipid moiety, diet, weight control, and drug therapy, regulation of blood pressure, and disuse of cigarettes. Relatively little attention has been directed to the control of physical fitness.

In the past several decades, the role of physical fitness in the genesis of diseases of the cardiovascular system has received increasing attention (2). Currently its role is being investigated in the treatment of the stricken subject and in a few areas in the prevention of coronary disease. Many epidemiologic studies have shown clearly that the incidence and prevalence of arteriosclerotic heart disease and hypertensive cardiovascular disease are lower in persons engaged in occupations requiring greater expenditures of energy than in those in sedentary occupations. The hypokinetic way of prosperous Western life apparently predisposes to an ever increasing incidence of coronary artery disease.

Attempts have been made to counteract the effects of this mode of life in other countries, notably in Germany and in Russia, by means of reconditioning centers and other positive programs. The efforts in the United States have been less striking. The beneficial effects of exercise have been amply substantiated in the past by reports on the training of normal fit and unfit subjects. Eckstein had demonstrated that exercise induced coronary collateral circulation in dogs with minimal narrowing of the coronary arteries (3). In other dogs with moderate and severe coronary narrowing, greater collateral circulation developed. Similar experimental work on the beneficial effect of exercise on experimental atherosclerosis has been performed on chickens and rabbits. Eckstein suggested, by extrapolation, that his findings perhaps could be applied to the treatment of subjects with coronary atherosclerosis by using exercise to improve their coronary collateral circulation and thereby to enhance the adequacy of their coronary circulation.

For the past decade, my associates and I in the United States have made a systematic study of the value of physical fitness enhancement

of normal, highly coronary prone subjects and on subjects with arteriosclerotic heart disease (2). At the time of my inital investigations,
I was aware of the emphasis that the ancient physicians and philosophers had placed on gymnastics and exercise for the preservation of
health. Indeed, in 1189 Maimonides wrote a brochure on the preservation of youth, for the son of the sultan of Egypt. In addition to
other good health practices, he advised that one should exercise daily
to the point of breathlessness. The importance of exercise for patients
with coronary disease was recognized almost 200 years ago by Heberden who in 1772 noted that one of his patients was nearly cured after a
six month period of sawing wood for one-half hour per day (4).
Apparently this was the first published observation of the benefical
effects of physical activity by subjects with coronary disease. Our initial
and subsequent encouraging reports have been confirmed and fortified
by recent studies by other American and European investigators. As a
result of the favourable reports of the value of physical training after
recovery from myocardial infarction, physical conditioning is currently
being applied even earlier in the illness, starting within the first week of
the acute myocardial infarct, in selected cases.

Thus, it would appear that physical conditioning may be important
and potentially beneficial in every phase of the illness, viz.: the acute
myocardial infarction with intensive care, the convalescent period, the
recovery and the return to work phases.

In a recent symposium on the value of exercise in the prevention,
evaluation and in the treatment of heart disease, a cautionary statement on exercise was proposed, in order to avoid excesses and misuses
(1). 'Epidemiologic and other studies have shown that physical fitness is
associated with a better state of well-being, enhanced quality of living,
and reduced morbidity from coronary heart disease. For these reasons,
we recommend that enhancement of physical fitness be part of comprehensive medical care which includes accepted good health practices
such as diet, weight control, disuse of cigarettes, and when indicated,
specific medical and surgical treatment. Physical conditioning can be
applied to normal subjects particularly those who are highly coronary
prone, and to selected patients of both sexes and of all ages. Like all
therapeutic measures, exercise and activity prescription for arteriosclerotic heart disease subjects and for normal coronary prone subjects,
particularly above the age of 30 to 35 years, exercise prescription
requires preliminary medical evaluation, exclusion of subjects with

specific contraindications, followed by the evaluation of cardiovascular status and function, particularly multi-level activity and when indicated exercise stress testing, precise prescription of the magnitude, frequency, and duration of effort, supervision, direction, and periodic re-evaluation'. A list of contraindications and indications are listed in table 1.

Table 1. Indications and contraindications for participation in programs planned to enhance physical fitness.

Indications	Contraindications	
	Cardiovascular	Others
Normal Subjects, especially highly coronary prone, general deconditioning, neurocirculatory asthenia, before and after surgery*	Severe (80-90%) stenosis of three major coronary arteries	Uncontrolled diabetes mellitus
		Marked obesity
	Rapidly progressing angina	
		Deforming arthritis*
Arteriosclerotic Heart Disease*	Impending infarction	
		Skeletal-muscle disorders
Intermittent claudication*	Massive ventricular aneurysm	
		Psychosis
Pulmonary disease*	Congestive failure	
		Recent pulmonary embolism
	Arrhythmias:	
		Severe varicose veins with thrombophlebitis, phlebo- thrombosis
	ventricular tachycardia 2nd, 3rd A-V block fixed ventricular rate pacemaker untreated atrial fibrillation ventricular premature beats at rest which in- crease with exercise	Anemia
		Central nervous system disease*
		CAUTION
	Valvular disease moderate to severe	*DRUGS*: reserpine, propranolol, guanethi- dine, ganglionic blockers, procaine amide, quini- dine
	Outflow obstruction	
	Uncontrolled hypertension	

* Selected cases.

This statement on exercise can be applied with slight modification to the various phases of coronary artery disease.

In order to understand the need for physical conditioning of the

coronary patient, it is important to review briefly the effects of myocardial ischaemia and of the clinical management on the subject and his
performance. When the blood supply to the myocardium is inadequate,
the number of contractile muscle units decreases and reduces the
power of the myocardium. The closure of a coronary artery or relative
or absolute inadequacy of blood flow frequently leads to arrhythmias
which fortunately can be controlled, to forestall 'mechanism death'.
However, during the stay in a coronary care unit and later in the
hospital, the effects of bedrest may be far greater than that of deletion
of heart muscle. Recent investigations have confirmed the fact that bed
rest and restriction of activity, reduces physical fitness, even in normal
subjects. Thus, the effects of the myocardial infarct and of bed rest and
restriction may be additive. For this reason, physical activity should not
be excessively or inordinately restricted. Throughout the care of the
patient one should attempt to prevent deconditioning and institute
measures to recondition the myocardium and the skeletal musculature.

REGULATION OF PHYSICAL ACTIVITY IN VARIOUS PHASES
OF THE ILLNESS

For convenience I have divided the process of rehabilitation after an
acute myocardial infarction into five phases (figure 1).
1. Acute illness – approximately one week in a Coronary Care Unit.
2. Remainder hospital stay, two to three weeks.
3. Convalescence, four to eight weeks.
4. Recovery – return to work.
5. Planned higher level physical fitness program.
The caloric expenditure or energy level increases gradually from a level
of 1 to 2 mets in the CCU phase, 2 to 3 mets in the remainder of the
hospital stay, 4 to 5 mets during convalescence and higher thereafter.
By the eight to twelfth week, in most coronary patients the fitness should
be enhanced so that approximately 80 to 85 per cent are able to return
to their old job particularly in an urban setting. Usually the job is unmodified. The preparation for the return to work should be systematic,
supervised and directed. Unfortunately, often this is random and ineffective. Many subjects are restricted excessively in a prolonged period
between the onset of illness and return to work.

METS, OXYGEN UPTAKE, AND CALORIES

In the subsequent discussion reference will be made to energy expend-

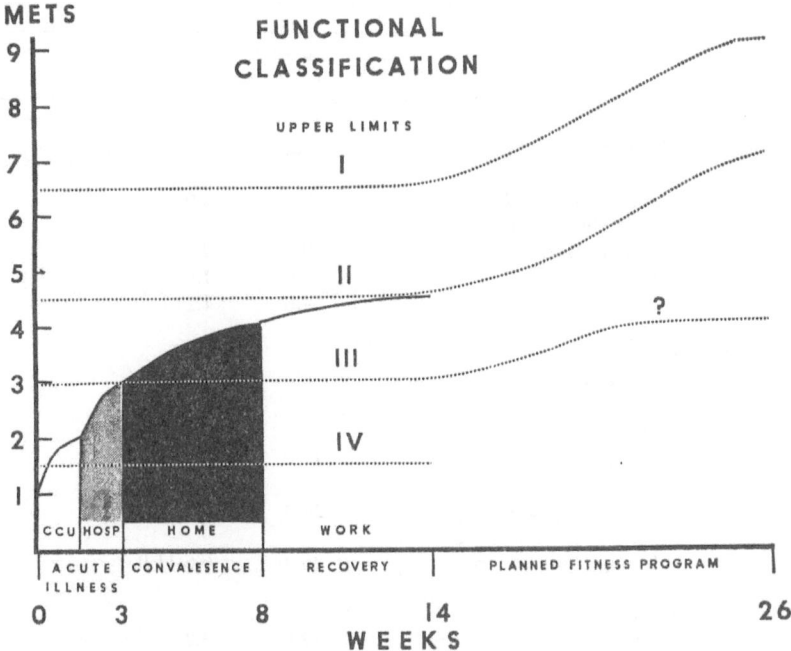

Fig. 1. Schematic representation of the activity level in Met units during 5 phases of myocardial infarction: acute illness in coronary care unit; remainder of hospital stay; convalescence; recovery with return to work, and planned higher level physical fitness program. The upper limits of energy expenditure are indicated by dotted lines for functional classifications (according to the New York Heart Association Criteria). Discussed in text.

iture and activities. The term 'Met' refers to the energy used per minute by a subject at rest, not necessarily basal. The term calorie refers to the heat produced, measured indirectly by oxygen uptake. In general, at rest but not in basal condition, an average 75 kg man uses approximately 1.5 calories per minute (300 ml O_2), which is equivalent to 4 cc oxygen/kg BW. Thus 1 met = 1.5 calorie or 4 ml O_2/kg BW. The aerobic power of normal subjects varies, ranging from 30 calories (25 mets) for champion athletes to 14 calories (12 mets) for healthy untrained young men. For most post-myocardial infarction subjects the aerobic power is about 10 to 11 calories (8 to 9 mets). For Class III cardiacs the maximal aerobic power is approximately 4 mets per minute.

It is important to relate the aerobic capacity of the individual subject to the energy demands of living and work activities. In table 2 the

Table 2. Mean energy expenditure of various activities (10).

Activity	ml O$_2$/ min/kg BW	Mets
Sleeping	3.2	0.8
Awake, lying at ease	3.4	0.9
Daily living activities		
Toilet-wash, dress, shave	8.4	2.1
Sit at ease	4.0	1.0
Stand at ease	4.8	1.2
Effort		
Walking on level at 3 mph	8.4	2.1
Walking uphill		
5% grade at 3 mph	12.0	3.0
Walking upstairs	24.0	6.0
Skiing cross country	26-44	6.6-11.0
Bicycling (mph)		
5.5	12.9	3.2
9.5	20.0	5.0
13.1	31.4	7.9
Swimming breast-stroke (yds/min)		
20	14.3	3.6
30	21.4	5.4
40	28.6	7.2
Dancing		
Foxtrot	14.9	3.7
Waltz	16.3	4.1
Rumba	20.0	5.0

mean energy expenditure of various activities is presented in ml O$_2$/min/kg BW and in metabolic units. There is an advantage in referring to the energy costs of an activity in terms of mets or ml O$_2$/kg BW rather than in calories, in order to obviate the effects of variations in the body weight between subjects.

In referring to figure 1, it becomes obvious that the aerobic power of Class I to Class III cardiacs is well above the energy required to sit and lie quietly, to move the arms and legs, and to perform active and passive movements in a bedside chair. For this reason it is highly inadvisable to restrict patients to complete bed rest in the absence of congestive heart failure or uncontrolled arrhythmias.

Within the first four to five days of acute illness the aerobic power of the majority of patients is sufficient to allow them to sit in a bedside chair and to take care of their ordinary needs (1). Fortunately with the monitoring electronic devices currently in use, the response of subjects can be evaluated objectively. The appearance of ventricular arrhythmias, or marked st-t displacement indicates that the activity at that level is excessive.

Phase I

This phase is instituted when the patient's clinical condition is relatively stable, usually within twenty-four hours after the acute myocardial infarct (1). Contraindications to this phase include severe heart failure, shock, intractable pain and uncontrolled arrhythmias.

In the uncomplicated cases there will be a gradual increase in activities which have a low energy requirement (in the range of one to two mets). This includes self-care, feeding, shaving, use of bedside commode or bathroom with assistance, active and passive body movements of the upper and lower extremities, approximately two to three minutes during each working hour. Also to be included are dangling and sitting in bedside chair. For the complicated cases passive movements of the upper and particularly lower extremities can be recommended. An activity can be considered to be excessive if there is an increase of a heart rate above 120 beats per minute, increase in the st-t displacement, appearance of significant arrhythmias such as ventricular premature beats, tachycardia, a-v block, increased chest pain and dyspnea, and marked changes in blood pressure above 20-30 mm of that at rest (1).

Phase II

This phase refers to the remainder of the hospital stay which ordinarily is 2 to 3 weeks. The range of the energy cost of allowed activities is approximately 2 to 3 mets.

During the first week out of the coronary care unit the patient is allowed to sit in a bedside chair for one to three hours per day. Body motion exercises are useful in preventing joint and muscular discomfort and immobility. In general, in uncomplicated cases, the patient should be able to be ambulatory in his room and by the third week (about the time of discharge from the hospital) he should be able to walk 50 to 100 feet, usually in a protected environment (usually in hospital corridors). The activities should be interspersed with periods of rest. In general higher energy activities should be avoided after a meal (1).

The same parameters as in Phase I may be monitored. Symptoms, signs, pulse rate, blood pressure, and ideally an electrocardiogram should be recorded before and after each new activity requiring a higher energy level.

Phase III – 4th to 8th week
In the absence of complications the activities of Phase III should be gradually increased to a level at which the patient would return to work by the end of the 8th to 12th week. This activity usually takes place in the patient's home or in a reconditioning center.

The activities include self-care, full activities in the house including stair climbing, and light housework. The patient should be encouraged to increase his activity so that by the fourth or fifth week he has increased his distance and speed of walking in a gradual and self-determined basis to approximately one or two miles a day, divided into two periods.

Prior to increasing the energy level at a higher magnitude in the sixth to eighth week, it is advisable that the cardiovascular function should be assessed by an effort test of a magnitude equal of that activity which the subject had been performing during the previous week at home, e.g., walking half a mile, climbing stairs, etc. Responses to this effort can serve as a useful guide to the physician to regulate the level of future activities. Some guidelines to reduce the magnitude of the activity would include post-exercise heart rate of more than 120 beats/minute, a drop in blood pressure of 20 to 30 mm two minutes after cessation of exercise, or appearance of chest pain. For the subsequent 6 to 8 weeks, the subject with a normal response can be advised to increase the duration and speed of walking to increase his endurance and strength in preparation for his return to work. In general, a reasonable goal is to attain the capacity to walk three to three and a half miles in one hour (approximately 4 to 5 mets).

Phase IV
In the fourth phase the majority of subjects have recovered sufficiently

to return to their previous occupation. In selected cases, where energy expenditure is higher than 4 to 5 mets, additional time to recover and recondition may be required. In some instances (approximately 20 per cent) work reclassification may be indicated. In the uncomplicated cases participation in a supervised physical fitness enhancement program may be desirable.

THE CASE FOR THE ENHANCEMENT OF THE FUNCTIONAL CAPACITY OF THE POST-CORONARY PATIENT

In our experience with approximately 3000 cardiac patients from 1950 to 1963, we found that they could work well and safely in a great variety of jobs. Doctor David Turell and I found in a long term follow-up study that the cardiacs who returned to work fared better than those with the same classification who did not return to work for emotional or financial reasons. We were impressed by the fact that those who worked improved more than those who did not work. Impressed that work seemed to enhance fitness, ten years ago my associates and I began a cautious program of reconditioning of coronary patients (5). We were unaware of Heberden's report in 1772, cited previously (3).

My associates and I have just completed an 8-year prospective feasibility study to which I will now refer. The objective of this study was to determine whether it was possible to interest habitually sedentary hypokinetic, endomesomorphic overweight males to adhere to a program of enhanced physical activity, and whether this program would be associated with evidence of some retardation of the effects of atherosclerosis, particularly in terms of the end point, death, or reduced morbidity and mortality. Details of this study have been presented elsewhere (2, 5, 6, 7).

The study population included both coronary stricken subjects and highly coronary prone subjects. The inclusion of ostensibly normal subjects, without manifest coronary disease, was predicated upon the findings of prospective epidemiologic surveys that certain host factors are consistently associated with a high risk of developing coronary disease, viz., elevated serum cholesterol, elevated blood pressure, obesity, cigarette smoking, physical inactivity, abnormal carbohydrate metabolism, and possibly psychologic patterns.

The design of our study was purposely comprehensive, with primary emphasis upon the enhancement of physical fitness. In recognition of the importance of nutrition, we attempted to persuade our patients to

attain a normal body weight by reducing the intake of saturated animal
fats. We also recommended that they abstain from the use of tobacco,
they continue a normal, social, and work mode of life, and lastly, that
they obtain an adequate amount of rest and sleep.

Methods

The subjects were white, middle-aged, middle and upper class businessmen, executives, managers, and free professions who were referred to
the program by their physicians.

The population of the study group consisted of 656 middle-aged
men, of whom 254 have coronary artery disease (ASHD). Sixty per cent
of the latter had angina pectoris. The ASHD have been followed for a
total of 697 subject years, with an average of 2.7 years. We have not
accepted subjects with uncompensated congestive heart failure or
severe vascular disease. In the study population there were subjects
with severe angina pectoris controlled by nitroglycerin, and some with
left bundle branch block. A few had complex arrhythmias, such as a
Wenckebach type of second-degree A-V block. One has an atrially
driven artifical pacemaker. Upon entry into the study the 402 normal
coronary-prone subjects had an average age of 45 years. The ASHD
subjects had an average age of 49 years. A historical review indicated
that since the age of 25 there had been an average gain in weight of
19 pounds. At the time of intake 28 per cent were more than 15 per
cent overweight. Thirty-two per cent were professionals, 20 per cent
business people, and 22 per cent of the managerial class. All were
employed in sedentary occupations. Their physical fitness was low
compared to Scandinavians of the same age and sex. Their lipids in
general were high. They worked more than 50 hours a week. Forty-
seven per cent of the subjects smoked cigarettes. In terms of personality
and the Minnesota Multiphasic Personality Inventory (MMPI) scores,
there was a high degree of depression, hypochondriasis, and hysteria.
According to the Rosenman-Friedman classification, 72 per cent of the
subjects were of the Type A variety (8).

The study plan included a detailed medical history, physical examination, somatotype according to the method of Sheldon and Dupertuis; standard 12 lead electrocardiogram at rest, Ekg response to Flack
and Valsalva maneuver, pulmonary function studies, serum cholesterol
and triglyceride, 7-day dietary diary, and 24 to 48 hour consecutive
monitoring of the electrocardiogram by means of a portable electro-

magnetic tape recorder (2, 6, 7). Determination of physical fitness was assessed by our modification of Åstrand bicycle ergometer exercise test (7).

The subject exercised for six minutes at each of several work levels with four minutes of rest in between, to a point that he attained a heart rate of approximately 150 beats/minute which represents approximately 85 per cent of age-determined maximal heart rate. Electrocardiograms were recorded at minute intervals and the blood pressure was recorded at the first and fifth minute of work and during the third minute of rest.

Physical fitness was characterized by the physiological variables, heart rate, blood pressure, and their derivatives HR × SBP (heart rate times systolic blood pressure), Work Load 150, and predicted maximal oxygen uptake. This was calculated according to the methods of Åstrand and Lange Andersen. The product of heart rate and blood pressure was calculated to provide an indirect measure of the myocardial oxygen consumption (7).

Our experiences indicate that untrained normal subjects and untrained cardiacs have higher blood pressure for the same level of work than trained normal subjects. This constitutes a clinical entity which we have called 'exertional hypertension'. Thus untrained normals and untrained cardiacs have a higher blood pressure for the same work level, which indicates that the myocardial oxygen need is greater than that which is imposed by the same work on the same subject when he is trained.

The exercise electrocardiograms were analyzed according to the method of Lester et al., namely, in terms of ST-J displacement and the slope of the first 0.08 seconds vector (2).

Psychological evaluation included a structured interview by a trained staff member, the Holzmann inkblot test, the Minnesota Multiphasic Personality Inventory, and the Rosenman-Friedman taped interview. Upon intake the study subjects had elevation of the so-called neurotic triad, (depression, hysteria and hypochondriasis scales) which has been shown in previous studies to be related to the severity of the disease (2, 9). In a study of 327 coronary patients the scores on the neurotic triad and on the psychasthenia scale increased with disability, as reflected by the therapeutic and functional classification (9). In the present study, these psychological scores showed significant improvement after conditioning (6).

Methods of conditioning

After each patient had been studied, a program was formulated to enhance his over-all fitness. Physical reconditioning was a part of a comprehensive positivist program, which included improvement of nutrition, attainment of normal body weight, adequate rest, abstinence from the use of tobacco, and continuation of gainful employment and of a normal social mode of life.

After the initial evaluation was completed each subject was counseled by a study physician, a dietician and a physical educator. A specialized program involving exercise, weight reduction, diet, and abstinence from smoking was formulated for each subject, with the approval of his personal physician.

Exercise prescription

The general principles of reconditioning that can be applied at all ages and in all states of health were followed. An exercise prescription was compounded to stress each subject to approximately 60 to 70 per cent of his aerobic capacity. This prescription was based upon the performance of steady-state multi-level bicycle ergometer exercise. For the subjects who did not develop electrocardiographic changes or arrhythmias with multi-level exercise, a target heart rate was determined which was 70 per cent of the predicted maximal heart rate for the age, with provisions that a heart rate of 85 per cent of the maximal heart rate be attained during the exercise sessions. In the prescription of target heart rates, one must take into account the fact that the maximal heart rate decreases with age. Thus the maximal heart rate at the age of 35 years is approximately 188 beats whereas the average maximal heart rate at the age of 55 is 165 beats. Thus, the minimal training target rate of 70 per cent in the former would be 132 beats, and the latter 115 beats. Seventy per cent of maximal heart rate corresponds to approximately 50 per cent of the maximal oxygen uptake; and 85 per cent maximal heart rate corresponds to approximately 75 to 80 per cent maximal oxygen uptake.

In the subjects who showed evidence of 'strain' (sт displacement 1 mm or more, ventricular tachyrhythms, A-v block, bundle branch block, hypotension, cerebrovascular insufficiency, severe chest pain) the target heart was determined as that rate below which the 'strain' appeared. The caloric value of the 'strain' level can be readily obtained from a plot of the work and heart rates (figure 2).

Example

In figure 2, the study subject (ASHD male, 90 kg body weight) developed 2 mm ST segment displacement and a heart rate of 143 at 750 kpm/min., equivalent to an uptake of 21 ml O_2/min/kg BW (5

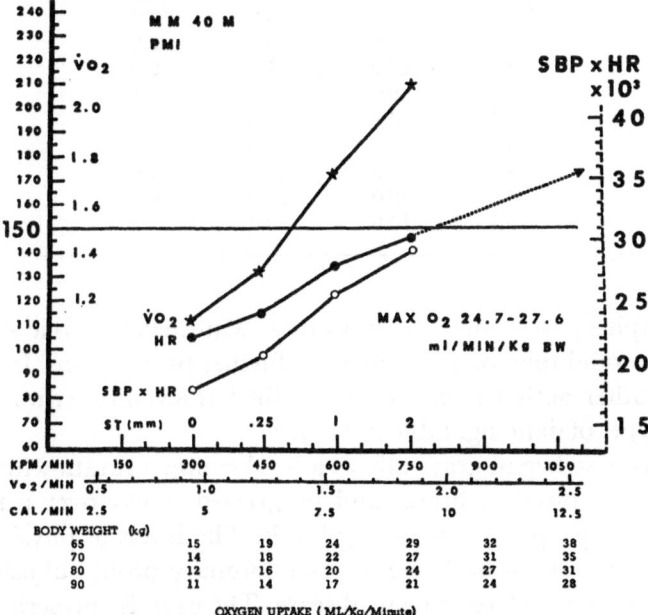

Fig. 2. Work diagram showing relationship of work load to heart rate, ST segment displacement, and oxygen uptake. Discussed in text.

mets). Obviously the initial exercise to be prescribed would be below 5 mets. The target heart rate (rate to be attained during exercise) would be the heart rate obtained below the level at which 'strain' appeared. A table of oxygen cost of walking at various speeds is useful in prescribing walking as exercise therapy (table 3).

In the subject cited above whose 'strain' level of oxygen uptake was 5 mets, the initial training level would be 60 to 70 per cent of this value (3.5 mets, 14 ml O_2/min/kg BW), equivalent to the heart rate of 115 produced at 450 kpm/min (figure 2) and equal to walking 3.5 mph (table 3). He would be started somewhat below this level (at 2.5 to 3.0 mph – 2.8 tot 3.1 mets) and the pace ordinarily increased in several weeks to 3.5 mph, as tolerated. His target heart rate would be 115 to 120. In 6 to 8 weeks, the majority of the patients would advance to

Table 3. Relationship between speed of walking (MPH) and energy expenditure (0_2 and mets) (10).

Speed MPH	Minutes Per Mile	Ml 0_2/min Per Kg BW	Mets
Rest	—	4.0	1.0
2.0	30.0	9.0	2.2
2.5	24.0	11.0	2.8
3.0	20.0	12.5	3.1
3.5	17.1	14.5	3.6
4.0	15.0	16.0	4.0
4.5	13.3	19.0	4.8
5.0	12.0	24.0	6.0
5.5	10.9	30.0	7.5

4 to 5 mph (4 to 6 mets) comfortably. Multilevel bicycle ergometer retesting would then be performed for further prescription. In a similar fashion, other activities can be prescribed (bicycling, swimming and certain types of dancing, table 2) (10).

The exercise began gradually at a level commensurate with the subject's state of physical fitness and progressed slowly over a period of months to more physically taxing levels. The levels of physical fitness initially were low in both the normal coronary prone subjects and in those with arteriosclerotic heart disease. The exercise prescription consisted of calishtenics for strength, run-walk sequences for endurance, and recreational exercise for fun. The calisthenics consisted of warm-up exercise involving the shoulders and arms; strenuous high-oxygen cost activities, i.e., hops, leg exercises, sit-ups and push-ups; and cooling-down arm and shoulder exercises. Upon entering the program most individuals began by performing one-half to two-thirds of each series of exercises. Exercises necessitating straining and the Valsalva maneuver were proscribed for men with coronary heart disease or documented hyperactivity of the carotid sinus reflex.

The caloric expenditure of full participation totalled approximately 400 calories per hour. Calisthenics required an expenditure of 200 calories over a 30-minute period, run-walk sequences 120 calories over a 15-minute period; and recreation, 80 calories over a 15-minute period. The design of the calisthenics sequence purposely included a warm-up period, work period, and a tapering off period. The mean maximal oxygen uptake per minute reached levels of 24 ml O_2 (6 mets) with an average of approximately 4.5 mets during the calisthenics period (7). For the subjects whose capacity was less than 4 mets per minute, or who developed signs of strain at a lesser level, the full sequence was not prescribed. On entering the program most subjects began by performing one-half to two-thirds of each series of calisthenics, reducing the expenditure to approximately 2 to 3 mets.

The average heart rate response during the calisthenics period was 120 beats per minute which represents approximately 70 per cent of the maximal heart rate for middle-aged men. This has been shown sufficient to induce training effects. During the run-walk sequence, higher heart rates were attained.

Monitoring the subjects

Heart rate with Ekg telemetry or by counting of the pulse has provided valuable information regarding current fitness and the validity of the exercise prescription based upon the performance of the bicycle ergometry. Initially many ASHD subjects showed arrhythmias and ST-T displacement of great magnitude. These usually subsided during continued effort. The prophylactic use of nitroglycerin was encouraged in symptomatic subjects. Recently, electronic equipment has been developed which provides an auditory signal to the subject when he has exceeded a desired heart rate; accordingly he then can reduce the magnitude of his effort.

Run-walk sequences were initially prescribed at low levels of work and were gradually increased until subjects could run a mile. Recreational activities including volleyball, swimming, bag punching were advocated but highly competitive team games demanding sudden spurts of energy were proscribed. In addition, the subjects were advised to climb stairs, not to use elevators; to walk, not ride and generally to be more vigorous in overall activities.

As mentioned in the introduction, an essential part of training has been supervision and follow-up. The subjects kept a record of their attendance and at monthly interval the staff physical educator and a study physician determined from the inspection of the records and the clinical and ergometric evaluations whether they were ready to progress to a more strenuous level. Complete re-examination of the subjects with coronary disease including bicycle ergometry and psychological testing were carried at 6-month intervals, or more frequently when indicated.

Results

The results of an active conditioning program on a subgroup of 100 of the 254 men with coronary disease were analyzed in greater detail (2). The average age was 48.8 years and the average body weight 81 kg. The subjects were followed for a period of 305 subject years with an average follow-up of 36 months. Seventy-five per cent of the subjects adhered to the program. There was an average weight loss of 2.5 kg of body weight, which was not considered to be biologically significant.

Physical fitness was significantly improved and sustained during this period in 65 per cent of the subjects. In the subjects who initially had an abnormal exercise EKG 63 per cent improved their exercise EKG. The electrocardiographic responses to exercise improved in 79 per cent of the subjects who improved their physical fitness.

Table 4. Changes in cholesterol and hemodynamic parameters of 100 ASHD subjects after training.

Item	Initial	Follow-up	p <
Cholesterol (mg/100 ml)	263.5	242.1	.01
Blood pressure (mm Hg)	s 129.9	121.7	.01
at rest	d 86.8	84.3	.05
during exercise	s 191.3	171.6	.001
Maximal O$_2$ uptake (ml O$_2$/kg BW/min)	23.2	28.9	.01
Work load 150 (kpm/kg BW/min)	8.1	9.8	.01
SBP × HR × 10^{-2} during exercise	248.3	192.7	.001
SBP × HR 25 × 10^{-3} (kpm/min)	496	609	.001

The changes in Work Load 150, maximal oxygen uptake, and blood pressure at rest and during exercise are listed in table 4. The WL 150 and maximal oxygen uptake rose significantly and the exercise systolic blood pressure decreased.

Heart rate X systolic blood pressure product (an approximation of the myocardial oxygen requirements). The improvement in the systolic blood pressure X heart rate product indicated that after training the subjects were able to perform more external work before the myocardial oxygen consumption attained a given level. For example, subjects who previously developed ischaemic changes at 600 kpm/min., with a heart rate of 150 and systolic blood pressure of 220 mm Hg, after training did not develop ischaemic changes at the same work load. Instead, characteristically they had a lower heart rate (125 beats) and lower blood pressure (180). However, if they exercised to a higher level, perhaps 900 kpm/min., the same HR × SBP product of his untrained performance at 600 kpm/min., would be attained and ischaemic changes would reappear.

Electrocardiographic changes
There were significant changes in the amount of ST displacement and 0.08 seconds vector. Prior to conditioning there was an average 1.74 mm displacement of the ST junction and the slope was 0.16 mV/sec. After training the ST junction displacement had decreased to 0.70 mm and the slope had increased to 0.91.

Adherence
There was a definite relationship between adherence to the training program and improvement of physical fitness and the exercise EKG. The subjects who adhered to the training program with 2.2 to three hours per week participation showed a significant greater improvement than the subjects who exercised less.

Psychological changes
Psychologically the group as a whole appeared to improve subjectively and objectively. The spouses of the subjects were enthusiastic because of the change in the personality and the greater ease of cohabitation, and the increased frequency of sexual activity! The decrease in the scores of the depression and psychasthenic scales was noteworthy. On a subjective basis, many subjects insisted that they had a more positive attitude to work, felt more energetic, accomplished more, and were less bored. They had an increased work output, felt more ambitious, met tense situations better, slept better, and needed less sleep. Improvement of the psyche after physical training has also been noted in normal subjects by other investigators.

Other factors which modify adherence included organization of the program design, the recreational aspects, the positive re-enforcement effect of the comradery of the group stimulus, and the regularity of the exercise sessions. The adherence was approximately twice as good in the subjects whose wife had a positive attitude toward the exercise program in contrast to the women who had a neutral or negative attitude. The reward system and recognition were also important, reinforced by public posting of performance in the exercise areas, distinctive symbols of participation, etc.

Other determinants of successful reconditioning

As indicated above adherence and motivation were important determinants. However, there was a small group of patients who failed to improve as manifested by relief of angina pectoris, decreased heart rate for the same work load and quicker recovery.

Cardiac catheterization has been performed on a small group of such subjects and has uniformly revealed multi-vessel involvement with severe (80 to 90 per cent) narrowing of two major arteries, and somewhat lesser narrowing of the third vessel. In such instances, physical training has been of limited value. Instead, a direct surgical approach has been employed successfully. In catheterization studies of subjects who have shown remarkable improvement with training, in general there has been significant involvement of only one major coronary artery.

In a series of ten cases studied by our associates, Doctors Cathel Macleod and Eugene Z. Hirsch, and in several other unreported series (Conner, Bay Pines, Florida) despite marked improvement in cardiovascular function, visible collateral vessels have not been detected. In our own experience with one patient and in several by Doctor A. Kattus, increased collateral vessels have been demonstrated.

Morbidity

In the present series and in other reports, marked relief of angina pectoris has been reported (2, 4, 12). The mortality rate in our series has been 2.1 per hundred patient years, which is below the mortality rate (4.5. to 5/100 subject years), of comparable subjects not undergoing training. In view of the fact that the present series was not randomized, we can not attribute statistical significance to this apparent reduction. We are certain, however, the mortality rate of physically conditioned patients is not greater than subjects who do not undertake such a program.

Discussion

The present study demonstrates that an active intervention program of conditioning including exercise, weight reduction, diet therapy and cessation of smoking is feasible, reasonably acceptable, and appears to be of benefit in the treatment of selected subjects with coronary heart disease.

The improvement in the parameters indicated that subjects with coronary artery disease who participated in an exercise program could be trained to do more work with fewer heart beats, lower heart rate and lower blood pressure, and greater stroke volume. Even during sleep fewer heart beats were required.

The adaptation of untrained and of highly coronary prone normal subjects and of coronary subjects appear to be similar qualitatively but not quantitatively. The data obtained on young men and athletes can not be transferred unreservedly to explain the improvement in the coronary subjects. Unfortunately, there have been no reports of the effects of training on animals with experimentally induced coronary atherosclerosis (13).

The mechanisms of the benefit of physical conditioning of coronary subjects have not been clarified adequately. However, on the basis of a review of the past 8 to 9 years of research on the effects of physical training after myocardial infarction, some insight has been gained. The amelioration in angina pectoris can result from a decrease of myo-cardial oxygen demand or from an increased myocardial oxygen supply or from both adjustments simultaneously. The decrease in the heart rate after exercise in the coronary subject is similar to the training response in healthy young and middle-aged men. According to a study by Frick and Katila, the left ventricular cavity does not increase in size, unlike the training response found in young men (14). Since the stroke volume has been shown to be increased after training, and since the heart size does not increase, one must assume that the augmented stroke volume occurs because of greater emptying rather than greater diastolic filling size. The functions of both the right and left ventricles are improved after training. Thus the increased stroke volume is prob-ably due to a more forceful contraction from fibers whose end diastolic fiber length has been unchanged. Perhaps this increase vigor of contraction may also be due to an improvement in the synchronized contractility of the myocardium. A possible additional factor is a change in the neurovegetative tone, i.e., a decrease in the sympathetic tone. Apparently training reduces sympathetic drive during exercise. Whether this is due to lesser norepinephrine content, or better storage in the myocardium has not been determined. In the preliminary experiments with mice, my associates and I have found that the heart of mice takes up less radio-active norepinephrine.

As mentioned above, the possible benefit of physical conditioning might be mediated through a change in the coronary blood flow. Unfortunately the present technique of coronary arteriography does not quantitate flow, particularly in small vessels. Studies are sadly needed to quantitate coronary flow before and after training (13).

There are other changes which are noteworthy. There is a reduction in serum triglyceride after training. It is unlikely that the reduction of serum cholesterol on our subjects was due to training by *per se*, in view of the fact that the subjects who adhered to a restricted animal fat diet showed a reduction in serum cholesterol regardless of whether they

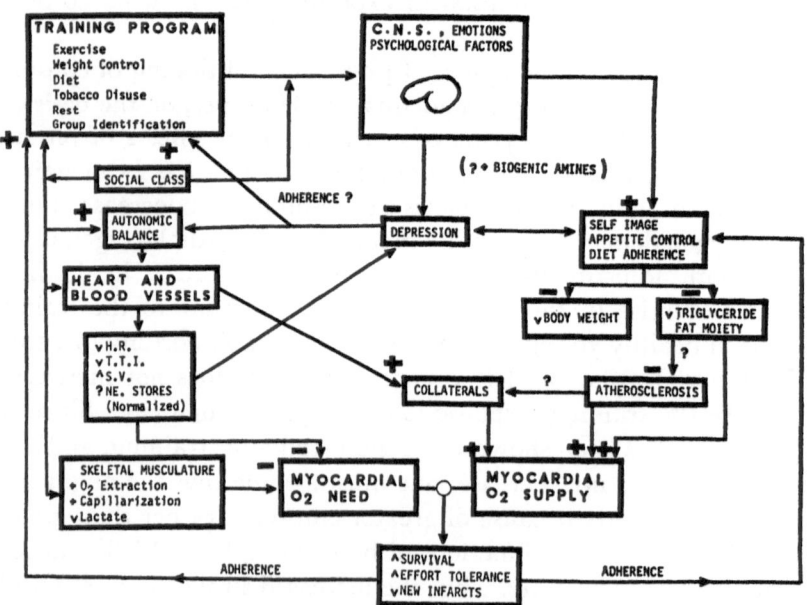

Fig. 3. Schematic representation of the effects of multifactoral intervention in coronary artery disease.

exercised or not. The effects of training on glucose tolerance have not yet been established. In our own unpublished experience there has been no significant change in serum insulin, growth hormone or glucose tolerance after training.

To explain the effects of multi-factorial intervention including physical conditioning, the systems approach has proved to be valuable. As indicated in figure 3, the relative adequacy of the myocardial oxygen supply versus oxygen need can be influenced by a multiplicity of inter-reacting factors.

In our study, the changes in the mood, in the functions of the cardio-vascular system, in nutrition, body weight, etc., indicate that the training program with its many facets (psychological, nutritional, physical conditioning, and group participation), has produced significant changes in both the cardiovascular and nervous systems.

SUMMARY

Exercise therapy has a place in coronary disease for rehabilitation and for secondary prevention. From the clinical viewpoint, it appears that an active supervised conditioning program can be used safely in the treatment of selected patients with coronary heart disease, infarction, and angina pectoris but not in congestive heart failure.

Our experiences with supervised training of coronary patients indicate that after training they were able to perform muscular work more efficiently than before training, i.e., with fewer heart beats, lower blood pressure, greater aerobic capacity, and lesser ischaemic ST changes in the exercise electrocardiogram. Important determinants of successful reconditioning include adherence to the training program, viable myocardium, and an available source of blood supply.

In all phases of the illness, including the acute illness, hospitalization, convalescence, recovery and return to work, the prescription of exercise and physical activity should be based upon the aerobic capacity of the individual and his physiologic and clinical responses. Like all therapeutic measures, exercise prescription requires preliminary medical evaluation, exclusion of subjects with contraindications, evaluation of the cardiovascular status and function by testing, precise prescription of the magnitude frequency and duration of effort, supervision, direction and periodic re-evaluation, all with the same care as the prescription of a potent drug.

ACKNOWLEDGMENT

I am pleased to acknowledge the support and cooperation extended to our research efforts by Professors Walter H. Pritchard and William Insull, and to my research colleagues who have contributed to the success of our research goals: Ira Bernstein, M. D., Alfredo Burlando, M. D., C. Wesley Dupertuis, Ph. D., George Feil, M. D., Ernst Friedman, M. D., Alberto Goldbarg, M. D., Eugene Z. Hirsch, M. D., Tom R. Hornsten, M. D., Herbert Maistelman, M. S., Sue Marik, B. S., Franklin Plotkin, M. D., John D. Radke, M. D., Raymond Ricklin, B. S., Stephen H. Salzman, M. D., and Oliver Winkler.

I am sincerely grateful to Miss Sandra Kuse, chief technician, Mrs. Edward J. Husselman, secretary, Case Western Reverve University, Mr. Herman A. Eigen and other members of the Cleveland Jewish Community Center, whose efforts have contributed immeasurably to the attainment of our research goals.

REFERENCES

1. Workshop of American Heart Association, President's Council on Fitness, and South Carolina Heart Association, May 6-8, 1969, Myrtle Beach, South Carolina.
2. Hellerstein, H. K., Exercise therapy in coronary disease. *Bull. N.Y. Acad. Med.* 44, 1028 (1968).
3. Eckstein, R. W., The effect of exercise and coronary artery narrowing on coronary collateral circulation. *Circ. Res.* 5, 230 (1957).
4. Heberden, W., Some account of a disorder of the breast. *Med. Trans. Roy. Coll. Physicians* 2, 59 (1772).
5. Hellerstein, H. K., E. Z. Hirsch, W. Cumler, L. Allen, S. Polster and N. Zucker, Re-conditioning of the coronary patient. A preliminary report. In: *Coronary Disease*, Likoff, W. and J. H., Moyer, eds. New York and London, Grune and Stratton (1963).
6. Hellerstein, H. K., T. R. Hornsten, A. W. Goldbarg, A. G. Burlando, E. H. Friedman, E. Z. Hirsch and S. Marik, The influence of active conditioning upon coronary athero-sclerosis. In: *Atherosclerotic Vascular Disease.* A Hahneman Symposium, Brest, A. W. and J. H. Moyer, eds. New York, Appleton – Century – Crofts (1967).
7. Hellerstein, H. K. and T. R. Hornsten, Assessing and preparing the patient for return to a meaningful productive life. *J. Rehab.* 32, 48 (1966).
8. Friedman, M. and R. Rosenman, Association of specific overt behavior pattern with blood and cardiovascular findings. *J.A.M.A.* 169, 1286 (1959).
9. Hellerstein, H. K., E. Friedman, P. Brdar, M. Weiss, C. W. Dupertuis, D. J. Turell and D. Rumbaugh, *A comparison of the personality of adult subjects with rheumatic heart disease and with arteriosclerotic heart disease.* Presented at the Meeting of Scientific Council on Re-habilitation of the International Society of Cardiology, Hohenried, Germany, June 18, 1969. In press.
10. Passmore, R. and J. V. G. A. Durnin, Human energy expenditure. *Physiol. Rev.* 35, 801 (1955).

11. Hellerstein, H. K. and E. H. Friedman, Sexual Activity and the Post Coronary Patient. *Medical Aspects of Human Sexuality* (March 1969).

12. Clausen, J. P., O. A. Larsen and J. Trap-Jensen, Physical training in the management of coronary artery disease. *Circulation.* In press.

13. Hellerstein, H. K., *Relationship of Exercise to Acute Myocardial Infarction (Therapeutic, Restorative, Preventive and Etiological Aspects)*. Presented at the Symposium on Research on Acute Myocardial Infarction. Phoenix, Arizona, March, 1969. In press.

14. Frick, M. H. and M. Katila, Hemodynamic consequences of physical training after myocardial infarction. *Circulation* 37, 192 (1968).

PANEL DISCUSSION ON TREATMENT AND SECONDARY PREVENTION

MODERATOR: C. L. C. VAN NIEUWENHUIZEN

Van Nieuwenhuizen: Does secondary prevention really exist, or do we merely have prevention, primary or secondary?

Hellerstein: Recently Professor Eugene Stead remonstrated strongly against the use of the terms secondary prevention and primary prevention. He felt that coronary disease was basically a continuum which continues through life. The difference between primary and secondary is only a matter of time.

Oliver: I think that it is a very unsatisfactory view to say that primary and secondary prevention are the same and to argue that coronary disease is a continuum. Since nearly 50 per cent of all who have their first heart attack are dead by 6 months, only about 50 per cent are available for any secondary trial. First, you have to assume that the risk factors that operate in those who die suddenly are exactly the same as in those who survive and this we don't know. Second, I suggest that the prognosis, after a myocardial infarct has occurred, may very well be more closely related to the functional impairment of the myocardium than merely to something like a high serum cholesterol level. Third, we have to consider the influence of a completely different set of forces: namely hemodynamic and thrombogenic ones. To assume that reduction in serum cholesterol after a coronary has occurred is necessarily going to have the same effect as reduction of serum cholesterol before the clinical disease has occurred, I think, is fallacious.

Hellerstein: Dr. Oliver and I are talking about two different things. Dr. Oliver is talking about the clinical manifestations of the disease. I am talking about the basic underlying disease process, I do not disagree that we may not be modifying arteriosclerosis but that we may be modifying the effects of arteriosclerosis.

Van Nieuwenhuizen: Dr. Oliver can you comment on therapy in cardiogenic shock, especially in the case of a spreading infarction?

Oliver: The present situation in regard to cardiogenic shock is extremely depressing. It is possible that one might contain the spreading type of infarct if one were able to restore adequate aërobic circulation to peripheral areas of this infarct. There are a number of attempts to do this. Counterpulsation is one of these attempts but it is not yet wholly worked out. Hyperbaric oxygenation has not yet proved to be satisfactory. More studies are needed, perhaps in the experimentally infarcted dog of the nature of the spreading infarct.

Van Nieuwenhuizen: I wonder, in view of the great variability of the pathological process in the coronary arteries and in view of the relatively smallness of the sample, whether it is justified to draw the conclusion that longterm anticoagulant therapy is necessary after myocardial infarction?

Loeliger: This question concerns the possibility of bias in clinical trials. The Leiden study included 250 patients treated with either coumarin or placebo. The two groups were comparable thanks to random allocation. All patients had proven to be capable of taking part in a clinical trial. Consequently, the differences in results can be due only to the difference in the two drugs. Although the differences are not large, they are statistically significant. Similar findings are published by other groups.

Frick: What can anticoagulant therapy offer to patients with 'crescendo angina'? These are patients who suddenly, within weeks, develop severe angina pectoris ending ultimately in myocardial infarction.

Loeliger: Personally, we have no evidence that anticoagulant therapy prevents the myocardial infarction; the data of Dr. Borchgrevink, however, are convincing. He found that anticoagulants can prevent myocardial infarction.

Varnauskas: The rate of sudden deaths after an acute myocardial infarction suggests that the ventricular arrhythmias are the major cause of the late mortality. An effective control of arrhythmias can thus markedly reduce the late mortality in analogy to what has happened with early deaths in coronary care units.

Antiarrhythmic therapy with conventional drugs appears to be effective only to a certain extent. For example quinidine may decrease or eliminate completely premature ventricular beats but the patient may still die in sudden death at home. It is quite obvious that we know too little about the mechanisms causing various electrical disturbances in ischaemic heart disease.

In our attempts to analyse the causes of these late deaths and causes of late severe arrhythmias we got involved in the question of post-infarction ventricular aneurysms.

In less than two years we have collected 39 cases of roentgenologically confirmed ventricular aneurysms. Patients presenting electrocardiograms suggestive of large transmural infarction, chest roentgenograms showing cardiac enlargement irrespective of configuration and the first week of myocardial infarction exhibiting a prolonged subfebrile course were submitted for cardioangiography. The injection of contrast material was made into the right atrium. All cardioangiograms confirmed clinical suspicion of left ventricular aneurysm.

Table 1 contains the mean values of the variables defining the material and their distribution with respect to mortality and surgical treatment. The selection of patients for surgery has been in most cases accidental due to the available surgical facilities. The total mortality in not operated cases during an average observation period of 20 months was 26%, which is obviously higher than expected from the follow-up investigations of uncomplicated post-infarction cases.

Three out of six patients with recurrent ventricular tachyarrhythmias died in sudden death. One out of three similar cases who were treated surgically did not survive operation. The operation of such cases is frequently refused because of high risks and because of uncertainty that a successful operation can be beneficial with respect to future arrhythmias. The results of the present pilot survey do not support such attitude. The surgical risks are high but as high as persistence of arrhythmia-attacks. Furthermore, these attacks most likely are prevented by a successful operation.

Figure 1 illustrates three electrocardiograms from a 61 years old

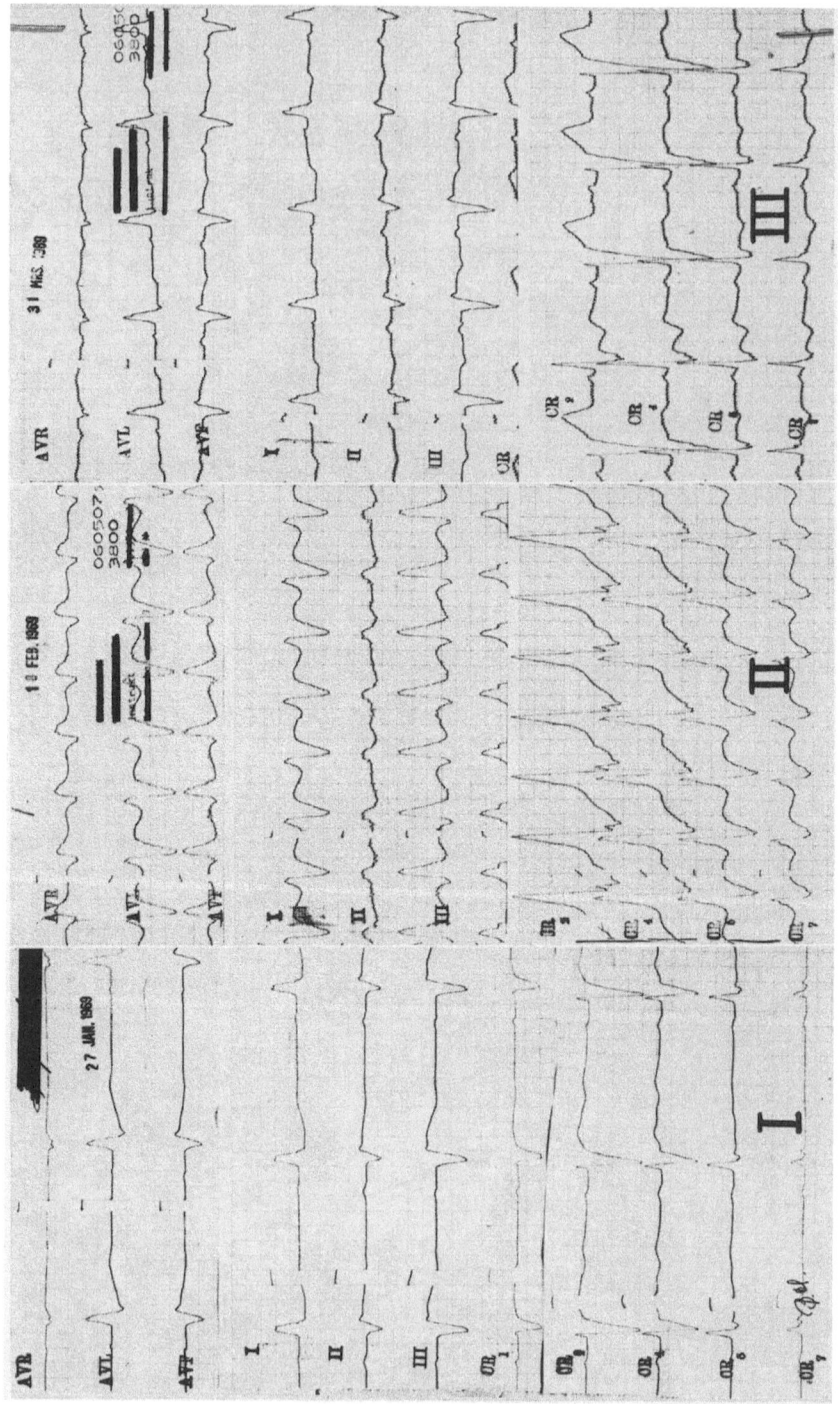

Fig. 1. Electrocardiograms before (I and II) and after (III) operation of a posteriorly located ventricular aneurysm.

man recorded before (I and II) and after surgical excision (III) of a posteriorly located ventricular aneurysm. The middle ECG (II) was recorded on 70 occasions despite intensive therapy with different anti-arrhythmic drugs. The patient was bed-ridden during the last two weeks before the operation; he experienced at least two such attacks daily. Postoperatively no arrhythmias were recorded during the entire observation period of 3 months. He can now perform 600 kmp per min. on a bicycle ergometer without symptoms and signs of cardiac failure and without any kinds of arrhythmias.

It seems obvious that our knowledge concerning late arrhythmias and their relation to post-infarction aneurysm is very limited. The detection of 39 cases can hardly be accidental as well as the occurrence of malignant ventricular arrhythmias in 9 of these cases.

It is quite possible that these malignant arrhythmias are preceded by for example frequent ventricular premature beats.

From the available data we have estimated that approximately 50 cases of ventricular aneurysm per year are to be expected in the city of Gothenburg (population equal to 450.000). Even if not all of these cases need to be considered as candidates for preventive or curative operation it is quite obvious that the problem might be great both from cardiological and surgical point of view.

Table 1. 39 Patients with postinfarction ventricular aneurysm.

	Alive	Dead	Operated
Number	23	8	8
Mean observation time in months	20	18	12
Mean age, years	60	60	54
Men/women	20/3	4/4	8/0
Heart size ml/m² BSA at 1 month after infarction	530	600	450
Increase of total heart size within 1 year, ml	170	240	220
Late ventricular tachyarrhythmias	3(13%)	3(43%)	3(37%)

Frick: We all know that nitroglycerin is the cornerstone of the treatment of angina pectoris. Recently we studied the average duration of anginal pain in our exercise test. The pain lasted two minutes on the average after the stopping of exercise at the onset of pain. One of the most clear-cut effects of nitroglycerin is a decrease in aortic pressure and this is probably the most relevant one to its pain relieving action. It requires 2.5 minutes to cause a pressure decrease of 5 mm Hg, the pressure was directly determined (1). Therefore the usual effect of sublingual nitroglycerin is prolonged over the period when the pain has vanished spontaneously. I would therefore say that the right way to take nitroglycerin is prophylactically.

All of us are familiar with β-blockading drugs. If we are unhappy with the response to propranolol in the usual dosage levels Prichard's experiments in London should us encourage to go a little further. The average dose that he is using for angina pectoris is 750 mg per day, his maximum dosage goes up to 4 gram propranolol per day (2).

I am advocating that you should not suspend the use of the drug because you get no response with 160 mg, you can easily increase the dose considerably if you carefully observe your patient.

REFERENCES

1. Heikkilä, J. and M. H. Frick, Rapidity of the hypotensive effect of short-acting nitrous compounds. *Ann. Clin. Res.* 1, 256-260 (1969).
2. Prichard, B. N. C., Personal communication (1969).

Van Nieuwenhuizen: I would like to ask Dr. Fisher to comment on the psychological aspects of rehabilitation.

Fisher:
Activities in Psychological Aspects of Cardiac Rehabilitation
An expert committee of the World Health Organization met in Warsaw in May, 1969, to discuss problems related to the Psychological Aspects of Cardiac Rehabilitation. This committee was concerned with the psychological aspects of the cardiac patient's rehabilitation from the time of onset of his cardiac disorder through his convalescence to the time he returned home as a member of society. When you take this kind of generalized view, you perceive a great number of psychological problems obviously that you don't see in an exercise program. We see an exercise program as only a small part of the total rehabilitation effort. The kind of problems that we were concerned at Warsaw were

the overwhelming fear that the patient had in the first three days of infarction. We were concerned with the behavioural manifestations that would cause the patient to be a management problem (acting negativistic and indeed doing things that would inhibit appropriate treatment). We were concerned with the patient as he came to consciousness and was surrounded by a great deal of equipment and how he would perceive this and how he would react. We saw these in relationship to how one manages a patient with these kinds of reactions so he can proceed through an appropriate program.

One of the major problems, and I have no answers for it, are those two groups of patients that I think will give the most trouble in most of the new rehabilitation programs that you are about to develop. The first group are those who refuse to participate and perceives his cardiac disorder as one which prohibits his doing any form of exertion. The others are those whom you know have cardiac disorders but who deny their limitations. How do we handle these patients and the problems that they present? This was the first time that psychology and cardiology got together even to discuss these problems. We have no set answers to the question. The important thing is that the problems have been recognized and that the WHO is taking a major step forward in attempting to resolve those problems involved in total cardiac rehabilitation. I think that the big problem that you will have in the need for psychological investigation will be focused on which patients will you have to send for therapy and which ones can you work with yourself in seeing that they proceed through a rehabilitation program. The WHO committee suggests that you have more problems than you can realize when you start considering the heart not as a pump but as an individual with a family who are victims of the cardiac episode. How do you send a patient back to work if his wife sees that any kind of exertion on his part will kill him? I think that you have a whole host of practical problems that sometimes get smothered over in anatomical considerations, especially if you are in practice, and you have these problems with your patients. What kind of work can the patient do? If he cannot do his former kind of work, what can you suggest? Rehabilitation makes vocational counsellors, psychologists, and perhaps even psychiatrists out of you. Are you trained for this? I suggest that you start calling in disciplines that may be able to help you in this kind of activity when you find it necessary.

Another international organization, the Rehabilitation Council of the International Society of Cardiology, is also doing work in behalf of cardiac rehabilitation. Last year the Council on Rehabilitation met for the first time. They recognized that there were psychological problems in cardiac rehabilitation. They initiated a world wide survey to find out about these psychological problems. Some questions in psychological aspects have been answered by your colleagues around the world. This survey was originated in March, 1969. To date we have collected material in 40 different countries. I will give the responses that other cardiologists have said in other countries.

Here are some of the items that appear on this questionnaire. What are the main psychological problems of the cardiac? What psychological variables do you find pose problems or barriers to cardiac individuals in returning to their former activity?

What test, techniques or methods are used in your country to evaluate the psychological factors of a cardiac? What percentage of cardiacs that you see return to their former activity?

Just think about your case load and decide. Dr. Hellerstein stated that we don't need a rehabilitation program because almost 90 per cent go back. What do you think, based on your own practice? What per cent of the cardiacs that you see return to certain activities when they should not do so because of cardiac limitations?

What percentage of your patients think they have heart disease but do not have heart disease? Are there any services or agencies available in your country to handle cardiacs with psychological problems? Are there any special psychological problems faced by the cardiac in your country that would be of interest to professionals in other countries?

The survey indicates an average of 71.9 when asked the percentage of patients that returned to their former work. One responded that most patients returned and another stated that all patients returned to work. They indicated an average of 15.5 per cent that did not return to their former activities because of psychological factors. They reported that 13.6 per cent of cardiacs returned to certain activities when they should not have done so. In response to the question what per cent of your patients think they have heart disease but do not have heart disease, the average was 17.5. These and other answers will be reviewed and serve as the basis for establishing hypotheses for research which perhaps will help us resolve a myriad of problems involved in the psychological aspects of cardiac rehabilitation. The WHO and International Society of Cardiology have opened up this area which will certainly feed back information to you as cardiologists to help your patients in their return to a fruitful life.

REFERENCES

1. Fisher, S., The cardiac work evaluation unit: A key to cardiac rehabilitation research. *Malattie Cardiovascolari*, vol. X, 1-2 (1969).
2. Fisher, S., *International survey on the psychological aspects of heart disease* (in press).
3. *WHO Report of committee on psychological aspects of cardiac rehabilitation.* Warsaw, May, 1969 (in press).

Hellerstein: Basically, the reaction of the patient depends upon the emotional and intellectual security of the doctor. Anxious patients have anxious doctors. If you deal with a catastrophic illness in a frightened and disorganized fashion you transfer to your patient your own fear and insecurity.

I think it important that in the private sector 66 per cent of cardiacs returned to their same job, 26 per cent to their same but slightly modified occupations, and 8 per cent did not go back to work. If you find this 8 per cent, get help from the social services and help these patients attain an optimal place in life.

I would urge you to recognize that the depression of the patient threatens his survival. Dr. Andrew Wallace found a positive correlation between mortality and catecholamine release during acute infarction. The change in catecholamine release appeared to be related to emotional factors, such as the wife's visit, remarks said in the coronary care unit and so on.

Van Nieuwenhuizen: Would you recommend that the general practitioner will be equipped with a transportable defibrillator?

Oliver: There might be some place for this if the practitioner is fully familiar, and I would think that he would have to be a cardiologist really, with arrhythmias and preferably has some form of monitoring system associated with the portable defibrillator.

Van Nieuwenhuizen: Is the reduction in case fatality in Coronary Care Units evenly distributed by sex and age?

Oliver: No, it is not. In both sexes under the age of 50, the mortality rate in those with ventricular fibrillation is 11 per cent. In the 50-59 age group it is 18 per cent, and in the 60-69 age group it is 23 per cent. This means therefore that we can do more for the younger age group, but I can't say anything about a sex difference.

Van Nieuwenhuizen: Does physical training influence risk factors?

Hellerstein: One of the coronary risk factors is ischaemic ST-T depression. According to surveys, people with ischaemic changes have a much higher chance of dying from coronary disease. Ischaemic change can be modified by physical training. I am sure that the change in cholesterol levels is not due to physical training at the level we are doing it. The reduction in exercise blood pressure may be another factor also.

Weeda: With regard to the level of physical training it is important to determine the maximal heart rate of each individual patient before you start the training program. Then it is possible to construct a training scheme adapted to the maximal heart rate of the particular patient. There is a large variation in maximal heart rates within the different age groups especially after myocardial infarction.

For instance we observed a range from 100 to 197 beats per minute in the 50-59 age group. Therefore one has to individualize with respect to the maximal heart rate and it is not correct to take a standard value from literature.

Van Nieuwenhuizen: There are pathologists who tell us that the scar is reasonably firm only four weeks after the infarction. Therefore you could argue that it would be dangerous after the occurrence of the myocardial infarction to start an exercise program before the end of this period. One of the dangers mentioned is the development of ventricular aneurysm.

Hellerstein: In a study that Drs. L. N. Katz, J. Schlichter and I published in 1955 (1) on 102 cases of ventricular aneurysm we found that a significant number of these patients were physicians who with a great element of denial remained ambulatory throughout the acute myocardial infarction. This report and that of Dr. P. D. White on patients in mental institutions (2) show that people who remain physically extremely active during the acute infarct have a higher risk of having a ventricular aneurysm or rupture.

REFERENCES

1. Schlichter, L., H. K. Hellerstein and L. N. Katz, Aneurysm of the heart: a correlative study of one hundred and two proved cases. *Medicine* 33, 43 (1954).
2. Jetter, W. W. and P. D. White, Rupture of heart in patients in mental institutions. *Ann. Int. Med.* 21, 783 (1944).

Van Nieuwenhuizen: If repetitive ventricular tachycardia is relatively frequent in patients with sinus bradycardia, can it be advocated that they should be treated beforehand with pacemakers?

Oliver: There are three types of ventricular tachycardia that we must consider here.

There is the type occurring on the basis of a sinus tachycardia. This is the common type of ventricular tachycardia after acute myocardial infarction and this requires treatment with lignocaïne etc.

The second type which is not so very uncommon is a type of accelerated idioventricular rate. There is a sinus rate of about 80 or 90. Then there is a switch to an idioventricular rate at about 90 or 100. This is a relatively benign arrhythmia.

The third type, and the least common type is the ventricular tachycardia occurring when there is a bradycardia, a brady-arrhythmia. This type responds very satisfactorily to atropine. It may well be that you will need to put a pacing catheter in such a patient, but in general a milligram or even more of atropine will cure this brady-arrhythmia.

Snellen: I would like to thank this panel, its moderator and also the members of all the other panels for the magnificent job they have done. A course like this can always be designed so that it looks well on paper, but its success depends on the participants. Moreover the co-operation of the Boerhaave Organisation with the Netherlands Heart Foundation and the interest shown by the Secretary of Health and by WHO have been of the greatest importance. Finally a course like this proves the truth of Dr. Hugenholtz' dictum that the Atlantic Ocean is rapidly becoming the Atlantic river, joining rather than dividing the people at both sides of it.